Plants and the Skin

To Robert Warin,
who inspired an enthusiasm for dermatology
and shared a love of plants

Plants and the Skin

Christopher R. Lovell MD, MRCP
CONSULTANT DERMATOLOGIST
ROYAL UNITED HOSPITAL, BATH

OXFORD
BLACKWELL SCIENTIFIC PUBLICATIONS
LONDON EDINBURGH BOSTON
MELBOURNE PARIS BERLIN VIENNA

© 1993 by
Blackwell Scientific Publications
Editorial Offices:
Osney Mead, Oxford OX2 0EL
25 John Street, London WC1N 2BL
23 Ainslie Place, Edinburgh EH3 6AJ
238 Main Street, Cambridge
 Massachusetts 02142, USA
54 University Street, Carlton
 Victoria 3053, Australia

Other Editorial Offices:
Librairie Arnette SA
2, rue Casimir-Delavigne
75006 Paris
France

Blackwell Wissenschafts-Verlag
Meinekestrasse 4
D-1000 Berlin 15
Germany

Blackwell MZV
Feldgasse 13
A-1238 Wien
Austria

All rights reserved. No part of this
publication may be reproduced, stored
in a retrieval system, or transmitted,
in any form or by any means,
electronic, mechanical, photocopying,
recording or otherwise without the
prior permission of the copyright
owner.

First published 1993

Set by Setrite Typesetters, Hong Kong
Printed and bound in Italy
by Vincenzo Bona s.r.l., Turin

Cover lettering by Tom Perkins

DISTRIBUTORS

Marston Book Services Ltd
PO Box 87
Oxford OX2 0DT
(*Orders*: Tel: 0865 791155
        Fax: 0865 791927
        Telex: 837515)

USA
Blackwell Scientific Publications, Inc.
238 Main Street
Cambridge, MA 02142
(*Orders*: Tel: 800 759–6102
        617 876–7000)

Canada
Times Mirror
Professional Publishing, Ltd
5240 Finch Avenue East
Scarborough, Ontario M1S 5A2
(*Orders*: Tel: 800 268–4178
        416 298–1588)

Australia
Blackwell Scientific Publications
Pty Ltd
54 University Street
Carlton, Victoria 3053
(*Orders*: Tel: 03 347–5552)

A catalogue record for this book
is available from the British Library

ISBN 0-632-02562-X

Contents

CONTRIBUTORS, vi

PREFACE, vii

ACKNOWLEDGEMENTS, viii

1 INTRODUCTION, 1

2 THE INDIVIDUAL AT RISK, 6
    2.1 Occupational exposure to plants (R.J.G. Rycroft), 6
    2.2 Plant products in perfumes and cosmetics (I.R. White), 15

3 IDENTIFICATION OF PLANTS (M.E. Hansen), 23
    3.1 The basics of plant taxonomy and nomenclature, 23
    3.2 Features used in plant identification, 24
    3.3 Collection of material for identification, 25
    3.4 Identification of plants, 26

4 URTICARIA DUE TO PLANTS, 29
    4.1 Introduction, 29
    4.2 Urticaria due to injection of toxins, 29
    4.3 Immunological contact urticaria, 35

5 IRRITANT PLANTS, 42
    5.1 Mechanical irritants, 43
    5.2 Chemical irritants, 50

6 PHYTOPHOTOTOXIC REACTIONS, 64
    6.1 Introduction, 64
    6.2 The naturally occurring psoralens and other plant photosensitizers and their mode of action (B.E. Johnson), 66
    6.3 Clinical features, 78
    6.4 Plants which cause phototoxic reactions, 86

7 ALLERGIC CONTACT DERMATITIS DUE TO PLANTS, 96
    7.1 Mechanisms of allergic contact dermatitis, 96
    7.2 Patch testing with plants and plant allergens, 97
    7.3 Preparation of plant extracts (M.G. Rowan), 101
    7.4 Poison ivy and poison oak dermatitis (C. Dannaker & H.I. Maibach), 105
    7.5 Other plant families causing allergic contact dermatitis, 121
    7.6 Allergenic conifers, 235
    7.7 Allergenic hardwoods, 246

8 EPILOGUE, 255
    8.1 Therapeutic uses of some plant products in dermatology, 255

INDEX, 259

Contributors

C. DANNAKER DO, MPH, *Department of Dermatology, University of California, California, USA*

M.E. HANSEN BPharm, MRPharmS, CBiol, MIBiol, *School of Pharmacy and Pharmacology, University of Bath, Bath, UK*

B.E. JOHNSON BSc, PhD, *Department of Dermatology, University of Dundee, Ninewells Hospital, Dundee, UK*

C.R. LOVELL MD, MRCP, *Department of Dermatology, Royal United Hospital, Bath, UK*

H.I. MAIBACH MD, *Department of Dermatology, University of California, California, USA*

M.G. ROWAN BSc, PhD, *School of Pharmacy and Pharmacology, University of Bath, Bath, UK*

R.J.G. RYCROFT MD, FRCP, FFOM, DIH, *St John's Institute of Dermatology, St Thomas's Hospital, London, UK*

I.R. WHITE BSc, MRCP, *St John's Institute of Dermatology, St Thomas's Hospital, London, UK*

Preface

Everyone comes into daily contact with plants. Even the urban dweller handles and eats vegetables and uses cosmetics, toiletries or medications containing plant products. Few houses or offices lack ornamental plants in pots or tubs. Gardening is an increasingly popular leisure activity; nursery gardeners are introducing new species and trouble-free, disease-resistant hybrids, enabling the amateur gardener to grow a wider range of plants than before.

This book gives a practical, profusely illustrated account of value to the dermatologist, general practitioner, physician, pharmacist or nurse confronted with an eruption which may be attributed to contact with a plant or plant product. The book is intended primarily for a medical or paramedical audience with no botanical training. Plants are described in layperson's terms, without confusing botanical jargon. In addition, it is hoped that the book will be a useful reference for the botanist, pharmacologist or chemist with an interest in plant toxicology.

The major types of eruption are described, with details of the plants that cause them. These include irritant reactions, contact urticaria and phototoxic reactions. In particular, plants which cause allergic dermatitis are reviewed comprehensively, with descriptions of the plants, clinical features and information on patch testing. There is a separate section on poison ivy and poison oak, the major cause of contact dermatitis in the USA. There are further chapters on plant identification and preparation of plant material for patch testing.

Other sections describe aspects of occupational exposure to plants, reactions to plants in food handlers and exposure to plant products in perfumes and cosmetics. There are several checklists of hazardous plants that should be considered in association with specific work or leisure pursuits, e.g. food handling or weeding. Finally, there is a brief outline of some of the plants and plant products that are used currently in treatment of skin diseases.

Christopher Lovell
Bath, 1992

Acknowledgements

Without the generous help and advice of many friends and colleagues, this book would never have been contemplated, let alone completed. In particular, I wish to thank those who have written chapters on specific topics, Penelope Guy for the line drawings and Steve Pitcher-Cumming for drawing the formulae.

I am indebted to the secretaries who coped nobly with my handwritten manuscript, in particular Glynis Dover and Janet Bryce, also Diana Barlow, Nikki Hopgood, Jennifer Jenkins and Diana Shelley.

I am grateful to Brian Mathew, of the Royal Botanic Gardens, for providing up-to-date lists of the current Kew classification of plants, to Michael Salmon and Noel Lothian for providing botanical information, and to Adelaide Botanic Garden for the herbarium specimen (Fig. 4.2.5).

I wish to acknowledge the help of the Medical Illustration and Histopathology Departments, Royal United Hospital, Bath, and the Medical Illustration Department, the Institute of Dermatology, in preparation of illustrations. I am grateful to the following individuals who have provided illustrations:

Jill Adams (Figs 6.3.1, 6.3.3, 6.3.5); Mike Beck (7.5.72, 7.5.124); Joe Boyle (7.5.29); John Burry (7.5.37, 7.5.38, 7.5.39, 7.5.46, 7.5.64); Bob Champion (7.5.2, 7.5.4); John Cook (6.3.4); Etain Cronin (4.3.2, 4.3.3); Chris Dannaker (7.4.7); Mike Davies (7.5.34, 7.5.35); Julia Ellis (6.3.6); John English (7.5.13); David Gledhill (6.4.3); Margaret Hansen (7.5.65); Roger Harman (7.5.60); Noel Lothian (7.5.23, 7.5.197); Robert McKenzie (7.5.108); Torquil Macleod (4.2.6, 5.1.2, 5.1.5, 5.1.7, 5.1.8, 5.2.3); Dick Mallett (7.5.1, 7.5.3, 7.5.4); Charles Parsons (7.5.5); Sheila Powell (7.4.4, 7.4.5); John Reeves (7.4.8, 7.4.9); Nick Reynolds (6.3.7); Richard Rycroft (2.1, 2.2, 2.3); Susan Shaw (6.3.9); the late Mark Smith (4.2.4); Bob Tan (6.3.8); Sue Young (7.5.132).

Finally, I am grateful to the staff of Blackwell Scientific Publications for their patient support and encouragement during the gestation of this book.

Christopher Lovell
Bath, 1992

1 Introduction

Gardening is the most popular leisure pursuit in Britain and many other temperate areas of the world. In a survey of patients in the patch test clinic at High Wycombe, 16% were professional gardeners or horticulturists (Shaw & Wilkinson 1987). In addition to professional and amateur horticulturalists and botanists, a surprisingly large number of occupations may involve exposure to plants or plant products (Table 1.1.1).

The frequency of skin reactions caused by plants is unknown. Many affected individuals never consult their general practitioner, let alone a dermatologist, since many reactions may be trivial and self-limiting or wrongly diagnosed. A major exception is poison ivy/oak dermatitis in the eastern seaboard of the USA (Chapter 7.4).

The major types of response are outlined in Table 1.1.2. The reader is referred to the relevant chapters for details of the plants or plant products known to cause the reactions. Table 1.1.3 lists some of the activities which lead to contact with toxic or allergenic plants and the species which may be encountered.

Other factors than plant exposure may contribute to, or may be the sole cause of, dermatitis. Plant growers, florists and food handlers are exposed to numerous physical and chemical irritants including water, detergents, wet cement and garden chemicals as well as allergens such as thiurams (in pesticides and rubber in gloves, boots), potassium

Table 1.1.1 Some occupations and activities involving plant exposure.

Gardeners, horticulturalists, nursery workers, fruit pickers
Farmers
Florists
Foresters, lumberjacks, sawyers, wood machinists, antique restorers, carpenters, builders
Botanists, naturalists
Herbalists, aromatherapists, homoeopaths
Pharmacists, pharmacologists, organic chemists, plant biochemists
Dentists, dermatologists, veterinary surgeons
Perfumiers, beauticians, cosmetologists
Food handlers, chefs, housewives, bar workers
Sports, especially golf, fishing
Military on exercise
Ramblers, hikers, climbers, campers
Children at play
Romantics (rolling in the hay)

Table 1.1.2 Cutaneous reactions to plants and plant products.

1 Contact urticaria (see Chapter 4)
   An immediate reaction (within minutes of contact)
   Itching, erythema and/or oedema

2 Irritant contact dermatitis (see Chapter 5)
   Skin dryness, often fissuring
   May be itchy
   Usually restricted to areas of skin contact
   Typically follows prolonged or extensive exposure to irritant
   Cactus glochids, in particular, may cause an extensive pruritic eruption simulating scabies

3 Phytophotodermatitis (see Chapter 6)
   Typically erythematous, streaky eruption, which may be vesicular or bullous, within 1–2 days of plant contact
   Reaction occurs precisely at sites of contact in sun-exposed areas
   Associated with, or followed by, brown hyperpigmentation at the same site; this persists for several weeks/months
   Common in children

4 Allergic contact dermatitis (see Chapter 7)
   Pruritic, often streaky, erythema, sometimes vesicular
   Starts at areas of contact but may spread outwards
   Develops, often progressively, within 1–3 days of exposure
   Recurrent episodes are typical, each lasting several days and usually followed by scaling; each episode may be worse than the last
   Minimal, if any, hyperpigmentation
   Airborne contact dermatitis typically affects face, neck, forearms and hands, simulating photosensitivity

dichromate (in cement and leather gloves) and nickel in tools (Shaw & Wilkinson 1987). The eruption may be due to fungi or other microorganisms in infected plant material (e.g. inoculation of *Mycobacterium* spp. inoculated via plant spines (see p. 49). Alternatively, an urticarial 'pseudo-phytodermatitis' may be induced by insects associated with the plants, e.g. irritant caterpillars such as the Pine Processionary Moth or the irritant papular eruption caused by mites such as *Pyemotes* spp. in grains (Hewitt *et al.* 1976, Rycroft & Kennedy 1981).

This book is intended to be a readable guide to the skin reactions produced by members of the plant kingdom. It is intended to supplement, rather than to replace, the excellent monographs which have been produced in recent years. In particular, the detailed account of Mitchell and Rook (1979) remains the ultimate source of reference; a new edition is awaited. The beautifully presented text by Benezra *et al.* (1985) is also invaluable. The reader who is fluent in German should also refer to Hausen (1988) and Frohne and Pfänder (1987).

Reference is made in the text to the famous herbals of Gerard (enlarged by Thomas Johnson in 1633) and Culpeper (1653). Both of these make delightful reading and are freely available in inexpensive

Table 1.1.3 Check lists of dermatitic plants and plant products.

Urticaria	Irritant	Phytophototoxic	Allergenic
1 Garden plants (ornamental) Loasa, Blumenbachia (only in specialist collections), Iris (rare), tulip (Tulipa)	Borage (Borago), forget-me-not (Myosotis), spurge (Euphorbia), bulbs, esp. hyacinth	Dictamnus albus (esp. USA), Queen Anne's lace (Ammi majus), Rue (Ruta)	Alstroemeria, chrysanthemum (X Dendranthema), Dahlia, elecampane (Inula helenium), feverfew (Tanacetum parthenium), Gaillardia, geranium (Pelargonium), Helenium, Humea elegans, Liatris spicata, marigolds (Tagetes), Phacelia, Rudbeckia hirta, tansy (Tanacetum vulgare), bulbs esp. Narcissus
2 Garden shrubs/trees/climbers Grevillea (esp. Australia)	Thorns, esp. rose, Berberis, Pyracantha, rose hip hairs		Gingko (fruit), Grevillea (Australia, southern USA), Hydrangea, ivy (Hedera helix), jasmine (Jasminum), Leyland cypress (X Cupressocyparis leylandii)
3 Weeds (see also 6) Nettles (Urtica)	Buttercup (Ranunculus), goose grass (Galium aparine), mayweed (Anthemis cotula), petty spurge (Euphorbia peplus)	Cow parsley (Anthriscus), cow parsnip (Heracleum), wild carrot (Daucus carota) (cause 'strimmer rash')	Dandelion (Taraxacum officinale), poison ivy/oak (Toxicodendron) (USA), yarrow (Achillea millefolium)
4 House plants (a) Flowering	Cacti		Chrysanthemum (X Dendranthema), Hoya carnosa, orchids (Cymbidium, Paphiopedilum), Primula obconica, Streptocarpus, tradescantia (Zebrina pendula)
(b) Foliage Monstera deliciosa	Codiaeum (croton) Dieffenbachia Synadenium grantii		Codiaeum (croton), Coleus, ferns (Arachnoides, Nephrolepis), Philodendron scandens, pick a back plant (Tolmiea menziesii) poinsettia (Euphorbia pulcherrima), Schefflera, Scindapsus
5 Herbs	Borage Chives Comfrey	Parsley Rue	Anise, caraway, chamomiles, coriander, dill, feverfew, lavender, mint, sage, tansy, thyme

Continued on p. 4

Table 1.1.3 Continued

Urticaria	Irritant	Phytophototoxic	Allergenic
6 *Countryside*			
(a) Woodland			
Lichens			
Dendrocnide (Australasia)			Ivy, lichens, liverworts, poison ivy/oak
(b) Hedgerows, fields, meadows, prairies, wasteland			
Nettles (*Urtica*)	Thorns inc. roses, blackthorn	*Anthriscus*	Capeweed (*Arctotheca*) (Australia), chamomiles,
	Tumbleweed (USA)	Hogweeds (*Heracleum*)	*Dittrichia viscosa* (Mediterranean), fleabane (*Conyza*)
	Soliva (Australia)	Weeds harmful to grazing animals	(Australia, USA), golden rod (*Solidago*) (USA),
	Pulsatilla (esp. USA)	(see p. 65)	*Larrea* (Argentina, USA) barbecues, mugwort (*Artemisia*)
			oxeye daisy (*Tanacetum cinerariifolium*), *Phacelia*
			(USA), ragweeds (USA)
(c) River banks, moist areas			
Nettles (*Urtica*)		*Angelica*	*Helenium* (USA)
		Hogweeds, esp.	
		H. mantegazzianum	
7 *Ointments/toiletries/cosmetics*			
Urticant fragrances in	Acne preparations – tea tree oil	Psoralens in essential oils and	Aromatherapy oils (e.g. neroli, lavender, geranium, eucalyptus,
toothpastes, henna, castor	Facial scrubs (e.g. apricot kernel)	suncare products	lemon grass, jojoba, sesame, *Tagetes*)
oil, cloves, sesame oil	Plant lipids → folliculitis		Ointments/liniments containing *Aloe*, *Arnica*,
	Fragrances		*Calendula*, *Centella*, *Hedera*, etc.
			Fragrances, balsams of Peru
8 *Occupational*			
(a) Florists	*Codiaeum*		*Alstroemeria*, chrysanthemum, *Codiaeum*,
	Dieffenbachia		X *Cupressocyparis leylandii* sprigs, ferns, globe
			artichoke (*Cynara scolymus*), *Helichrysum* (dried
			flowers), orchids (*Cymbidium*, *Paphiopedilum*), *Primula*
			obconica (rare), bulbs – daffodil, jonquil, tulip
(b) Food handlers			
Lettuce, many fruits, nuts,	Garlic/onion/chives/leeks	Celery, carrot, parsnip, parsley,	Asparagus shoot, bayleaf, carrot, cashew, cauliflower, chicory,
spices, coffee, castor beans,	Peppers, prickly pears, chicory,	figs, citrus fruit	cinnamon, citrus fruit, endive, galangal, garlic, ginger, globe
cereals	lettuce, cereals, pineapples,		artichoke, lettuce, mango, mustard, nutmeg, okra, onion,
	tomato plants		peppers, star anise, sunflower, turmeric, vanilla
(c) Wood handlers			
Lichens, red cedar, birch,	Several hardwoods		Lichens, liverworts, softwoods e.g. deal, pine (Chapter 7.6),
larch, a few tropical	(see Chapter 7.7)		numerous hardwoods (Chapter 7.7)
hardwoods			

modern editions. In addition, the writings of Dioscorides are quoted. His herbal *De materia medica libri quinque,* compiled in the first century AD, had a fundamental influence on early medicine. The English botanist, John Goodyer, translated it between 1652 and 1655 and this translation is used here.

I hope the reader will not only gain a clearer perception of the varied effects of plants on the skin but also enjoy the challenge of investigating a patient with suspected plant dermatitis.

References

Benezra C., Ducombs G., Sell Y. & Foussereau J. (1985) *Plant Contact Dermatitis.* B.C. Decker, Toronto.
Frohne D. & Pfänder H.J. (1987) *Giftpflanzen. Ein Handbuch für Apotheker, Ärzte, Toxikologen und Biologen Wissenschaftliche.* Verlagsgesellschaft mbH, Stuttgart.
Hausen B.M. (1988) *Allergie pflanzen-Pflanzenallergene: Handbuch und Atlas der allergie-induzierenden Wild- und Kulturpflanzen.* Teil I. Kontakt allergene. Ecomed, Landsberg, München.
Hewitt M., Barrow G.I., Miller D.C. & Turk S.M. (1976) A case of *Pyemotes* dermatitis with a note on the roles of those mites in skin disease. *British Journal of Dermatology* **94**: 423–30.
Mitchell J.C. & Rook A. (1979) *Botanical Dermatology: Plants and Plant Products Injurious to the Skin.* Greengrass, Vancouver.
Rycroft R.J.G. & Kennedy C. (1981) *Pyemotes* dermatitis in display artists. *Clinical and Experimental Dermatology* **6**: 629–34.
Shaw S. & Wilkinson J.D. (1987) Contact dermatitis in the garden. In Verbov J.L. (ed.) *Current Concepts in Contact Dermatitis.* MTP Press, Lancaster, pp. 33–48.

2 The individual at risk

2.1 Occupational exposure to plants
R.J.G. RYCROFT

2.1.1 Introduction and definition

Occupational contact dermatitis from plants is common and disabling: medically, psychologically, socially and financially. Its broad definition is dermatitis due wholly or partly to plant contact at work. A stricter definition is dermatitis that would not have occurred at all without plant contact at work. Occupational contact dermatitis in general accounts for 90–95% of occupational dermatoses. Occupational dermatoses that are not contact dermatitis include contact urticaria, which can also be caused by certain plants.

2.1.2 Occupations and frequency

Horticulture and floristry ranked 11th for women and 13th for men in Fregert's (1975) listings of the commonest occupations causing contact dermatitis in southern Sweden. In the same study of nearly 1500 patients with occupational contact dermatitis, agriculture ranked ninth for men, though it did not feature in the 12 leading occupations for women.

In the USA, agriculture has been identified as the industry with the highest risk of occupational skin disease (O'Malley *et al.* 1988). Nearly 50% of the cases were due to plants, trees and naturally occurring vegetation, with an additional 10% being due to food products, mainly vegetables and fruits. In contrast, a mere 20% of the total were considered attributable to agricultural chemicals.

A recent review of workers' compensation claims for occupational skin disease in Ohio (Mathias *et al.* 1990) identified forestry as the major source of such claims, with agricultural crop production third in the ranking order of occupations.

In the Netherlands, agriculture was ranked fourth by Coenraads *et al.* (1983) among occupations yielding cases of eczema of the hands and forearms in men.

Agriculture, horticulture, forestry and floristry between them therefore account for a very sizeable proportion of the total burden of occupational skin disease, with plants and plant products being the commonest causes of contact dermatitis within these industries.

2.1.3 Aetiology

Allergy and irritancy

Fregert (1975) found an unusual predominance of allergic contact dermatitis over irritant contact dermatitis for women in horticulture and floristry. This contrasted with the finding that, in nine out of the 12 occupations most commonly causing occupational contact dermatitis in women, irritant contact dermatitis was considered to be either as common or more common than allergic contact dermatitis. Allergic contact dermatitis also predominated in men, though this was also the case in the majority of their commonest causal occupations.

Major causes

The major scourges of outdoor workers of all kinds are poison oak and poison ivy sensitization in areas such as the western USA (Epstein 1974), and Compositae (Asteraceae) sensitization in many other land masses, including the midwestern USA, southern Australia (Burry et al. 1973), India (Lonkar et al. 1974) and, increasingly being recognized, Europe (Diepgen et al. 1989). Allergic contact dermatitis from *Frullania* growing on trees has been established as a cause of serious occupational disability among forestry workers in northwestern North America (Mitchell 1981), as well as in southern Europe. Lichen harvesters in Scandinavia are frequently sensitized by *Cladonia alpestris* (Salo et al. 1981) and other lichens sensitize in southern Europe (Gonçalo et al. 1981). Airborne contact dermatitis occurs in all these occupational dermatoses.

Tulip fingers (Klaschka et al. 1964) is perhaps the most recognized allergic contact dermatitis among horticulturalists, and daffodil itch or lily rash (Gude et al. 1988) the most widespread irritant (usually) contact dermatitis. Tulip fingers occurs mainly in those who handle the bulbs and occasionally in those who pick and trim the flowers, whereas its close 'cousin' alstroemeria dermatitis is mainly sustained from handling the flowers (Fig. 2.1.1). Daffodil itch is endemic among those who cut, bunch and pack daffodils (or narcissi and jonquils), but bulb packers and florists are also at risk.

Hausen and Oestmann (1988) reported a study of 71 patients, recruited by questionnaire, who were mainly market gardeners and wholesale florists, plus a few retail florists. The most frequent allergens were the Compositae (Asteraceae), followed by the Liliaceae and Primulaceae. Chrysanthemums were responsible for most cases of Compositae dermatitis. Tulips and *Alstroemeria* cultivars were the next most common causes of allergic contact dermatitis. Thiboutot et al. (1990) also found

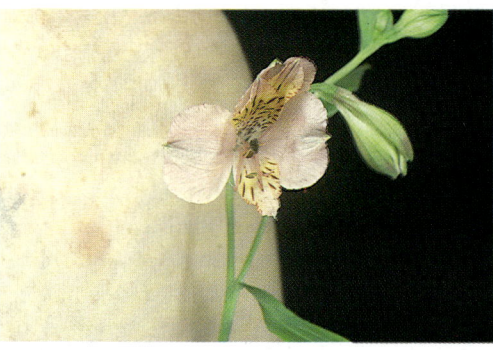

Fig. 2.1.1 An *Alstroemeria* cultivar and the positive patch test elicited in a sensitized retail florist by its leaf. (Courtesy of St John's Institute of Dermatology.)

alstroemerias to be common sensitizers in retail florists. Allergic reactions to daffodils and primulas were rarely observed by Hausen and Oestmann; more than 90% of skin reactions to *Narcissus* species were irritant and the risk of primula allergy seemed to them to be well known in the industry, the majority of sensitizations being non-occupational. Domestic, rather than occupational, sensitization to primula was also emphasized in a recent Danish study (Ingber & Menné 1990).

Other Anacardiaceae

Plants of the Anacardiaceae other than poison oak and poison ivy have a similar potential to sensitize, putting a wide variety of other occupations at risk. Such occupations include: mango pickers (*Mangifera indica*), operatives processing cashew nuts (Pasricha *et al.* 1988), cashew nut shell oil (CNSO) (Reginella *et al.* 1989), or exposed to CNSO in the manufacture of varnishes and impregnating materials, phenolic resins, plasticizers, germicides and insecticides, colouring materials and indelible inks, lubricants and preservatives (*Anacardium occidentale*); oriental lacquer craftspeople (Kawai *et al.* 1991) using the product of the Japanese lacquer tree (*Rhus verniciflua*); and woodworkers (Goh 1988) exposed to the wood of the Rengas tree (various species).

Other allergic causes

Among other common occupational causes of allergic contact dermatitis from plants are the following: *Codiaeum variegatum*, confusingly known as 'croton' but to be distinguished from *Croton* which is highly irritant, increasingly implicated among florists and market gardeners (van Ketel 1979) and recently reported in a plant and flower delivery driver (Cleenewerck & Martin 1989); colophony (rosin) in Pinaceae such as X *Cupressocyparis leylandii* (Lovell *et al.* 1985), the popular fast-growing conifer, and Christmas trees (Macfarlane 1987); and garlic, onion, chives and leeks (Alliaceae) in food handlers (Lautier & Wendt 1985).

Other irritant causes

Other important causes of irritant contact dermatitis from occupational contact with plants include the raphids of *Dieffenbachia* (Ippen *et al.* 1986) (Fig. 2.1.2), and the glochids of *Opuntia* (sabra dermatitis) (Banerjee 1977). The sap of chicory (*Cichorium intybus* var. *foliosum*) can be irritant, as well as sensitizing, during its intensive processing (Rycroft *et al.* 1987) (Fig. 2.1.3); endive and lettuce cross-react. Plants belonging to the Cruciferae (Brassicaceae) contain highly irritant isothiocyanates (mustard oils), but a rare case of sensitization in a cauliflower grower was reported by van Ketel and Bruynzeel (1987). The irritancy of the Euphorbiaceae is illustrated by the case of a teacher of flower arrangement with acute irritant contact dermatitis from snow-on-the-mountain (*Euphorbia marginata*) (Urishibata & Kase 1991).

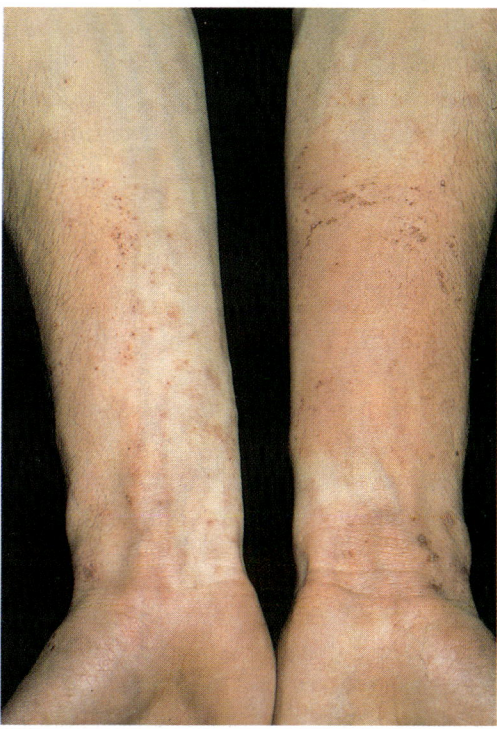

Fig. 2.1.2 Acute irritant contact dermatitis contracted from manually transporting a large number of *Dieffenbachia* plants. (Courtesy of St John's Institute of Dermatology.)

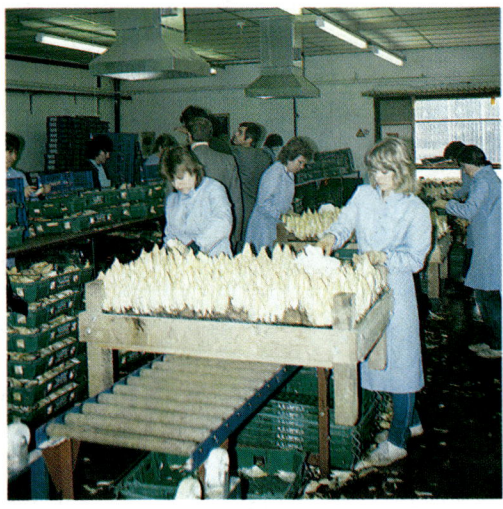

Fig. 2.1.3 Intensive processing of chicory (*Cichorium intybus* var. *foliosum*) leading to irritant contact dermatitis from its sap.

Staple crops

The staple cereal crops can cause dermatitis both on the farm and during later processing and transportation. Sensitization to rolled oats, malt flour (prepared from barley) and barley dust has been described (Cronin 1979) and irritant contact dermatitis may also occur (Seligman & Key 1968). Another staple crop, tobacco, commonly causes irritant erythema, urticaria and mild dermatitis, the much rarer cases of sensitization mainly occurring in cigarette and cigar factories (Rycroft *et al.* 1981).

Phytophotodermatitis

The Rutaceae and Apiaceae (Umbelliferae) are both well known for causing phototoxicity, and phytophotodermatitis has recently been described from a member of the former family in a university botanist on a field trip (*Ruta corsica*) (Ena & Camarda 1990), and from a member of the latter family in two gardeners in a university botanic garden *Heracleum mantegazzianum* (giant hogweed) (Goitre *et al.* 1987). Phototoxicity among celery (Apiaceae) harvesters occurs particularly when it is diseased, usually with the fungus *Sclerotinia sclerotiorum* (although another fungus *Septoria apii* and a bacterium *Erwinia carotovora* have also been implicated), which greatly increases the levels of psoralens in the plant (Ashwood Smith *et al.* 1985), though an outbreak in grocery workers has been ascribed to naturally occurring high levels (Cronin 1989). String trimming of weeds has been identified as an occupation particularly at risk of phytophotodermatitis from plants such as *Heracleum sphondylium* (cow parsley) (Oakley et al. 1986).

Contact urticaria and protein contact dermatitis

Contact urticaria occurs from a wide variety of plants and plant products met with occupationally, including lettuce, potato and citrus fruits, and may be either irritant (non-immunological) or allergic (immunological) (von Krogh & Maibach 1981). Protein contact dermatitis from Type I allergies to fruits and vegetables occurs in food handlers (Cronin 1989). Strawberry pickers' rash can be an allergic contact urticaria (Grattan & Harman 1985).

2.1.4 **Diagnosis**

More than simply ascertaining the patient's occupation, the dermatologist needs to acquire a mental picture of precisely how the patient carries out his or her work with plants, which parts of which plants come into contact with the skin as a result, and to what extent such contact occurs. In addition, accurate botanical identification of plants is frequently required.

Other lines of enquiry that often contribute to the diagnosis include the following: the time of onset of the earliest signs; the primary site of onset; the sites (and timing) of any secondary spread; whether the rash improves away from work and worsens on return to work (how much? how quickly?); whether fellow-workers have experienced similar symptoms; and whether sun exposure appears to be an aggravating factor.

Patch, and sometimes also photopatch and monochromator, testing are crucial in suspected occupational cases, given the multiplicity of plants with which such patients are often in contact and the notorious difficulty in distinguishing clinically between airborne contact dermatitis, photocontact dermatitis and photosensitivity. The differential diagnoses of allergic contact dermatitis from pesticides and, in outdoor workers, phototoxic drug eruptions are particularly important to remember. While repetition, serial dilution of plant extracts and control testing are the keys to avoiding false positive patch test reactions, false negatives can only be avoided by constant vigilance; the offending plant is easily missed.

Prick, scratch, scratch-chamber, and open and rub tests may be used in the diagnosis of occupational contact urticaria from plants and plant products (Hannuksela 1987). These tests also need to be repeated in control subjects if false positive reactions are to be avoided. Open and rub tests are more sensitive on previously involved than on uninvolved skin.

Workplace visits or, as a second best, communication with medical, nursing, employer and employee representatives by letter or telephone, are a 'requisite for adequate solving of problems of occupational dermatology' (Fregert 1963) and suspected cases involving plants are no exception (Rycroft et al. 1987). Sometimes an epidemiological survey may even be required.

There are three textbooks and three chapters of other textbooks that are particularly useful in diagnosing occupational plant dermatitis (Mitchell & Rook 1979, Mitchell 1980, Benezra et al. 1985, Mitchell & Fisher 1986, Hausen 1988, Schmidt 1990).

2.1.5 Treatment

Occasionally it is necessary to advise that a patient stays away from work during the acute phase of an occupational plant dermatitis. The prime aim in preventing long-term disability, however, is to enable the patient to remain in the same work and to restrict sickness absence to the minimum. Exceptions to this general policy arise when patients have isolated uncomplicated allergic contact dermatitis from plants or when individuals with sensitive skins find themselves in certain types of wet work, such as catering; then a change of occupation may hold out the only reasonable chance of clearance, or at least improvement, of the dermatitis.

2.1.6 Prevention

Because of the poor prognosis associated with certain forms of occupational plant dermatitis, such as that from Compositae (Asteraceae), and the partial, or even total, loss of livelihood that a change of occupation may involve, prevention is of great importance.

Those with a history of severe childhood eczema, especially if with hand involvement, should generally be advised against occupations such as horticulture, food processing or catering, because of their increased risk of irritant contact dermatitis (Rystedt 1986). Atopics do not incur a correspondingly increased risk of allergic contact dermatitis.

The occupational hygiene in many industries where plants are intensively handled is poor. Retail florists' premises, for example, were found in a survey to be generally small, poorly designed and unhygienic (Merrick et al. 1991).

Protective gloves have a role to play but are subject to three main problems:
1   This is simply their tendency to be punctured by many of the sharp

implements and materials used by plant handlers, as well as by some of the plants themselves.

2 The more subtle choice of their material; Marks (1988) has demonstrated, for example, that the allergen tuliposide A (tulips and alstroemerias) readily penetrates vinyl (PVC) gloves, while nitrile rubber (NBR) gloves resist it.

3 A small percentage of rubber glove wearers develop an allergic contact dermatitis from their processing chemicals or, from natural rubber (NR) gloves, an allergic contact urticaria from the latex itself (Turjanmaa & Reunala 1988).

'Barrier' creams are in general all too fallible, though a barrier cream containing cysteine has been suggested as protective against tulipalin A (Thiboutot et al. 1990). Clinical experience suggests that the application of emollient creams or lotions after hand washing or at the end of the working day may be beneficial in prevention, though this has yet to be scientifically established.

The various strategies for prevention of poison oak and poison ivy dermatitis have been reviewed by Epstein (1990). Hyposensitization, though theoretically possible, is too critical a procedure to be recommended routinely for outdoor workers.

References

Ashwood Smith M.J., Ceska O. & Chaudhury S.K. (1985) Mechanism of photosensitivity reactions to diseased celery. *British Medical Journal* **290**: 1249.
Banerjee K. (1977) A case report of sabra dermatitis. *Indian Journal of Dermatology* **22**: 159–62.
Benezra C., Ducombs G., Sell Y. & Foussereau J. (1985) *Plant Contact Dermatitis*. B.C. Decker, Toronto.
Burry J.N., Kuchel R., Reid J.G. & Kirk J. (1973) Australian bush dermatitis: Compositae dermatitis in South Australia. *The Medical Journal of Australia* **1**: 110–16.
Cleenewerck M.-B. & Martin P. (1989) Occupational contact dermatitis due to *Codiaeum variegatum* L., *Chrysanthemum indicum* L., *Chrysanthemum* X *hortorum* and *Frullania dilatata* L. In Frosch P.J., Dooms-Goossens A., Lachapelle J.-M., Rycroft R.J.G. & Scheper R.J. (eds) *Current Topics in Contact Dermatitis*. Springer-Verlag, Berlin, pp. 149–57.
Coenraads P.J., Nater J.P. & van der Lende R. (1983) Prevalence of eczema and other dermatoses of the hands and arms in the Netherlands. Association with age and occupation. *Clinical and Experimental Dermatology* **8**: 495–503.
Cronin E. (1979) Contact dermatitis from barley dust. *Contact Dermatitis* **5**: 196.
Cronin E. (1989) Dermatitis in food handlers. In Callen J.P., Dahl M.V., Golitz L.E., Schachner L.A. & Stegman S.J. (eds) *Advances in Dermatology. Vol. 4*. Year Book, Chicago, pp. 113–23.
Diepgen T.L., Häberle M. & Bäurle G. (1989) Fallstricke in der Berufsdermatologie: Das aerogene Kontaktekzem auf Pflanzen. *Dermatosen in Beruf und Umwelt* **37**: 23–5.
Ena P. & Camarda I. (1990) Phytophotodermatitis from *Ruta corsica*. *Contact Dermatitis* **22**: 63.
Epstein W.L. (1974) Poison oak and poison ivy dermatitis as an occupational problem.

Cutis **13**: 544–8.
Epstein W.L. (1990) Poison oak and poison ivy dermatitis. In Adams R.M. (ed.) *Occupational Skin Disease*, 2nd edn. W.B. Saunders, Philadelphia, pp. 536–42.
Fregert S. (1963) The organization of occupational dermatology in Lund. *Acta Dermato-Venereologica*. **43**: 203–5.
Fregert S. (1975) Occupational dermatitis in a 10-year material. *Contact Dermatitis* **1**: 96–107.
Goh C.L. (1988) Occupational allergic contact dermatitis from Rengas wood. *Contact Dermatitis* **18**: 300.
Goitre M., Roncarolo G., Bedello P.G. *et al*. (1987) Occupational phytophotodermatitis from *Heracleum mantegazzianum*: isolation of furocoumarins. *Bollettino di Dermatologia Allergologica e Professionale* **2**: 177–84.
Gonçalo S., Born M. & Pereira dos Santos A. (1981) Contact dermatitis to lichens. *Contact Dermatitis* **7**: 118–20.
Grattan C.E.H. & Harman R.R.M. (1985) Contact urticaria to strawberry. *Contact Dermatitis* **13**: 191–2.
Gude M., Hausen B.M., Heitsch H. & König W.A. (1988) An investigation of the irritant and allergenic properties of daffodils (*Narcissus pseudonarcissus* L. Amaryllidaceae). *Contact Dermatitis* **19**: 1–10.
Hannuksela M. (1987) Tests for immediate hypersensitivity. In Maibach H.I. (ed.) *Occupational and Industrial Dermatology*, 2nd edn. Year Book, Chicago, pp. 168–78.
Hausen B.M. (1988) *Allergie pflanzen-Pflanzenallergene: Handbuch und Atlas der allergie-induzierenden Wild- und Kulturpflanzen*. Kontakt allergene. Ecomed, Landsberg, München.
Hausen B.M. & Oestmann G. (1988) Untersuchungen über die Häufigkeit berufsbedingter allergischer Hauterkrankungen auf einem Blumengrossmarkt. *Dermatosen in Beruf und Umwelt* **36**: 117–24.
Ingber A. & Menné T. (1990) Primin standard patch testing: 5 years experience. *Contact Dermatitis* **23**: 15–19.
Ippen I., Wereta-Kubek M. & Rose U. (1986) Haut- und Schleimhautreaktionen durch Zimmerpflanzen der Gattung Dieffenbachia. *Dermatosen in Beruf und Umwelt* **34**: 93–101.
Kawai K., Nakagawa M., Kawai K. *et al*. (1991) Hyposensitization to urushiol among Japanese lacquer craftsmen. *Contact Dermatitis* **24**: 146–7.
Klaschka F., Grimm W.W. & Beiersdorff H.U. (1964) Tulpenkontaktekzem als Berufsdermatosen. *Hautarzt* **15**: 317–21.
Lautier R. & Wendt V. (1985) Kontaktallergie auf Alliaceae. Fallbeschreibung und Literaturübersicht. *Dermatosen in Beruf und Umwelt* **33**: 213–15.
Lonkar A., Mitchell J.C. & Calnan C.D. (1974) Contact dermatitis from *Parthenium hysterophorus*. *Transactions of the St John's Hospital Dermatological Society* **60**: 43–53.
Lovell C.R., Dannaker C.J. & White I.R. (1985) Dermatitis from X *Cupressocyparis leylandii* and concomitant sensitivity to colophony. *Contact Dermatitis* **13**: 344–5.
Macfarlane A.W. (1987) Cross reaction to a Christmas tree. *British Medical Journal* **295**: 1660–1.
Marks J.G. (1988) Allergic contact dermatitis to *Alstroemeria*. *Archives of Dermatology* **124**: 914–16.
Mathias C.G.T., Sinks T.H., Seligman P.J. & Halperin W.E. (1990) Surveillance of occupational skin diseases: a method utilizing workers' compensation claims. *American Journal of Industrial Medicine* **17**: 363–70.
Merrick C., Fenney J., Clarke E.C., Hodnett T. & Fletcher G. (1991) A survey of skin problems in floristry. *Contact Dermatitis* **24**: 306.
Mitchell J.C. (1981) Industrial aspects of 112 cases of allergic contact dermatitis from *Frullania* in British Columbia during a 10-year period. *Contact Dermatitis* **7**: 268–9.

Mitchell J.C. & Fisher A.A. (1986) Dermatitis due to plants and spices. In Fisher A.A. (ed.) *Contact Dermatitis*, 3rd edn. Lea & Febiger, Philadelphia, pp. 418–53.

Mitchell J.C. & Rook A. (1979) *Botanical Dermatology: Plants and Plant Products Injurious to the Skin*. Greengrass, Vancouver.

Mitchell J.N.S. (1980) Plants. In Cronin E. (ed.) *Contact Dermatitis*. Churchill Livingstone, Edinburgh, pp. 461–547.

Oakley A.M.M., Ive F.A. & Harrison M.A. (1986) String trimmer's dermatitis. *Journal of the Society of Occupational Medicine* **36**: 143–4.

O'Malley M., Thun M., Morrison J., Mathias C.G.T. & Halperin W.E. (1988) Surveillance of occupational skin disease using the supplementary data system. *American Journal of Industrial Medicine* **13**: 291–9.

Pasricha J.S., Srinivas C.R., Krupa Shankar D.S. & Shenoy K. (1988) Contact dermatitis due to cashew nut (*Anacardium occidentale*) shell oil, pericarp and kernel. *Indian Journal of Dermatology, Venereology and Leprology* **54**: 36–7.

Reginella R.F., Fairfield J.C. & Marks J.G. (1989) Hypo-sensitization to poison ivy after working in a cashew nut shell oil processing factory. *Contact Dermatitis* **20**: 274–9.

Rycroft R.J.G., Smith N.P., Stok E.T. & Middleton K. (1981) Investigation of suspected contact sensitivity to tobacco in cigarette and cigar factory employees. *Contact Dermatitis* **7**: 32–8.

Rycroft R.J.G., Lovell C.R., Harries P.G., Winter P. & Mallet A.I. (1987) Occupational irritant contact dermatitis from chicory. *Bollettino di Dermatologia Allergologica e Professionale* **2**: 77–82.

Rystedt I. (1986) Atopy, hand eczema and contact dermatitis: summary of recent large scale studies. *Seminars in Dermatology* **5**: 290–300.

Salo H., Hannuksela M. & Hausen B. (1981) Lichen picker's dermatitis (*Cladonia alpestris* (L.) Rab.). *Contact Dermatitis* **7**: 9–13.

Schmidt R.J. (1990) Plants. In Adams R.M. (ed.) *Occupational Skin Disease*, 2nd edn. W.B. Saunders, Philadelphia, pp. 503–24.

Seligman E.J. & Key M.M. (1968) Corn dermatitis. *Archives of Dermatology* **97**: 664–6.

Thiboutot D.M., Hamory B.H. & Marks J.G. (1990) Dermatoses in floral shop workers. *Journal of the American Academy of Dermatology* **22**: 54–8.

Turjanmaa K. & Reunala T. (1988) Contact urticaria from rubber gloves. *Dermatologic Clinics* **6**: 47–51.

Urishibata O. & Kase K. (1991) Irritant contact dermatitis from *Euphorbia marginata*. *Contact Dermatitis* **24**: 155–6.

Van Ketel W.G. (1979) Occupational contact dermatitis due to *Codiaeum variegatum* and possibly to *Aeschynantus pulcher*. *Dermatosen in Beruf und Umwelt* **27**: 141–2.

Van Ketel W.G. & Bruynzeel D.P. (1987) Contact dermatitis due to plants in Amsterdam. *Bollettino di Dermatologia Allergologica e Professionale* **2**: 132–8.

von Krogh G. & Maibach H.I. (1981) The contact urticaria syndrome — an updated review. *Journal of the American Academy of Dermatology* **5**: 328–42.

2.2 Plant products in perfumes and cosmetics

I.R. WHITE

2.2.1 What is a cosmetic?

Products applied to the skin, for non-medicinal reasons, are variously known by terms such as cosmetics, toiletries or skin care preparations. Whatever term is used all are cosmetics as the word has a legal definition. By a directive of the European Commission published in

1976* with subsequent amendments, the term 'cosmetic' has a statutory meaning and is defined as:

> ...any substance or preparation intended for placing in contact with the various external parts of the human body (epidermis, hair system, nails, lips and external genital organs) or with the teeth and the mucous membranes of the oral cavity with a view to cleaning them, perfuming them or protecting them to keep them in good condition, change their appearance and/or correct body odours.

Within this definition are included products such as:
- soaps, shampoos, toothpastes, cleansing and moisturizing creams for regular care;
- colour cosmetics such as eye-shadows, lipsticks and nail varnishes;
- hair colourants and styling agents;
- fragranced products such as deodorants, aftershaves and perfumes;
- ultraviolet light-screening preparations.

Excluded from the definition are any products intended for use because of pharmacological activity. A moisturizer intended as part of the treatment of an eczema is still a cosmetic preparation although it is being used medically. If a product has pharmacological activity but is being used for cosmetic purposes, then legislation covering pharmaceuticals† takes priority to the exclusion of the rules applicable to cosmetic products.‡

2.2.2 Historical overview of use of plants in cosmetics

Plants and substances derived from them have been used in cosmetics since historical times. Woad was used by the ancient Britons to dye their skin and henna in Asia to colour hair and stain skin for religious rites, olive oil by the ancient Greeks to cleanse their skin and the Phoenicians made soap by boiling animal fat with wood ash. Throughout the centuries the pleasant smells of many plants have been used and blended to make fragrances for personal application which paralleled their use in medicinal remedies and for religious purposes (Guin 1982). Many of these fragrance ingredients are now made synthetically.

---

* Council Directive 76/768/EEC of 27 July 1976 on the approximation of the laws of the Member States relating to cosmetic products.
† Council Directive 65/65 EEC of 26 January 1965 on the approximation of provisions laid down by law, regulation or administrative action relating to proprietary medicinal products.
‡ The Upjohn Company and Another v. Farzoo Inc. and Another. Case C-112/89; European Law Reports, *The Times*, 3 June 1991, p. 24.

2.2.3 **Current uses of plant material in cosmetics**

Plant-derived products used in cosmetics have many uses quite apart from the obvious one of smell imparted by essential oils. Many lipids or oils (Table 2.2.1) used are of vegetable origin as well as some colours (e.g. anatto, carotene, chlorophyll, henna), abrasives (e.g. ground almond and walnut shells), humectants (e.g. aloe vera, glycerol), absorbants (e.g. starches), thickening and other agents (e.g. gum arabic, guar gum, pectin, xanthan gum, colophony and karaya gum).

Table 2.2.1 Lipids of plant origin used in cosmetics.

Almond oil	Linseed oil
Apricot kernel oil	Olive oil
Avocado oil	Peach kernel oil
Castor oil	Peanut oil
Cocoa butter	Safflower oil
Coconut oil	Sesame oil
Corn oil	Soybean oil
Cottonseed oil	Wheatgerm oil
Grape seed oil	

The recent popular trend in using cosmetics which have been made from substances not of animal origin has resulted in many important cosmetic ingredients now being made from vegetable sources rather than traditional animal sources. Examples of these are stearic acid and glycerol. Similarly, major cosmetic components are synthesized from coconut and palm nut oils to produce an array of ingredients such as many surfactants used in cleansers. This industry and its diversity is reminiscent of the petrochemical industry.

There is often no functional rationale for the inclusion of some plant extracts in cosmetics. They are added for marketing reasons so that claims such as 'with extracts from nature' or 'with herbal extracts' can be made to nurture consumer interest in the perceived benefits of 'natural ingredients' on the skin. Products with such plant extracts have an enormous market share. Some cosmetic ranges have contained whole stems and leaves from plants such as ivy, thyme and rosemary. Most, however, contain trivial amounts, often 0.1% of commercial aqueous extracts, so that a valid claim for their inclusion can be made. The incorporation of these extracts often has a transient trend so that, for example, seaweed extract may be used in a cosmetic range for one season to be changed for cucumber the next but with little alteration in the basic formulation of the product; the packaging and image change. Consumer and media interest in herbalism encourages such use.

Table 2.2.2 Examples of plant extracts (often aqueous) used in cosmetics.

Aloe vera	Juniper
Birch	Lemon
Calendula	Pine needles
Capsicum	Quince seed
Clover	Rose water
Comfrey	Rosemary
Cucumber	Sage
Fennel	St John's Wort (*Hypericum*)
Gentian	Thyme
Hops	Witch hazel
Horse chestnut	Yarrow
Horsetail	

Some performance cosmetics contain large numbers of plant extracts which are marketed with a high and expensive media profile. Examples of the plant extracts used in one range of performance cosmetics are:
- *cleansing milk with alpine herbs*: sweet almond oil, wheat germ oil, chamomile, carrot, gentian, arnica, balm mint, juniper, pine needle, horsetail, corn poppy;
- *toning lotion*: aloe, rosemary, pansy, sage, bilberry, horsetail, pine needle;
- *facial peel*: burdock, mallow, coltsfoot, marsh mallow, sambucus;
- *breast cream*: hops, cypress, fennel, lemon, peppermint oil.

An exhaustive list of such extracts has been published (Nater & de Groot 1985) but an abridged list appears in Table 2.2.2.

Despite the huge quantities of such extracts (as opposed to essential oil extracts from some of the same materials) used by the cosmetic industry, adverse reactions to them among consumers is very rare. This rarity of reactions is probably a manifestation of the low concentrations present in the finished product. Adverse reactions have been more frequently reported from the use of some extracts, e.g. horse chestnut, or calendula, in pharmaceuticals.

2.2.4 Extraction of plant materials

Fixed or non-volatile oils (e.g. castor oil, almond oil) and waxes (e.g. carnauba wax from the leaves of *Copernicia cerifera*) of vegetable origin are obtained by expression in hydraulic presses. Essential oils (volatile oils) are the odorous principles found in various plant parts. These essential oils may be extracted in several ways depending on the type of plant material to be extracted and the stability of the oil. Distillation with water, water and steam, or direct steam are used to extract oils such as cinnamon, clove, peppermint and spearmint. Those volatile oils which cannot be distilled without decomposition, e.g.

lemon grass oil, are obtained by expression. Citrus oils are obtained by rolling the fruit over a trough lined with sharp projections; the oil globules collect in the trough. The volatile oil content of flower petals may be so small that extraction is not possible by large-scale methods. In such circumstances a bland oil is placed on a glass plate which is then covered with the petals. After the oil has absorbed as much fragrance as possible the oil is removed and extracted with alcohol.

Most essential oil production for the perfume industry is now accomplished by solvent extraction with petroleum distillates. The advantage of this method over distillation is that extraction occurs at low temperature which reduces chemical decomposition and gives a product with a more natural odour.

Substances often called 'plant extracts' may be obtained by nothing more than steeping plant material in water.

2.2.5 Fragrance materials

Up to 3000 fragrance materials are in current use. A single fragrance may contain up to 500 different ingredients but most of these are present in only trace amounts. Fragrance ingredients are derived from plant, animal and synthetic sources.

Details of the composition of a particular fragrance are closely guarded by industry which maintains that secrecy of the formulae is fully commensurate with investment in the development and marketing of a product (International Fragrance Association statement). The industry also maintains that disclosure of the nature of the fragrance materials used in a product is detrimental to the interest of the consumer and that it would not improve the safety of fragrances.

In the USA, where ingredient labelling of cosmetics has existed since 1977, fragrance details are not disclosed and in the proposed sixth amendment of the 1976 Cosmetic Directive of the European Commission, the industry will again be spared formula disclosure but it will be required to catalogue the most frequently used ingredients.

A perfume compound will normally be present at a concentration of <0.5% in a general cosmetic, about 4% in colognes and 20% in fine perfumes. In aromatherapy, fragranced essential oils are greatly diluted with corn or other fixed oils before application to the skin.

Fragrances account for a major part of allergic contact reactions to cosmetics. About one third of investigated cases of cosmetic allergy are identified as being due to fragrances (de Groot 1988). Currently, in patch testing the fragrance mix, colophony and balsam of Peru are used as 'standard' indicators for fragrance sensitivity. These indicators may detect fragrance sensitivity in only about 70–80% of cases (Larsen & Maibach 1982) and up to 12% of individuals with eczema react to

Table 2.2.3 Fragrance materials often present at a concentration of >1% in fine perfumes (alphabetically).

Amyl cinnamic aldehyde	Isobornyl acetate
Amyl salicylate	Lilial
Benzyl acetate	Linalool
Benzyl salicylate	Linalyl acetate
Citronellol	Lyral
Coumarin	Methyl ionone gamma
Eugenol	Musk ketone
Galaxolide 50*	Phenyl ethyl alcohol
Geraniol	Terpineol
Hedione	Terpinyl acetate
Heliotropine	Vertenex*
Hexyl cinnamic aldehyde	Vertifix*
Hydroxycitronellal	

* Trade-named aroma chemicals.

them. The fragrance mix, consisting of eight ingredients (eugenol, isoeugenol, oak moss absolute, geraniol, cinnamic aldehyde, amyl cinnamaldehyde, hydroxycitronellal, and cinnamic alcohol, emulsified with sorbitan sesquioleate), was defined from the investigation of a small number of fragrance-sensitive individuals. The mix is currently being developed to increase its usefulness.

Balsam of Peru (derived from *Myroxolon pereirae*, q.v., a tree native to El Salvador) is no longer used in cosmetic preparations although it is in some topical medicaments. It is useful as a screening agent in patch testing because of the numerous fragrance substances that it contains.

Table 2.2.3 gives a list of those fragrance ingredients said to be commonly present at a concentration of >1% in fine fragrances (Fenn 1989).

There is a belief in the fragrance industry that mixing fragrance ingredients together can reduce the sensitizing potential of a compound (International Fragrance Association). The sensitizing potential of cinnamic aldehyde is said to be reduced by mixing with equal parts of eugenol or D-limonene, a process known as 'quenching'.

Although allergic contact dermatitis to fragrance materials is common, contact urticaria, normally of the non-immunological (irritant) type, is not rare and is partially responsible for the transient irritation caused by some perfumes on topical application. Fragrance materials causing contact urticaria are listed in Table 2.2.4 (Emmons & Marks 1985, de Groot 1988).

The pleasant tingling sensation associated with contact urticaria has resulted in many fragrance compounds causing the reaction to be used as flavouring agents in toothpastes to give 'tingling freshness' (Table 2.2.5).

Table 2.2.4 Plant-derived fragrance materials causing contact urticaria.

Anisyl alcohol	Eugenol
Balsam of Peru	Geraniol
Benzoic acid	Menthol
Camphor	Terpinyl acetate
Capsicum	
Caraway oil	Other plant products causing contact urticaria:
Cinnamic acid, alcohol, aldehyde	Henna
Coumarin	
Ethyl vanillin	

Table 2.2.5 Examples of plant-derived contact allergens and urticants in toothpastes.

Anethole (from aniseed)	Menthol
Carvone (from dill)	Oil of anise
Cinnamic aldehyde	Peppermint oil
Cinnamon oil	Spearmint oil
Laurel oil	Thymol

Essential oils and fragrance ingredients have caused unintentional pigmentary problems on the skin from direct staining or post-inflammatory reactions (Table 2.2.6). Additionally, a number of essential oils contain furocoumarins which can cause phototoxicity, such as in

Table 2.2.6 Plant-derived substances causing unintentional colour changes on the skin.

	Example	Reaction
Essential oils	Juniper Lemon Lime Orange	Red discoloration by terpenes
Cinnamic alcohol		Post-inflammatory depigmentation
Perfume ingredients	Benzyl alcohol Benzyl salicylate Cananga oil Cinnamic alcohol Geraniol Hydroxycitronellal Jasmine absolute Lavender oil Methoxycitronellal Sandalwood oil Ylang-ylang oil	Post-inflammatory depigmentation Pigmented cosmetic dermatitis

Table 2.2.7 Plant-derived cosmetic products reported to have caused phototoxicity.

Balsam of Peru
Carotene
Cinnamic aldehyde
Essential oils (e.g. bergamot, cedar, citron, lavender, lime, neroli, petitgrain, sandalwood)
Furocoumarins (e.g. in oil of Bergamot)
Oak moss

Berloque dermatitis. In the European Community there is now a maximum permitted concentration of bergapten (5-methoxypsoralen) and other psoralens of 1 ppm in all cosmetics (including perfumes) except for one suncare product which presently contains it at a level of up to 50 ppm. Some other plant-derived compounds have also caused phototoxicity (Table 2.2.7).

2.2.6 Other problems

Some oils have caused cosmetic acne and folliculitis (Table 2.2.8). Ground kernels (e.g. apricot kernel), used in exfoliating scrubs, have caused irritant contact reactions. Henna has caused anaphylaxis.

Table 2.2.8 Plant-derived lipids causing acne/folliculitis.

Cocoa butter	Peanut oil
Coconut oil	Pine tar
Corn oil	Safflower oil
Linseed oil	Sesame oil
Olive oil	

References

Emmons W.W. & Marks J.G. (1985) Immediate and delayed reactions to cosmetic ingredients. *Contact Dermatitis* **13**: 258–65.

Fenn R.S. (1989) Aroma chemical usage trends in modern perfumery. *Perfumer Flavorist* **14**: 1–7.

De Groot A.C. (1988) *Adverse reactions to cosmetics.* Thesis, State University of Groningen, The Netherlands.

Guin J.D. (1982) History, manufacture, and cutaneous reactions to perfumes. In Frost P. & Horwitz S.N. (eds) *Principles of Cosmetics for the Dermatologist.* C.V. Mosby, St Louis, pp. 111–29.

Larsen W.G. & Maibach H.I. (1982) Fragrance contact allergy. *Seminars in Dermatology* **1**: 85–90.

Nater J.P. & de Groot A.C. (1985) *Unwanted Effects of Cosmetics and Drugs Used in Dermatology.* Elsevier, Amsterdam.

3 Identification of plants

M.E. HANSEN

3.1 The basics of plant taxonomy and nomenclature

Numerous systems for the classification of plants have been proposed, all of them being based in some way upon a hierarchical grouping according to certain shared features and characteristics. Earlier systems, pre-dating evolutionary theory, relied upon a few easily observed features, and this often resulted in rather artificial and spurious groupings (phenetic systems). Modern taxonomy aims to produce systems that reflect likely evolutionary relationships (phylogenetic systems) and are based upon comparisons of numerous features of whole plants.

It should be recognized that there is never complete agreement between taxonomists as to correct classification and nomenclature, and that there may be some differences in systems used by different authorities. Moreover, with the development of new techniques for examining all aspects of plant biology, changes are continuously occurring in the grouping and naming of species.

A complete taxonomic scheme involves a large number of sub-divisions and groupings of increasingly close affinity, but for most practical purposes it is only necessary to be familiar with a few of them.

Almost all of the plants dealt with in this book belong to the group termed Spermatophyta, or seed plants. There are two divisions of these, the large group of flowering plants, or angiosperms, and the smaller group, termed gymnosperms, which includes all the conifers.

Within each of these divisions, the most important sub-group is the family, for example Umbelliferae, Compositae (Asteraceae), which is further divided into genera. Some families consist of only one genus, but there are generally a number, sometimes several hundred. Within each genus are listed individual species of plants, occasionally with further differentiation into varieties or sub-species.

The scientific Latin name of a plant is binomial, consisting of the generic name, shared by all members of the genus, and the specific name which is unique to that plant. By convention, generic names have an upper case initial, and specific a lower case, and the whole name is italicized. The family name should also be cited, for example, *Ricinus communis* (Euphorbiaceae). The binomial system was devised by Linnaeus in the 18th century, and the fact that a large proportion of his original names are still in use is reflected by the use of 'Linn' or 'L.' after the scientific name in many publications. Other names or initials indicate other botanists who first used the nomenclature and, although to be strictly correct they should be included in the name, it is generally acceptable to omit them.

The use of English names for plants may seem a simpler alternative, but can lead to confusion and ambiguity. Despite some differences of opinion regarding classification, the scientific name accurately defines one particular plant and is universally understood.

There are often regional variations in common names, and the same plant may have a very large number of names. Conversely, the same trivial name may be used for several different plants. Interesting examples of this are given in *The Englishman's Flora* by Geoffrey Grigson (1975).

Caution should therefore be exercised when a plant's identity is reported using an English name, and it should always be authenticated. Most reference books use names listed in *English Names of Wild Flowers* (Dony et al. 1980) published by the Botanical Society of the British Isles.

3.2 Features used in plant identification

The description of characteristics of the various morphological parts of plants has its own technical vocabulary, which is outside the scope of this book. However, it is, in most cases, possible to make an identification from a simple illustrated description.

The various identification guides referred to all include some form of glossary, often illustrated, which defines the botanical terms used in the text and is designed for the non-specialist.

It is, however, useful to know, at the time of collection or observation, what are the most important identifying features. Some of these are listed below.

3.2.1 Flowers

1   Whether solitary, or in clusters, heads or spikes.
2   Whether open, with petals, or bell-shaped, lipped, daisy-like or some other shape.
3   Number of petals.
4   Colour, and any variation in colour.

There are numerous other details of flower structure that might need expert examination, but the above are sufficient for most identifications.

3.2.2 Leaves

1 Whether simple or compound (composed of a number of smaller leaflets).
2 Relationship to one another and to the stem, for example growing alternately.
3 Surface, whether smooth, hairy, prickly, shiny, etc.
4 Shape — there are a number of terms used to describe leaf shape, and reference should be made to a glossary for correct definitions. However, a general note can be made of whether leaves are broad, narrow, pointed, etc., and whether the margin is smooth or jagged.
5 Differences between basal leaves (those immediately next to the ground) and leaves growing further up the stem.

3.2.3 Stems

1 Whether smooth, hairy or prickly.
2 Presence of spots or markings.
3 Whether cylindrical, angled or ridged.

3.2.4 Fruit and seeds

If these are present, they will be a useful aid to identification. There is an enormous variety in form of fruits and seeds and the features used will depend upon the type of fruit. Comparison should be made with the published descriptions.

3.3 Collection of material for identification

The general rule regarding plant identification is 'take the book to the plant, not vice versa', and it should be remembered that it is illegal to dig up any wild plant without the permission of the owner of its habitat (Conservation of Wild Creatures and Wild Plants Act 1975). Moreover, the collection of flowers, even without uprooting the plant, will remove potential seeds. It may be possible to record all the necessary information photographically and using sketches and notes, without disturbing the plant.

However, the majority of plants dealt with in this book are not of rare or endangered species, and it is usually acceptable to collect reasonable quantities of material from the above-ground parts in order to make an identification, or to provide an expert with the means to do so. It should not be necessary to remove the roots or other underground portions of wild plants.

Photographs or sketches to indicate the habitat, and the size and shape of the whole plant, often provide useful supplementary information.

It will be seen from any reference book that identification schemes are primarily based upon the flowering parts of plants, so, ideally, the specimens collected should include fully formed flowers. The whole flowering stalk should be collected if possible, since the arrangement of flowers on the stem may be as important as their shape and colour.

When the plant is not in flower, then a representative sample should be taken of leaves and stems. If flowering is over, some of the fruits and seeds, at various stages of development, should be collected. In some cases, for instance the family Umbelliferae, examination of the fruits is one of the best ways of distinguishing between members of a difficult group.

It is obviously easier to identify a fresh plant in good condition than a wilted, shrivelled or dried-up specimen. Collected material should be handled carefully, without crushing, transported in a suitable container, kept moist and put into water as soon as possible.

If it is impossible to keep a specimen alive, or if it is desirable to preserve it after identification, then careful pressing and drying is the usual procedure. This may be done using a special plant press, but satisfactory results can be obtained by arranging the various plant parts carefully between sheets of thick absorbent paper and pressing under heavy books. When completely dry, the specimens are mounted on sheets of paper or card and labelled with the relevant details.

For the identification of entire plants or undamaged parts, observation of key features by the naked eye is generally adequate. A useful aid, however, is a simple hand or pocket lens, giving approximately $\times 10$ magnification. This will enable a closer scrutiny of features such as hairs, flower structure, or fine markings.

If the only material available is in the form of small fragments, or is damaged or shrivelled beyond recognition, then microscopic examination of the tissues may be necessary. It is often possible to make an identification from very small samples, even in the form of powder. Expertise in this technique may be available in university or college pharmacy or botany departments.

3.4 Identification of plants

3.4.1 Wild plants

The identification of a plant may be carried out in a number of ways, the strategy used depending very much upon the level of botanical knowledge and vocabulary of the identifier.

For the expert, the standard work is Clapham, Tutin and Moore's *Flora of the British Isles* (1987), in which keys based on the observation of a number of botanical features are used to assign the specimen to the correct family, genus and species.

However, there is a large number of popular guides that do not require a great deal of background knowledge, and that enable the amateur to identify a plant fairly easily. Almost all of them incorporate an illustrated glossary of botanical terms used in the text, and this should generally be sufficient for the non-specialist.

Many are arranged according to family, for example *The Concise British Flora in Colour* (Keble Martin 1965), and although this presupposes some knowledge of classification, in practice the excellent illustrations make it fairly easy to locate most species by simply leafing through the colour plates.

The Wild Flower Key (Rose 1981) provides keys based on both flower and vegetative characteristics, as well as habitats, which enable assignment to the correct family, from which an identification can be made from the illustrations.

Other guides, such as Fitter and Blamey's *Wild Flowers of Britain and Northern Europe* (1974) use flower colour and shape to establish the identity of a specimen, without the need for preliminary assignment to a family.

The Collins Pocket Guide to Wild Flowers (McClintock & Fitter 1965) and some more recent publications use colour illustrations as the starting point, with plants grouped according to flower colour.

As a rule, identification can be made with more certainty from coloured drawings and paintings, rather than from photographs. Botanical illustrations deliberately include, and may highlight, those characteristics that are important in identification, and these may not always show clearly in a photograph.

3.4.2 Garden and house plants

The identification of non-indigenous plants, such as cultivated varieties grown in gardens and greenhouses, and house plants, may present some problems.

A very comprehensive guide is the Royal Horticultural Society's *Gardeners' Encyclopaedia of Plants and Flowers*, which includes 4000 photographs. On a more modest scale, but with excellent illustrations, is the 'Expert' series by Dr D.G. Hessayon (pbi Publications), providing separate books on flowers, house plants, and trees and shrubs.

It is important to realize that variation in cultivated plants, in the form of numerous hybrids and named varieties, can produce biochemical differences as well as the more obvious ones of shape, size and colour and that this may be significant when studying dermatological effects. It may be necessary when attempting an accurate identification to enlist the help of a horticultural expert.

References

Clapham A.R., Tutin T.G. & Moore D.M. (1987) *Flora of the British Isles*, 3rd edn. Cambridge University Press, Cambridge.

Dony J.L., Perring F.H. & Rob C.M. (1980) *English Names of Wild Flowers*. Botanical Society of the British Isles, London.

Fitter R., Fitter A. & Blamey M. (1974) *Wild Flowers of Britain and Northern Europe*. Collins, London.

Grigson G. (1975) *The Englishman's Flora*. Paladin, St Albans.

Hessayon D.G. *The Flower Expert, The House Plant Expert, The Tree and Shrub Expert* and others in the 'Expert' series. pbi Publications, Waltham Cross, Herts.

Keble Martin W. (1965) *The Concise British Flora in Colour*. Ebury Press & Michael Joseph, London.

McClintock D. & Fitter R.S.R. (1965) *Collins Pocket Guide to Wild Flowers*. Collins, London.

Rose F. (1981) *The Wild Flower Key*. Warne, London.

Royal Horticultural Society (1989) *Gardeners' Encyclopaedia of Plants and Flowers*. RHS, London.

4 Urticaria due to plants

4.1 Introduction

'Urticaria' (hives) describes areas of cutaneous erythema and oedema affecting the dermis and subcutis. A typical urticarial weal is short-lived (less than 24 h), associated with itch or tingling, and resolving without trace. If these features develop within an hour of exposure to an agent at the site of contact, the term 'contact urticaria' is used.

Contact urticaria due to plants may be induced by pharmacological mechanisms; a classic example is the eruption induced by stinging nettles (*Urtica dioica*) from which the term 'urticaria' ('nettle rash') is derived. Alternatively, an individual may develop a specific Type I hypersensitivity to a specific molecular component of the plant ('immunological urticaria'). Some atopic individuals develop an acute vesicular response within minutes after handling plant or animal material; this has been called 'protein contact dermatitis' and is especially important in food handlers (Hjorth & Roed-Petersen 1976, Cronin 1989). Repeated exposure to such stimuli may lead to a persistent eczematous state (von Krogh & Maibach 1982).

References

Cronin E. (1989) Dermatitis in food handlers. *Advances in Dermatology* **4**: 113–24.
Hjorth N. & Roed-Petersen J. (1976) Occupational protein contact dermatitis in food handlers. *Contact Dermatitis* **2**: 28–42.
Von Krogh G. & Maibach H.I. (1982) The contact urticaria syndrome. *Seminars in Dermatology* **1**: 59–66.

4.2 Urticaria due to injection of toxins

Minor forms of this eruption are extremely common, and do not involve hypersensitivity mechanisms. Several plant species possess sharp hairs (strictly 'emergences') on the surface of the leaves and stem. These deliver a cocktail of irritant chemicals into the skin or mucous membranes after contact, as a defence mechanism against browsing animals. (Some caterpillars employ a similar strategy to avoid predation.) The common stinging nettle (*Urtica dioica*) (Fig. 4.2.1) is a familiar example. This plant is native to Europe but naturalized in temperate areas worldwide. It enjoys rich nitrogenous soil in moist areas. Light trauma (e.g. brushing against the plant) shears off a protec-

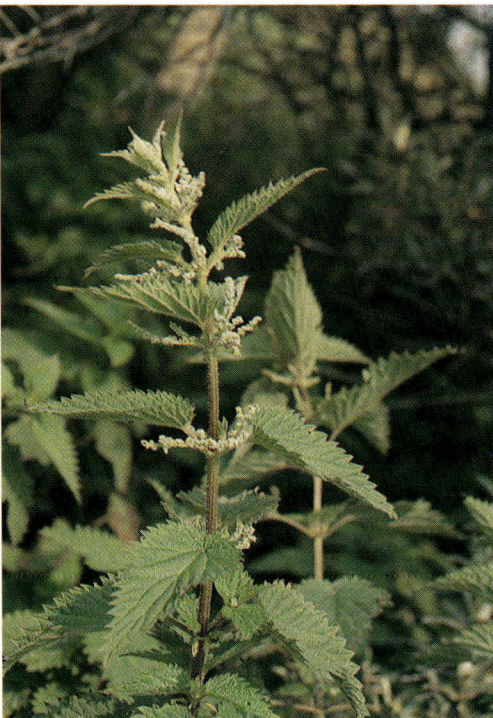

Fig. 4.2.1 The stinging nettle, *Urtica dioica*.

tive cap from the hair, revealing a sharp bevelled hollow structure resembling a hypodermic needle (Fig. 4.2.2). The walls of this structure are rigid and silicaceous (Thurston 1974). Plants grown in a silica-free medium have considerably reduced capacity to sting (Barber & Shone 1966). After puncture, an irritant liquid is released into the skin. Studies of *Urtica* species, and the allied genus *Girardinia*, have show that this liquid contains several pro-inflammatory mediators, including histamine, acetylcholine (Emmelin & Feldberg 1947) and 5-hydroxytryptamine (Collier & Chesher 1956, Saxena *et al.* 1966).

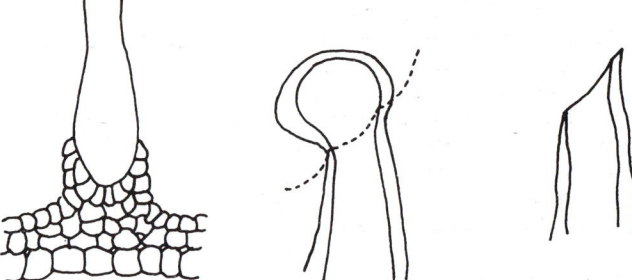

Fig. 4.2.2 Development of the stinging trichome in *Urtica dioica*, showing the site of fracture at the tip (after Thurston & Lersten 1969).

These substances cause the immediate reaction following a nettle sting. However, a stinging reaction occurs at the site for more than 12 h, even when clinical features of urticaria have disappeared. This suggests the presence of other substances capable of secondary release of inflammatory mediators; a possible histamine releaser in *Urtica parviflora* was noted by Saxena et al. (1965). Alternatively, nettles may contain neurotoxic substances (Oliver et al. 1991). The persistence of implanted silicaceous hairs may also cause continued irritation (Mitchell & Rook 1979).

Plants with stinging hairs have been recorded in four main families, Urticaceae (including stinging nettles and stinging trees), Euphorbiaceae (Spurges — also contains many irritant species), Loasaceae and Hydrophyllaceae (*Wigandia*) (Thurston & Lersten 1969). The genera are listed in Table 4.2.1. The vast majority are tropical plants and extremely rare in cultivation. *Wigandia* is grown as an ornamental tree in warmer

Table 4.2.1 Plants possessing urticating hairs.

URTICACEAE
Urtica (stinging nettles) *dioica, urens, pilulifera* (worldwide), *parviflora* (Himalaya), *ferox* (New Zealand), etc.
Dendrocnide (stinging trees) (Australia, New Guinea, Timor)
Fleurya aestuans (Trinidad)
Girardinia (tropical Africa)
Gyrotaenia (West Indies)
Hesperocnide (California, Hawaii)
Laportea (nettle tree) (northeast USA, Asia); see also *Dendrocnide* and *Fleurya*
Nanocnide (eastern Asia)
Obetia (tropical Africa)
Urera/Scepocarpus (tropical Africa, Central America and Hawaii)

Loasaceae (Central and South America)
Some species cultivated as ornamentals: *Blumenbachia, Caiophora, Cevallia, Eucnide, Fuertesia, Gronovia, Loasa*

EUPHORBIACEAE
Acidoton urens (tropical America)
Caperonia palustris (pantropical)
Cnesmone (Himalaya, Far East)
Cnidoscolus (spurge nettle, tread softly) (tropical America)
C. stimulosus (southeast USA)
Dalechampia (tropical America)
Jatropha urens (Ortiga) (tropical America, Africa, south USA)
Pachystylidium (South-East Asia)
Platygyna hexandia and *pruriens* (Cuba)
Sphaerostylis (East Africa, Malaysia)
Tragia (tropics and sub-tropics)

HYDROPHYLLACEAE
Wigandia caracasana (some forms) (Central America) — also allergenic (see pp. 190–1)

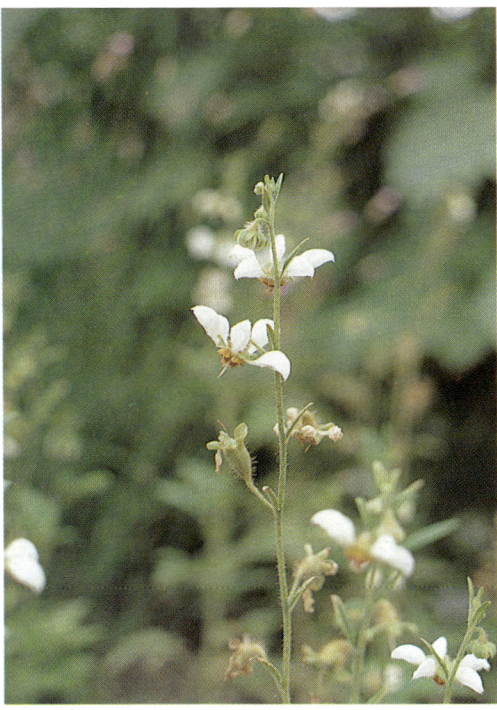

Fig. 4.2.3 *Loasa vulcanica*.

areas of the USA (see pp. 190–1). *Loasa* (Fig. 4.2.3) and *Blumenbachia* spp. (Loasaceae) are occasionally grown in specialist collections as ornamentals.

Most reactions are annoying but trivial. Squeezing a nettle firmly ('grasping the nettle') is (usually) less likely to cause stinging. The value of dock leaves, popular in folk lore, is unproven. Vigorous massaging or cold compresses will often reduce symptoms. Some reactions are more severe; dogs which come into contact with *Urtica* species in southern USA were reported to 'stagger, salivate profusely, gag and vomit' (Thurston & Lersten 1969). *Urtica gigas* (?*Dendrocnide gigas*), 'the tree of the settlers', has caused death in horses in New Zealand (Aston 1923). *Urtica ferox* (Fig. 4.2.4) has caused death in humans (Gilles & Wright 1966).

In Australia, the toxicity of *Dendrocnide* (Figs 4.2.5, 4.2.6) (previously referred to as *Laportea*), the stinging tree, has been recognized since the mid 19th century. Bailey and Gordon (1887) reported that 'the stinging hairs have frequently caused the death of horses' (quoted in Gilles & Wright 1966). Three species of *Dendrocnide* are found in eastern Australia, chiefly in rain forests. *Dendrocnide gigas* and *D. photinophylla* are trees, up to 40 m; the young shoots and branchlets are covered with stiff stinging hairs, which disappear from older trees. *Dendrocnide moroides* (Gympie bush), a tall shrub, is the

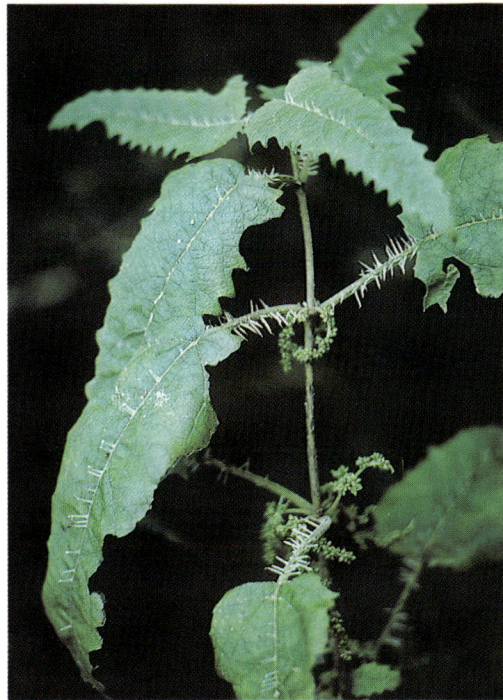

Fig. 4.2.4 *Urtica ferox* (photographed by Dr Mark Smith in Akarua, New Zealand).

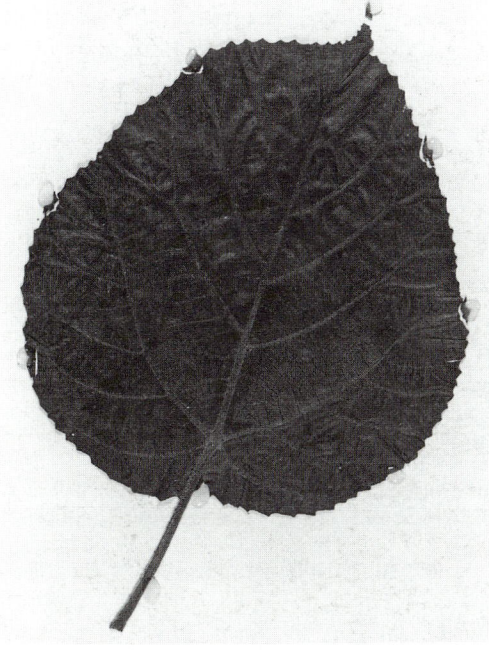

Fig. 4.2.5 Herbarium specimen of the leaf of *Dendrocnide excelsa*, a 'stinging tree'. (Courtesy of Adelaide Botanic Gardens.)

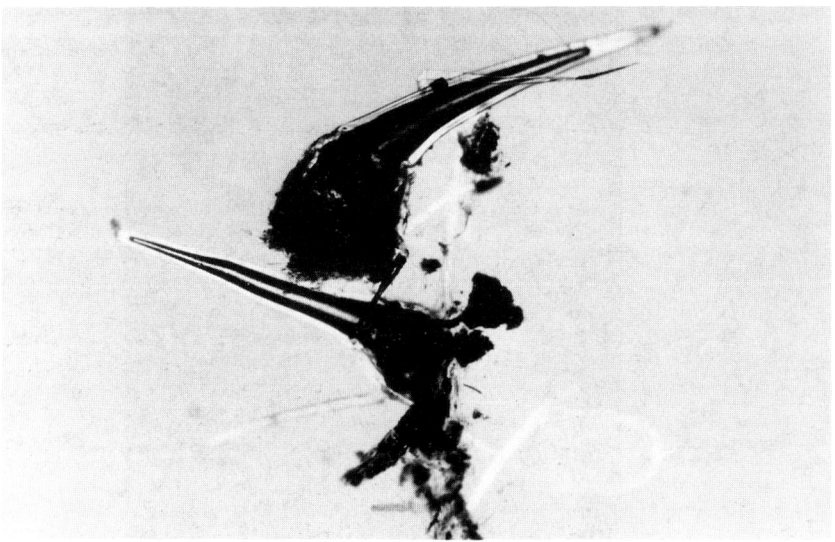

Fig. 4.2.6 Photomicrograph of stinging emergence of *Dendrocnide excelsa*. (Courtesy of Dr T.I. Macleod.)

most virulent species in Australia (Francis & Southcott 1967). Urticaria, from contact with the hairs, is severe, persisting for days or even weeks. Initially, slight pruritus is followed by severe, intermittent, stabbing pains, particularly along the course of lymphatics. Robertson and Macfarlane (1957) isolated a stable, heat-resistant non-dialysable substance which induced the pain. This material has a molecular weight of over 1000 (Macfarlane 1963) and has been purified (Oelrichs & Robertson 1970). A related species, *D. cordata*, has caused a human death in New Guinea (Winkler 1922).

References

Aston B.C. (1923) The poisonous, suspected and medicinal plants of New Zealand. *New Zealand Journal of Agriculture* **26**: 149–56.
Barber D.A. & Shone M.G.T. (1966) The absorption of silica from aqueous solution by plants. *Journal of Experimental Botany* **17**: 569–78.
Collier H.O.J. & Chesher G.B. (1956) Identification of 5-hydroxytryptamine in the sting of the nettle *Urtica dioica*. *British Journal of Pharmacology* **11**: 186–9.
Emmelin N. & Feldberg W. (1947) The mechanism of the sting of the common nettle (*Urtica dioica*). *Journal of Physiology* **106**: 440–5.
Francis D.F. & Southcott R.V. (1967) *Plants Harmful to Man in Australia*. Miscellaneous Bulletin No. I. Botanic Garden Adelaide, South Australia.
Gilles R.G. & Wright A.S. (1966) Laportea, the stinging tree. *North Queensland Naturalist* **33**: 2.
Macfarlane W.V. (1963) The stinging properties of *Laportea*. *Economic Botany* **17**: 303–11.
Mitchell T. & Rook A. (1979) *Botanical Dermatology*. Greengrass, Vancouver.
Oelrichs P.B. & Robertson P.A. (1970) Purification of pain-producing substances from *Dendrocnide* (*Laportea*) *moroides*. *Toxicon* **8**: 89–90.

Oliver F., Amon E.U., Breathnach A. et al. (1991) Contact urticaria due to the common stinging nettle (*Urtica dioica*) — histological, ultra-structural and pharmacological studies. *Clinical and Experimental Dermatology* **16**: 1–17.

Robertson P.A. & Macfarlane W.V. (1957) Pain producing substances from the stinging bush *Laportea moroides*. *Australian Journal of Experimental Biology* **35**: 381–94.

Saxena P.R., Pant M.C., Kishor K. & Bhargava K.P. (1965) Identification of pharmacologically active substances in the Indian stinging nettle, *Urtica parviflora* (Roxb). *Canadian Journal of Physiology and Pharmacology* **43**: 869–76.

Saxena P.R., Tangri K.K. & Bhargava K.P. (1966) Identification of acetylcholine, histamine and 5-hydroxytryptamine in *Girardinia heterophylla* (Decne). *Canadian Journal of Physiology and Pharmacology* **44**: 621–7.

Thurston E.L. (1974) Morphology, fine structure, and ontogeny of the stinging emergence of *Urtica dioica*. *American Journal of Botany* **61**: 809–17.

Thurston E.L. & Lersten N. (1969) The morphology and toxicology of plant stinging hairs. *Botanical Review* **35**: 393–412.

Winkler H. (1922) Die Urticaceen Papuasiens. *Botanische Jahrbuch* **57**: 501–8.

4.3 Immunological contact urticaria

An immediate Type I contact reaction occurs in an individual who has previously become sensitized to a plant or plant product. Molecules of the contact sensitizer penetrate the epidermis, and then react with specific immunoglobulin E (IgE) bound to mast cells, leading to release of vasoactive mediators (Lahti 1986a). Histamine appears to be the major protagonist; pre-injection of compound 48:80 blocks the response and it is reduced by concurrent injection of an antihistamine (Larko et al. 1983). Other pharmacologically active substances, such as prostaglandins, kinins, leukotrienes, etc., may amplify the inflammatory response.

Irritant hairs on the surface of the plant enhance penetration of the antigen(s). A good example is tumbleweed (*Salsola kali*) which possesses sharp floral bracts, causing an irritant reaction in all individuals. A few become sensitized to the plant and subsequently develop contact urticaria (Powell & Smith 1978). Doubtless, the wet working conditions and resultant maceration of the skin explain the high incidence of Type I reactions to foodstuffs in food handlers (Hjorth & Roed-Petersen 1976). Any plant is probably capable of inducing immunological contact urticaria; the list in Table 4.3.1 may reflect frequency of exposure rather than an inherent sensitizing property of the plant.

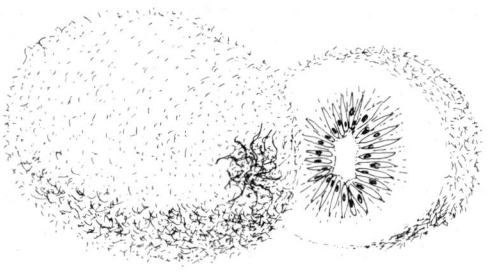

Fig. 4.3.1 Kiwi fruit (*Actinidia chinensis*).

Table 4.3.1 Plants and plant products reported to cause immunological contact urticaria or anaphylaxis (Lahti 1986a, Cronin 1987).

VEGETABLES AND HERBS
Beans — alfalfa, chick peas (Acciai *et al.* 1991), runner bean (Marshman & Lovell 1991), winged bean; cabbage; carrot; cauliflower; celery; chives; coriander; cucumber; dill; endive; garlic; green pepper; leek; lettuce; mustard; onion; parsley and parsley root; parsnip; potato; rapeseed; shallot; spinach; tomato; watercress

FRUITS
Apple; apricot; banana (flesh); grapefruit; kiwifruit (Fig. 4.3.1) (Veraldi & Schianchi-Veraldi 1990); lemon flesh and peel; lime (Picardo *et al.* 1988); mango; melon; orange flesh and peel; pineapple flesh; strawberry

SPICES
Caraway; cinnamon

NUTS
Almond; brazil; hazel

BEVERAGES
Coffee

OTHER ECONOMIC PLANTS
Cannabis indica (hemp) (Lindemayr *et al.* 1980); *Gossypium* spp. (cotton) (Harris & Shure 1950); *Hevea brasiliensis* (rubber tree); *Humulus lupulus* (hop); *Lawsonia inermis* (henna) (Cronin 1979, Nigam *et al.* 1988); *Linum usitatissimum* (flax); *Ricinus communis* (castor oil bean) (Fakhri & Erwa 1988); *Semecarpus anacardium* (source of Dhobi (launderer) mark) (Krupa Shankar 1992)

ESSENTIAL OILS
Sesame seed oil (Torsney 1964)

COSMETIC INGREDIENTS
Balsam of Peru; lime extract in shampoos (Picardo *et al.* 1988)

GRASSES AND CEREALS
Wheat; maize; barley; rye

HERBACEOUS PLANTS
Blumea gariepina (native to Southern Africa); *Iris* spp.; *Tanacetum cinerariifolium*; *Monstera deliciosa* (edible fruit in tropics; foliage house plant in northern Europe); *Salsola kali* (tumbleweed) (Powell & Smith 1978); *Trifolium pratensis* (red clover); *Tulipa* cultivars (Lahti 1986b); Bougainvillea (Fischer 1991) Chrysanthemum cultivars (see p. 162)

SHRUBS
Agave americana; *Cornus sanguineus* (bloodtwig dogwood); *Cotoneaster* spp.; *Crataegus monogyna* (hawthorn); *Grevillea juniperifolia* and *Hakea suaveolens* (Apted 1988a, b)

ALGAE
(Esp. *Lyngbya majuscula*)

LICHENS

HORSETAILS
Equisetum arvense (an immediate eruption resembling seborrhoeic dermatitis — Sudan 1985)

TREES AND WOODS
Betula verrucosa (birch); *Dalbergia latifolia* (Indian rosewood); *Eucalyptus* spp. (gums); *Larix decidua* (larch); *Shorea* (Philippine red mahogany); *Tectona grandis* (teak); *Terminalia superba* (Limba tree); *Thuja plicata* (arborvitae, western red cedar); *Triplochiton scleroxylon* (abachi, obeche)

4.3.1 Testing for Type I hypersensitivity

Type I reactions are best elicited by *prick tests* (Figs 4.3.2, 4.3.3). A sliver of the material is placed on the flexor forearm and superficial pricks are made through it using a blood lancet or a sterile hypodermic needle with the bevel facing upwards. The needle should be introduced almost parallel with the skin, barely tenting up the skin and taking care not to draw blood. After an immediate reading, the plant material is then secured in place with tape and left for 15–20 min. Care should be taken to avoid known irritants or urticants. Positive prick tests with an unusual plant or foodstuff should be checked by screening the material in control subjects (e.g. the clinic staff!) (Cronin 1987). Different parts of a vegetable should be tested, e.g. tomato peel and flesh, as the allergens may differ. In the *scratch test*, a 5 mm scratch is made on the forearm or back and the test material applied for 15–20 min. More positive reactions are obtained using the *scratch-chamber* method, where the test material is occluded with an aluminium patch test chamber. Dry foods can be attached to the chambers using

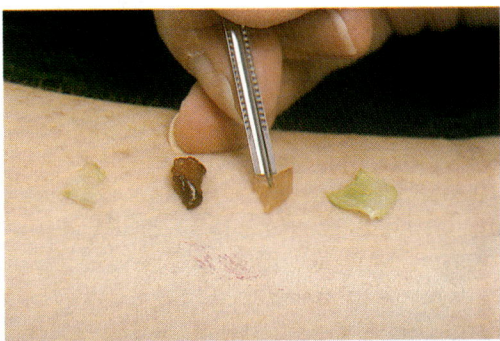

Fig. 4.3.2 Prick testing with foods using a blood lancet. (Courtesy of Dr E. Cronin.)

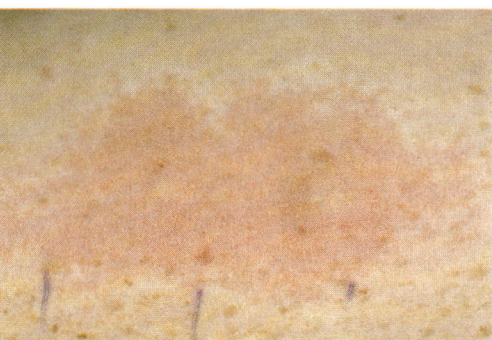

Fig. 4.3.3 Positive prick test reaction to cucumber skin and flesh. (Courtesy of Dr E. Cronin.)

moistened blotting paper. After the 20-min reading, the chambers can be replaced to test for delayed hypersensitivity at 2 and 4 days (Niinimäki 1987). Prick testing appears to be remarkably safe. Even in patients with anaphylactic reactions to rubber, there were no adverse reactions even when multiple prick tests were performed simultaneously. In contrast, scratch testing or use tests with rubber gloves may cause life-endangering reactions (Turjanmaa & Reunala 1988).

Serological tests, e.g. the *radioallergosorbent* (RAST) *test*, do not usually convey as much information as prick testing although RAST inhibition tests and crossed radioimmunoelectrophoresis (CRIE) and its inhibition may help in the investigation of possible cross-sensitivity (Lowenstein & Eriksson 1983).

Hjorth and Roed-Petersen (1976) investigated the causes of dermatitis in chefs and sandwich makers. They found that application of certain foods to eczematous skin caused irritation, redness and sometimes vesiculation. They termed this phenomenon 'protein contact dermatitis'. Although the fingertips of the non-dominant hand are typically affected, the clinical features are not characteristic and the diagnosis can only be made by testing with foodstuffs.

The major Type I plant sensitizers are listed in Table 4.3.1. Except where stated, the references are given in the excellent reviews of Lahti (1986a) and Cronin (1987).

4.3.2 Clinical features

Clinical features of Type I hypersensitivity may range from relatively trivial symptoms and signs such as pruritus, erythema or weals localized to the site of contact (e.g. fingers or oral mucosa) to a generalized urticarial eruption, bronchospasm and even death due to anaphylaxis. The severity of reaction may depend on the dose of allergen as well as the site of contact. Certain plants, including celery, appear to be more likely to cause a generalized reaction (Forsbeck & Roos 1979). Similarly, Type I reactions to henna (*Lawsonia inermis*) in hair dye, although rare, can be severe (Cronin 1979, Starr *et al.* 1982). Fatal anaphylaxis to rubber latex has been reported, e.g. following a barium enema using a rectal catheter with a latex cuff (Ownby *et al.* 1991). Histological features of contact urticaria include lymphocytes and monocytes in the epidermis together with a lymphohistiocytic infiltrate with mast cells in the dermis (Daroczy & Temesvari 1988).

Immunological contact urticaria is commoner in atopics, and in individuals who have increased exposure to the allergen. Of 42 Finnish patients with latex contact urticaria, 36 (86%) had a personal history of atopy (Turjanmaa & Reunala 1988). As the authors suggest, this high incidence is not necessarily due to an immunological defect in atopics; individuals with atopic eczema are more likely to wear rubber gloves and the latex allergens can penetrate eczematous skin more easily than intact skin. Similarly, up to 64% of food handlers with 'protein contact dermatitis' may give a history of atopy (Cronin 1987). Occupational exposure to the allergen increases greatly the risk of developing Type I hypersensitivity, e.g. castor bean sensitivity in growers (Fakhri & Erwa 1988) and rubber glove latex sensitivity in surgeons (Turjanmaa & Reunala 1988).

The same allergen may cause Type I and Type IV hypersensitivity. Examples include mustard (Panconesi et al. 1980) and castor beans (Kanerva et al. 1990). In addition, there appears to be a higher incidence of delayed hypersensitivity to other components of the allergenic material; thus patients with latex hypersensitivity are more likely to exhibit positive patch test reactions to rubber chemicals, notably thiurams (Turjanmaa & Reunala 1988). Cross-reactions can occur between botanically unrelated species (which presumably possess similar allergens) such as the cross-sensitivity between birch pollen and raw fruit (White & Calnan 1983, Lowenstein & Ericksson 1983).

The plant constituents causing Type I reactions have not been precisely identified. Usually, the allergens are proteins or protein complexes (Lahti 1986a). Morales et al. (1989) obtained positive prick tests using washings from rubber gloves in patients with latex hypersensitivity; at least four soluble polypeptides from natural latex (derived from *Hevea brasiliensis*) were able to bind specific human IgE from these patients. Thorough washing of the gloves before wearing prevented further episodes of contact urticaria (Morales et al. 1989). Many allergens in fruit or vegetables are destroyed by cooking or processing; crushing apples in a liquidizer reduces their allergenicity, possibly due to chemical reactions between the allergens and phenolic compounds in apple flesh (Bjorksten et al. 1980).

'Protein contact dermatitis' presents as urticarial weals or as an acute vesicular eczema at the site of contact (Hjorth & Roed-Petersen 1976). An eczematous response may occur within 30 min after the suspected material is applied to an area already affected by eczema. Histological studies reveal spongiosis, papillary oedema and a mononuclear perivascular infiltrate in the superficial dermis (Tosti et al. 1990). The mechanism is unclear, although the speed of reaction suggests that cell-mediated immunity is unlikely to be the principal mechanism (Tosti et al. 1990).

References

Acciai M.C., Brusi C., Francalanci S., Gola M. & Sertoli A. (1991) Skin tests with fresh foods. *Contact Dermatitis* **24**: 67–8.

Apted J. (1988a) Acute contact urticaria from *Hakea suaveolens* (L). *Contact Dermatitis* **18**: 126.

Apted J. (1988b) Acute contact urticaria from *Grevillea juniperina* (L). *Contact Dermatitis* **18**: 126.

Bjorksten F., Halmepuro L., Hannuksela M. et al. (1980) Extraction and properties of apple allergens. *Allergy* **35**: 671–7.

Cronin E. (1979) Immediate-type hypersensitivity to henna. *Contact Dermatitis* **5**: 198–9.

Cronin E. (1987) Dermatitis of the hands in caterers. *Contact Dermatitis* **17**: 265–9.

Daroczy J. & Temesvari E. (1988) Light microscopic and electron microscopic (EM) examination of contact urticaria. *Contact Dermatitis* **19**: 156–8.

Fakhri Z.I. & Erwa H.H. (1988) Skin test survey in castor bean allergic working population in eastern Sudan, with frequency responses of first dilutions giving skin reactions. *Journal of the Society of Occupational Medicine* **38**: 128–33.

Fischer T. (1991) Bougainvillea contact urticaria. *Contact Dermatitis* **24**: 376.

Forsbeck M. & Roos A.M. (1979) Anaphylactoid reaction to celery. *Contact Dermatitis* **5**: 191.

Harris C. & Shure N. (1950) Sudden death due to allergy tests. *Journal of Allergy* **21**: 208.

Hjorth N. & Roed-Petersen J. (1976) Occupational protein contact dermatitis in food handlers. *Contact Dermatitis* **2**: 28–42.

Kanerva L., Estlander T. & Jolanki R. (1990) Long-lasting contact urticaria from castor bean. *Journal of the American Academy of Dermatology* **23**: 351–5.

Krupa Shankar D.S. (1992) Contact urticaria induced by *Semecarpus anacardium*. *Contact Dermatitis* **26**: 200.

Lahti A. (1986a) Contact urticaria to plants. *Clinics in Dermatology* **4**: 127–36.

Lahti A. (1986b) Contact urticaria and respiratory symptoms from tulips and lilies. *Contact Dermatitis* **14**: 317–19.

Larko O., Lindstedt G., Lundberg P.A. & Mobacken H. (1983) Biochemical and clinical studies in a case of contact urticaria to potato. *Contact Dermatitis* **9**: 108–14.

Lindemayr H. & Jäger S. (1980) Beruflich erworbene Typ-I-Allergie durch Hanfpollen und Haschisch. *Dermatosen in Beruf und Umwelt* **28**: 17–19.

Lowenstein H. & Eriksson N.E. (1983) Hypersensitivity to foods among birch pollen-allergic patients. *Allergy* **38**: 577–87.

Marshman G. & Lovell C.R. (1991) Contact urticaria from runner bean (*Phaseolus multiflorus*). *Contact Dermatitis* **24**: 76.

Morales S.C., Basombra A., Carreira J. & Sastre A. (1989) Anaphylaxis produced by rubber-glove contact. Case reports and immunological identification of the antigens involved. *Clinical and Experimental Allergy* **19**: 425–30.

Nigam P.K. & Saxena A.K. (1988) Allergic contact dermatitis from henna. *Contact Dermatitis* **18**: 55–6.

Niinimaki A. (1987) Scratch-chamber tests in food handler dermatitis. *Contact Dermatitis* **16**: 11–20.

Ownby D.R., Tomlanovich M., Sammons N. & McCullough J. (1991) Fatal anaphylaxis during a barium enema associated with latex allergy (abstract). *Journal of Allergy and Clinical Immunology* **87**: 268.

Panconesi E., Sertoli A., Fabbri P., Giorgini S. & Spallanzini P. (1980) Anaphylactic shock from mustard after ingestion of pizza. *Contact Dermatitis* **2**: 294–5.

Picardo M., Rovina R., Cristaudo A., Cannistraci C. & Santucci B. (1988) Contact urticaria from *Tilia* (lime). *Contact Dermatitis* **19**: 72–3.

Powell R.F. & Smith E.B. (1978) Tumbleweed dermatitis. *Archives of Dermatology* **114**: 751–4.

Starr J.C., Yunginger J. & Brashser G.W. (1982) Immediate type-I asthmatic response to henna following occupational exposure in hairdressers. *Annals of Allergy* **48**: 98.

Sudan B.J. (1985) Seborrhoeic dermatitis induced by nicotine of horsetails (*Equisetum arvense* L.). *Contact Dermatitis* **13**: 201–2.

Torsney P.J. (1964) Hypersensitivity to sesame seed. *Journal of Allergy* **35**: 514–19.

Tosti A., Fanti P.A., Guerra L., Piancastelli E., Poggi S. & Pileri S. (1990) Morphological and immunohistochemical study of immediate contact dermatitis of the hands due to foods. *Contact Dermatitis* **22**: 81–5.

Turjanmaa K. & Reunala T. (1988) Contact urticaria from rubber gloves. *Dermatologic Clinics* **6**: 47–51.

Veraldi S. & Schianchi-Veraldi R. (1990) Contact urticaria from kiwi fruit. *Contact Dermatitis* **22**: 244.

White I.R. & Calnan C.D. (1983) Contact urticaria to fruit and birch sensitivity. *Contact Dermatitis* **9**: 164–5.

5 Irritant plants

The term 'irritant contact dermatitis' is used to describe a cutaneous inflammatory response to a physical and/or chemical injury. It is not immunologically mediated; potentially anyone can be affected and the severity of the response depends on the barrier function of the individual's skin as well as upon the potency and duration of the irritant stimulus. It may take the form of an acute toxic reaction, such as to strong acids or alkalis; some plant saps may cause such a reaction, sometimes even causing haemorrhagic bullae and necrosis. Alternatively, repeated exposures to a milder irritant can cause a chronic (cumulative) dermatitis. Initial exposure may produce subliminal damage to the skin. If the skin is re-challenged before full recovery of barrier function, the resulting damage will be greater until eventually clinical dermatitis is apparent. Despite apparent clinical improvement, the skin's defence against future irritants may be impaired (Malten 1981). Irritant contact dermatitis may be caused by more than one factor, e.g. physical trauma from handling narcissus bulbs may enhance the chemical trauma from oxalate crystals. Hot or wet working conditions contribute to the injury. The severity may range from a mild 'irritant reaction' with erythema and perhaps fissuring, to a severe dermatitides which renders the individual unable to work. In common with other irritant dermatitides (e.g. induced by soluble oils), the eruption affects areas of contact, especially where the stratum corneum is thinner, e.g. fingerwebs and backs of hands, fingertips and under the free edge of the nails. Skin damage by irritants renders the individual more susceptible to allergic sensitization, which may lead to a confused clinical picture.

Plants can irritate the skin by mechanical and/or chemical means (Table 5.1.1). The irritancy of a plant is often a defence mechanism. Ferocious spines or hooks or a bitter taste are a deterrent against predators. Some plants have devised specialized 'stinging hairs' which cause contact erythema or urticaria; this is discussed in more detail in Chapter 4. Almost any plant or plant product is capable of irritancy. This chapter surveys some of the major irritant plant families.

The incidence of irritant contact dermatitis due to plants is difficult to determine because of the frequency of mild reactions. Almost any gardener who handles tomato plants will notice a mild irritation. The frequency of occupational irritant dermatitis is discussed in Chapter 2, Section 1.3.

Table 5.1.1 Irritant plants.

Injury	Example
Mechanical/physical	
Blunt trauma	Falling branches, nuts, etc.
Thorns	Rose family (Rosaceae)
Sharp-edged leaves and leaf hooks	Holly, *Agave*, *Yucca*, etc.
Spines and glochids	Cacti, esp. *Opuntia*
Stem/leaf hairs	Borage family (Boraginaceae), compositae (*Bidens*) (Fig. 5.1.3)
Irritant fibres	Rose hips (Figs 5.1.4, 5.1.5), tulip bulbs
Chemical	
Stinging hairs (see Chapter 4)	
Irritant sap/latex	Spurge family, (Euphorbiaceae) buttercup family, (Ranunculaceae), etc.
Calcium oxalate crystals	Bulbs

Irritant plants often cause confusing positive patch test results, sometimes even causing chemical burns. *Do not* patch test with a species which is a known irritant. If additional allergic sensitization is strongly suspected, it is advisable to use serial dilutions of an extract, confirming the irritant threshold in control subjects.

Reference

Malten K.E. (1981) Thoughts on irritant contact dermatitis. *Contact Dermatitis* 7: 238–47.

5.1 Mechanical irritants

5.1.1 Hairs and hooks

Penetration of the skin by hairs, spines or thorns typically produces a papular irritant eruption which may sometimes mimic scabies or the eruption caused by fibreglass. Many plant species bear hairs (or trichomes) on the stems or leaves. These may play a defensive role or permit trapping and absorption of water. Several members of the borage family (Boraginaceae) are covered in coarse, stiff hairs. These include borage itself (*Borago*) (Figs 5.1.1, 5.1.2), cultivated as a herb and bee plant. Mass cultivation can cause irritant contact dermatitis. Other irritant members of the family include familiar garden plants such as forget-me-not (*Myosotis* spp.), viper's bugloss (*Echium* spp.), hound's tongue (*Cynoglossum* spp.), comfrey (*Symphytum officinale*) and lungwort (*Pulmonaria officinalis*) (Woods 1962). The hairs of the Mexican species *Malphigia urens* induce a stinging reaction entirely

44   IRRITANT PLANTS

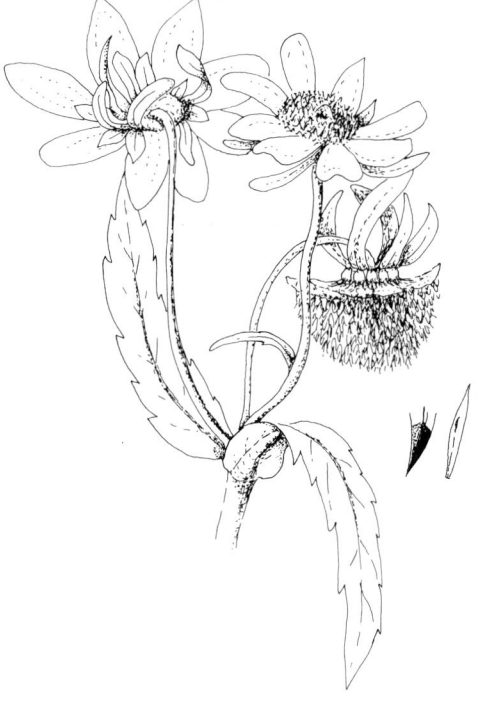

Fig. 5.1.1 *Bidens cernua* (burweed).

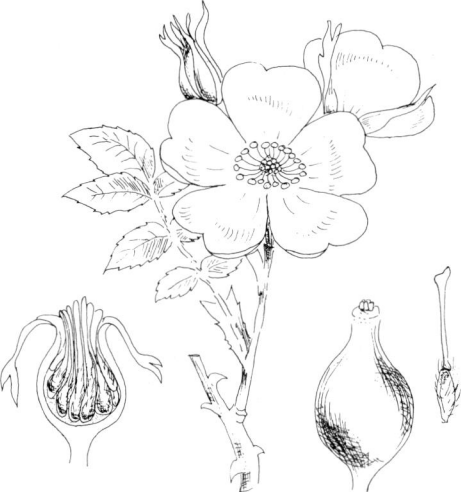

Fig. 5.1.2 *Rosa canina* (dog rose) showing hip containing hairs.

due to mechanical trauma (Thurston & Lersten 1969). Other plants bear hooks or spines on their stems or fruits which aid dispersal by grazing animals (Howes 1974). Many gardeners will recognize goose-grass (*Galium aparine*, Rubiaceae) a straggling or climbing plant bearing fruit with hooked prickles. Similar hooks occur on some tropical

MECHANICAL IRRITANTS 45

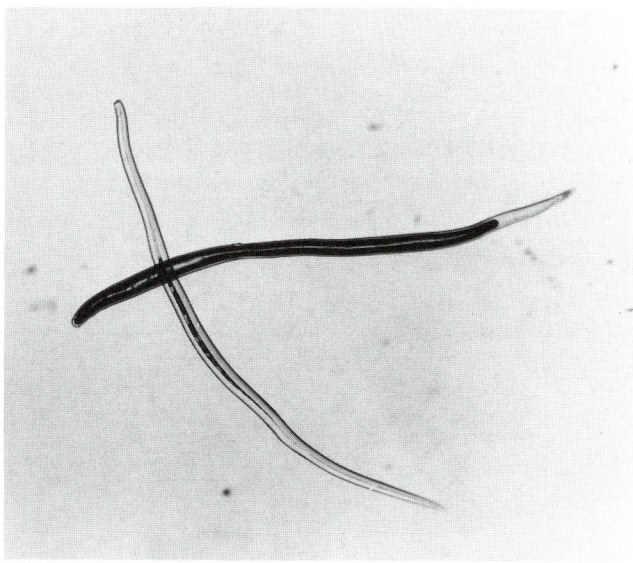

Fig. 5.1.3 Photomicrograph of irritant hairs from rose hip. (Courtesy of Dr T.I. Macleod.)

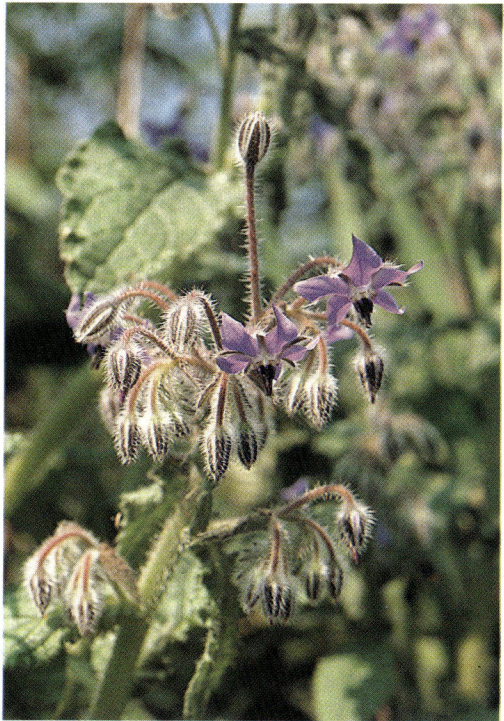

Fig. 5.1.4 *Borago officinalis* (borage).

46 IRRITANT PLANTS

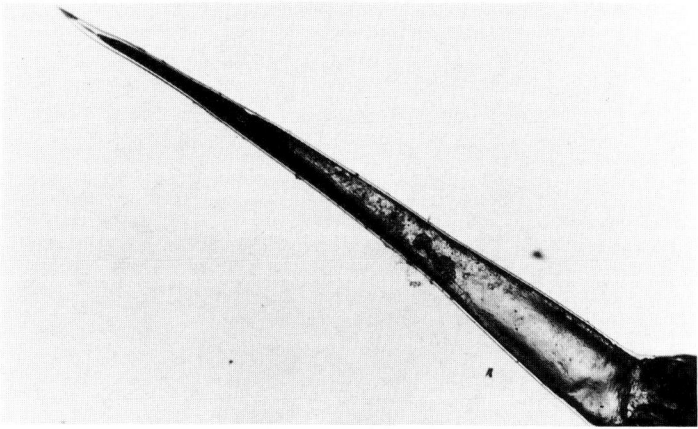

Fig. 5.1.5 Photomicrograph of irritant hair from borage. (Courtesy of Dr T.I. Macleod.)

palms and on bindii (*Soliva pterosperma*), an Australian weed (see p. 175). The Russian thistle (*Salsola kali*) possesses wedge-shaped floral bracts which induce a papular urticarial rash on contact (Powell & Smith 1978). Awns of cereal grasses, including barley, produce a similar eruption or pruritus and erythema of the interdigital clefts (Faninger 1960). The American dogwoods (*Cornus* spp.) have T-shaped hairs which cause erythema and urtication when the leaf is rubbed on the skin in the direction of its long axis (Woods 1962). Coarse fibres in bulb tunics contribute to 'tulip finger' (see p. 225). The hairs in rosehips are currently used in itching powders.

5.1.2 Spines, glochids and thorns

Implantation of cactus spines or hooks is an occupational hazard in growers. The term sabra dermatitis (Shanon & Sagher 1956) was coined in Israel to describe a pruritic papular eruption, prevalent among prickly pear pickers. The prickly pear (*Opuntia ficus indica*) (Fig. 5.1.6) is native to central America but is widely cultivated and naturalized in temperate areas. These large, bush-forming cacti form an effective burglar-proof garden fence in Africa and many Mediterranean areas. The species was cultivated for its edible fruit, particularly in Israel ('sabra' — a native-born Israeli; the term is colloquially applied to the fruit). In addition to obvious spines, the pads and fruit of *Opuntia* bear tufts of shorter hooked hairs, termed glochids (Fig. 5.1.7) which appear innocuous but cause mechanical injury. The glochids are transferred to clothing and to any part of the skin, particularly softer areas such as the genitalia and between the fingers. The oral mucosa and hard palate

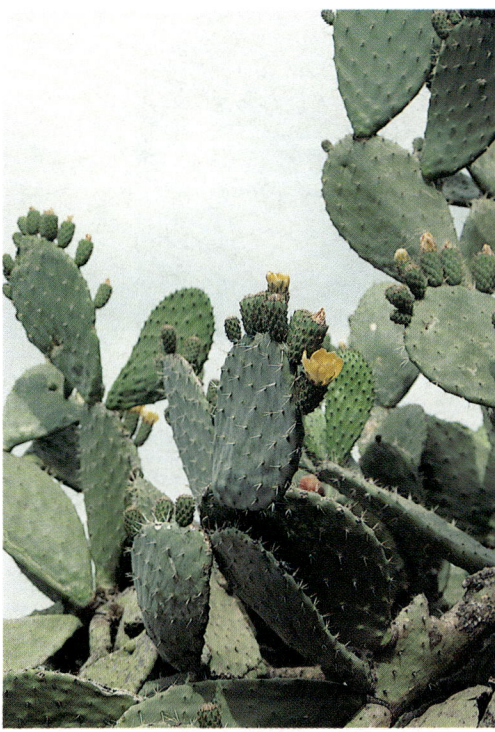

Fig. 5.1.6 The prickly pear, (*Opuntia ficus-indica*) grown as a boundary plant in Greece.

are sometimes affected. Other features include nasal furunculosis and burning irritation, particularly at night. The eruption can closely resemble scabies. Isolated lesions may superficially resemble a comedo naevus (Banerjee 1977). In Israel, it occurs during the fruit picking season (July–October) (Shanon & Sagher 1956). With increased prosperity in the Mediterranean area, it is now rarer but more recently it has been described in India (Banerjee 1977). The fruits which appear in

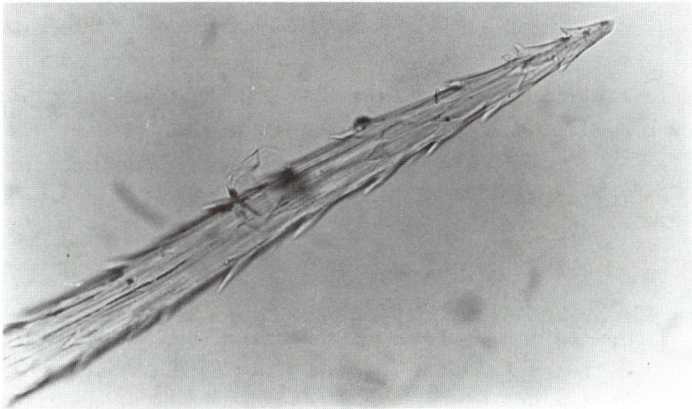

Fig. 5.1.7 Photomicrograph of barbed glochid from an *Opuntia* species. (Courtesy of Dr T.I. Macleod.)

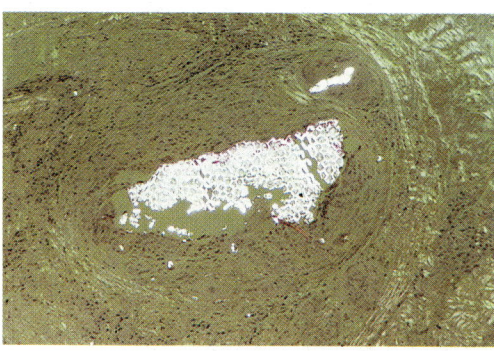

Fig. 5.1.8 Photomicrograph (using polarized light) of a dermal granulomatous reaction to a bamboo spine. (Courtesy of Dr T.I. Macleod.)

the shops are usually shaven, although they can still cause irritation. Glochids or fine cactus spines are best removed from the skin by the application of warm wax, glue, sticking plaster or sellotape to the irritating area, followed by quickly ripping it off (Watt & Breyer-Brandwijk 1962, Gelbard 1984). Other ingenious techniques include the use of facial gels (Putman 1981) and masks (Lawton 1985).

Spines and glochids also cause foreign body granulomata. Glochids of the Cholla cactus, *Opuntia lingularis* cause immediate pain after penetrating the skin followed by erythema and swelling. If the spine remains *in situ*, plaques resembling granuloma annulare may follow, persisting for several months (Winer & Zeilenga 1955, Karpman *et al.* 1980). Schreiber *et al.* (1971) obtained positive prick tests with extracts of glochids in these patients, suggesting that granuloma formation requires immediate hypersensitivity to a constituent. Alternatively, it might be argued that a continued antigenic stimulus induces hypersensitivity in the affected individual.

Thorns and splinters may also induce deep granulomata (Fig. 5.1.8). The spines of the Canary date palm are radiolucent and may be missed (Morton 1962). Maylahn (1952) reported three cases of osteolytic and osteoblastic lesions which radiologically resembled bone tumours. Surgical removal of the thorns (rose, yucca (Fig. 5.1.9) and date palm) was followed by rapid recovery in each case.

Additionally, spines and thorns introduce infective organisms, including *Clostridium tetani*, into the skin and subcutaneous tissues. Shrikes and other birds of prey impale their 'kills' on the thorns of blackthorn (*Prunus spinosus*) (Fig. 5.1.10), a common species in hedgerows. This may explain the high incidence of persistent infected lesions following skin penetration. Buhr (1960) reported an illustrative case in a thatcher who developed a purulent tenosynovitis after blackthorn injury. *Staphylococcus aureus* was isolated from the wound. The long, brittle, jagged thorns snap off easily at the tips (Brimble 1940, quoted in Buhr 1960).

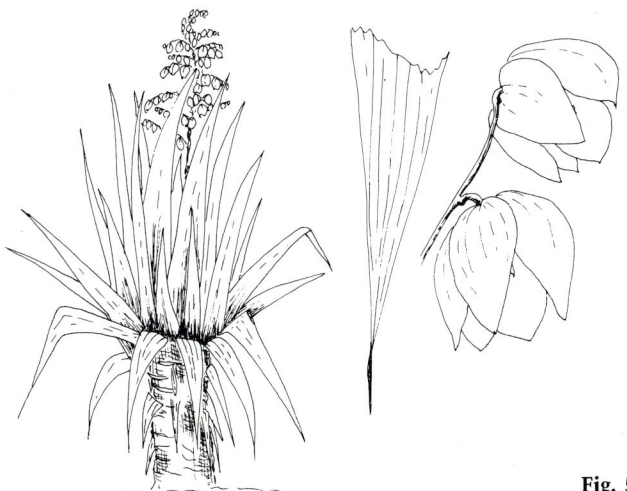

Fig. 5.1.9 *Yucca* species.

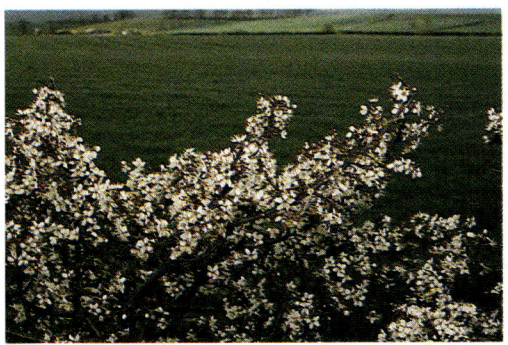

Fig. 5.1.10 Blackthorn, *Prunus spinosus*.

More exotic infections following mechanical injury from plants include sporotrichosis (Foerster 1926). *Sporothrix schenckii* is found on several plants, including grasses and sphagnum moss (Grotte & Younger 1981). *Berberis* (barberry) is another important vector (Foerster 1926). Vegetable fragments and barley awns have been observed in lesions of actinomycosis (Lampe & Fagerström 1968).

Numerous species of *Mycobacterium* can be inoculated by plant thorns, including *M. kansasii* in a patient who was picking blackberries (Grange *et al.* 1988), and *M. marinum* from cactus spine injury (McManigal & Henderson 1986). The organism causing Buruli ulcer (*M. ulcerans*) is probably inoculated into the skin by spiky vegetation in the tropics (Barker 1973).

References

Banerjee K. (1977) A case report of sabra dermatitis. *Indian Journal of Dermatology* **22**: 159–62.

Barker D.J.P. (1973) Epidemiology of *Mycobacterium ulcerans* infection. *Transactions of the Royal Society of Tropical Medicine and Hygiene* **67**: 43–50.
Buhr A.J. (1960) The thorn in the flesh. *Lancet* **i**: 309–10.
Faninger A. (1960) Berufsdermatosen durch trichome von Cereallen. *Berufsdermatosen* **8**: 313–18.
Foerster H.R. (1926) Sporotrichosis: occupational dermatosis. *JAMA* **87**: 1605–9.
Gelbard M.K. (1984) Removal of small cactus spines from the skin. *JAMA* **252**: 3368.
Grange F.M., Noble W.C., Yates M.D. & Collins C.H. (1988) Inoculation mycobacterioses (review article). *Clinical and Experimental Dermatology* **13**: 211–20.
Grotte M. & Younger B. (1981) Sporotrichosis associated with sphagnum moss exposure. *Archives of Pathology and Laboratory Medicine* **105**: 50–1.
Howes F.N. (1974) *A Dictionary of Useful and Everyday Plants and Their Common Names*. Cambridge University Press, Cambridge.
Karpman R.R., Spark R.P. & Fried M. (1980) Cactus thorn injuries to the extremities: their management and etiology. *Arizona Medicine* **37**: 849–51.
Lampe K.F. & Fagerström R. (1968) *Plant Toxicity and Dermatitis*. Williams & Wilkins, Baltimore.
Lawton M.B. (1985) Resourceful women unmask cactus spines. *JAMA* **253**: 2830.
McManigal S.A. & Henderson J.C. (1986) *Mycobacterium marinum* infection associated with cactus spine injury. *Journal of Medical Technology* **3**: 235–6.
Maylahn D.J. (1952) Thorn-induced 'tumors' of bone. *Journal of Bone and Joint Surgery* **34A**: 386–8.
Morton J.F. (1962) Ornamental plants with toxic and/or irritant properties. II. *Journal of the Florida State Horticultural Society* **78**: 484–91.
Powell R.F. & Smith E.B. (1978) Tumbleweed dermatitis. *Archives of Dermatology* **114**: 751–4.
Putman M.H. (1981) Simple cactus spine removal. *Journal of Pediatrics* **98**: 333.
Schreiber M.M., Shapiro S.I. & Berry C.Z. (1971) Cactus granulomas of the skin: an allergic phenomenon. *Archives of Dermatology* **104**: 374.
Shanon J. & Sagher F. (1956) Sabra dermatitis: an occupational dermatitis due to prickly pear handling simulating scabies. *Archives of Dermatology* **74**: 269–75.
Thurston E.L. & Lersten N.R. (1969) The morphology and toxicology of plant stinging hairs. *Botanical Review* **35**: 393–412.
Watt J.M. & Breyer-Brandwijk M.G. (1962) The medicinal and poisonous plants of southern Africa, 2nd edn. E. & S. Livingstone, Edinburgh.
Winer L.H. & Zeilenga R.H. (1955) Cactus granulomas of the skin. *Archives of Dermatology* **49**: 566.
Woods B. (1962) Irritant plants. *Transactions of the St John's Hospital Dermatological Society* **48**: 75–82.

5.2 Chemical irritants

(see also non-immunological contact urticaria, Chapter 4)

Several plants contain chemical irritants. The major families, together with the causative chemicals (if known) are listed in Table 5.2.1. Many plants possess irritant hairs or spines as well as chemical irritants, exacerbating their harmful effect. Chemical irritation is caused by either crystalline calcium oxalate, which has an additional physical irritant effect, or a wide range of chemicals dissolved or suspended in the plant (latex) or housed in specific organelles. Table 5.2.1 and **5.I** (p. 57) give an idea of the range of substances invoked.

CHEMICAL IRRITANTS 51

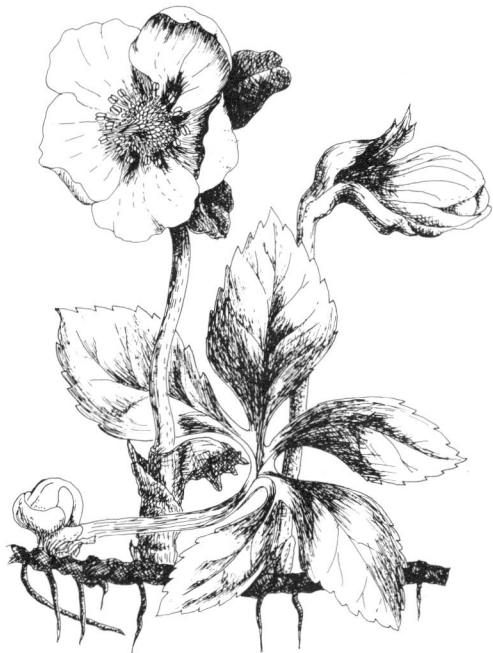

Fig. 5.2.1 *Helleborus niger*, Christmas rose.

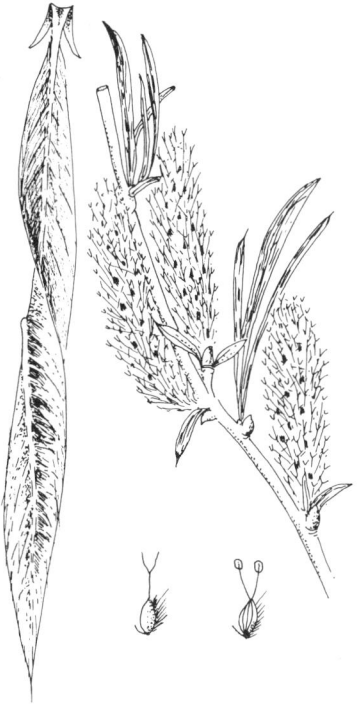

Fig. 5.2.2 *Salix vimminalis*, osier.

Table 5.2.1 Some important plants causing chemical irritation to skin.

Family	Genus	Species	Common name(s)	Toxin(s)	Comments/references
Ranunculaceae	Pulsatilla (Anemone)	patens	Prairie crocus	Protoanemonin	(See text)
	Pulsatilla	vulgaris	Pasque flower		Vance 1982
	Ranunculus	species	Buttercup		Aaron and Muttitt 1964
	Clematis	vitalba	Clematis		Woods 1962
	Helleborus	spp. esp. corsicus	Hellebore (Fig. 5.2.1)		
Cruciferae (Brassicaceae)	Brassica	nigra	Black mustard	Thiocyanates derived from sinigrins	Also allergenic (see p. 128)
	Raphanus	sativus	Radish		Also allergenic (rarely) (see p. 129)
	(also horseradish, broccoli, nasturtium, etc.)				
Leguminosae	Mucuna	pruriens	Cowhage Buffalo bean	Mucunain, an endopeptidase	Dried trichomes previously used as itching powder. Shelley and Arthur 1955
Rosaceae	Agrimonia	eupatoria	Agrimony Beggars' ticks	?	Irritant dermatitis resembling phototoxicity. O'Donovan 1942
Compositae	Anthemis	cotula	Stinking mayweed		Woods 1962
	Arctium	lappa	Burdock		Several other Compositae may be irritant and many are allergenic (see pp. 147–81) Rycroft et al. 1987
	Cichorium	intybus	Chicory		
Asdepiadaceae	Calotropis	spp.	Crownflower	Mudarin, a proteolytic enzyme	Very caustic latex – has caused blindness in Hawaii (Wong 1949)
Solanaceae	Capsicum	spp.	Pepper	Capsaicin	Used as a rubefacient. Lundblad et al. 1985
	Nicotiana	tabacum	Tobacco	Nicotine, etc.	Also allergenic (see p. 193)
Polygonaceae	Polygonum	spp.	Knotweeds		Several spp. irritant (Hjorth & Mitchell 1974)

Family	Genus	Species	Common name	Irritant	Comments
Lauraceae	*Cryptocarya*	*pleurosperma*	Poison walnut	Cryptopleurine (an alkaloid)	A rainforest tree in north Queensland. Causes a vesicular dermatitis (Francis & Southcott 1967)
Euphorbiaceae	Several genera (see Table 5.2.2 and text)				
Buxaceae	*Buxus*	*sempervirens*	Boxtree		Acid juice in leaves and stems
Salicaceae	*Salix*	*vimminalis*	Osier (Fig. 5.2.2)	Salicylic acid	Irritant dermatitis in women packing glass bottles with macerated branches (Goncalo et al. 1986)
Bromeliaceae	*Ananas*	*comosus*	Pineapple	Bromelin (a proteolytic enzyme) plus calcium oxalate	Causes occupational dermatitis affecting the hands Polunin 1951
Agavaceae	*Agave*	spp.	Century plant		Irritant eruption after chopping down dead flower stem. Severe irritation recorded after using sap as a 'hair restorer'! (Kerner et al. 1973)
Hyacinthaceae	*Hyacinthus*	*orientalis* cvs	Hyacinth	Calcium oxalate	May also be allergenic (see p. 217)
Amaryllidaceae	*Narcissus*	spp. and cvs	Daffodil, narcissus Pheasant eye, jonquil	Calcium oxalate	Also rare sensitizer (see pp. 220–21)
Araceae	*Dieffenbachia*	*picta*	Dumb cane Mother in law's tongue	Calcium oxalate plus ?proteolytic enzyme	A severe irritant. May cause severe mucosal oedema and blindness (see text)
(Several other aroids are irritant; see Table 7.5.12, pp. 230–1)					

5.2.1 Irritant crystals

Many bulbs and some other plants, notably *Dieffenbachia*, the dumb cane, and rhubarb, contain calcium oxalate. This water-insoluble salt forms bundles of needle-like crystals (raphides), which are surrounded by a mucilaginous liquid and held in cells. After contact with water, the cell ejects the crystals into the skin or mucosa (Lampe & Fagerström 1968). Calcium oxalate crystals are found in other forms, including styloids (elongated crystals with pointed or ridged ends) and prisms (Fig. 5.2.3); small sand-like crystals may be massed together or form a spherical aggregate (druse) (Franceschi & Herner 1980). Crystals may be important in the ionic equilibrium of the plant or simply represent a means of disposal of waste products; again they help to protect against foraging animals (Franceschi & Herner 1980). Some cacti, such as *Cephalocereus senilis*, contain up to 85% calcium oxalate by dry weight! (Cheavin 1938).

The dumb cane (*Dieffenbachia*), a popular house plant (Fig. 5.2.4) in the arum family (Araceae), has an evil reputation for causing severe local effects if the leaf or fruit is chewed. These include increased salivation, a burning sensation, oedema and occasionally blisters on the oral mucous membranes, sometimes causing hoarseness and even aphonia. If the plant material is swallowed, oedema and erosions also occur in the upper gastrointestinal tract (Pohl 1961). Death may follow (Arditti & Rodriguez 1982). Splashes of plant tissue juice in the eye cause immediate severe pain, lacrimation and blepharospasm. Large numbers of calcium oxalate crystals penetrate the cornea (Ellis *et al.* 1973).

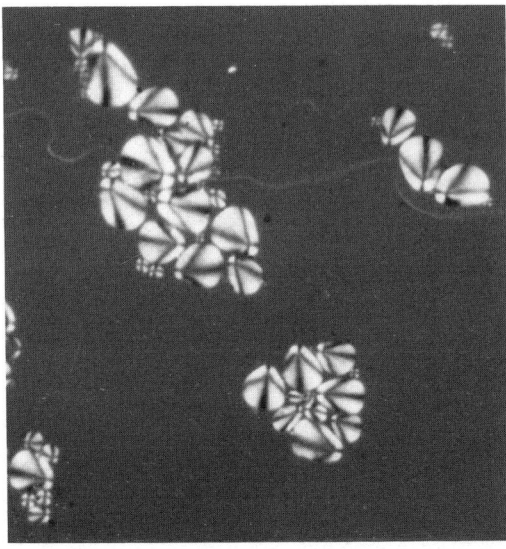

Fig. 5.2.3 Photomicrograph of prism-like crystals of calcium oxalate in a tulip bulb. (Courtesy of Dr T.I. Macleod.)

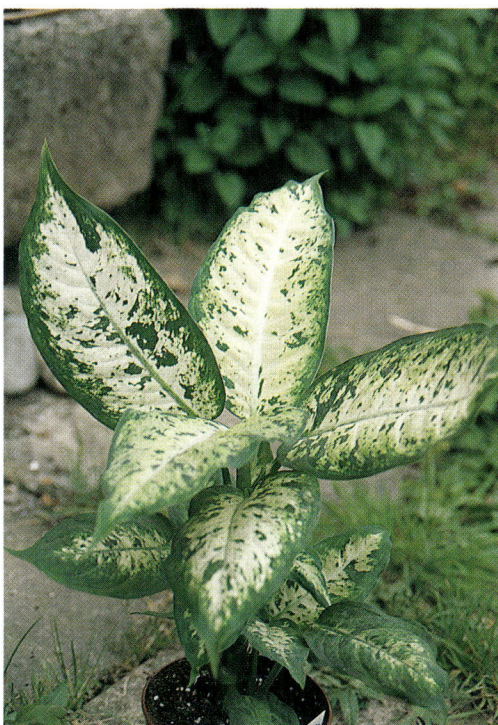

Fig. 5.2.4 *Dieffenbachia picta*, the dumb cane.

Irritant dermatitis caused by bulbs (Fig. 5.2.5) is much less dramatic but much commoner and economically more important. Bulbs contain a high concentration of calcium oxalate, up to 6% in hyacinths (Hjorth & Wilkinson 1968). Sap from daffodil stems was reported to be the most commonly suspected cause of rashes in florists (Merrick *et al.* 1991) and irritant reactions are the commonest cause of daffodil dermatitis (Gude *et al.* 1988). Bulb dermatitis is chiefly an occupational hazard of nursery gardeners, bulb planters and those cutting the flowers. Skin lesions affect chiefly the fingers (especially the tips) (Fig. 5.2.6), hands and forearms; often there is subungual hyperkeratosis. If dust containing oxalate crystals penetrates clothing, the eruption can be more extensive and there may be fingertip contamination of the face, neck and genitalia (Van der Werff 1959, Hjorth & Wilkinson 1968).

Irritancy is in part due to the structure of the crystals themselves. A detailed study by Snyder *et al.* (1979) showed that the crystals isolated from the fishtail palm (*Caryota mitis*) retained their irritant potential even when subjected to chemical processes aimed to inactivate enzymes or remove organic substances. However, irritancy was lost when the physical structure of the crystal was altered. Similarly, crystals were found to be irritant only if barbed or if longer than 180 μm (Sakai *et al.* 1984).

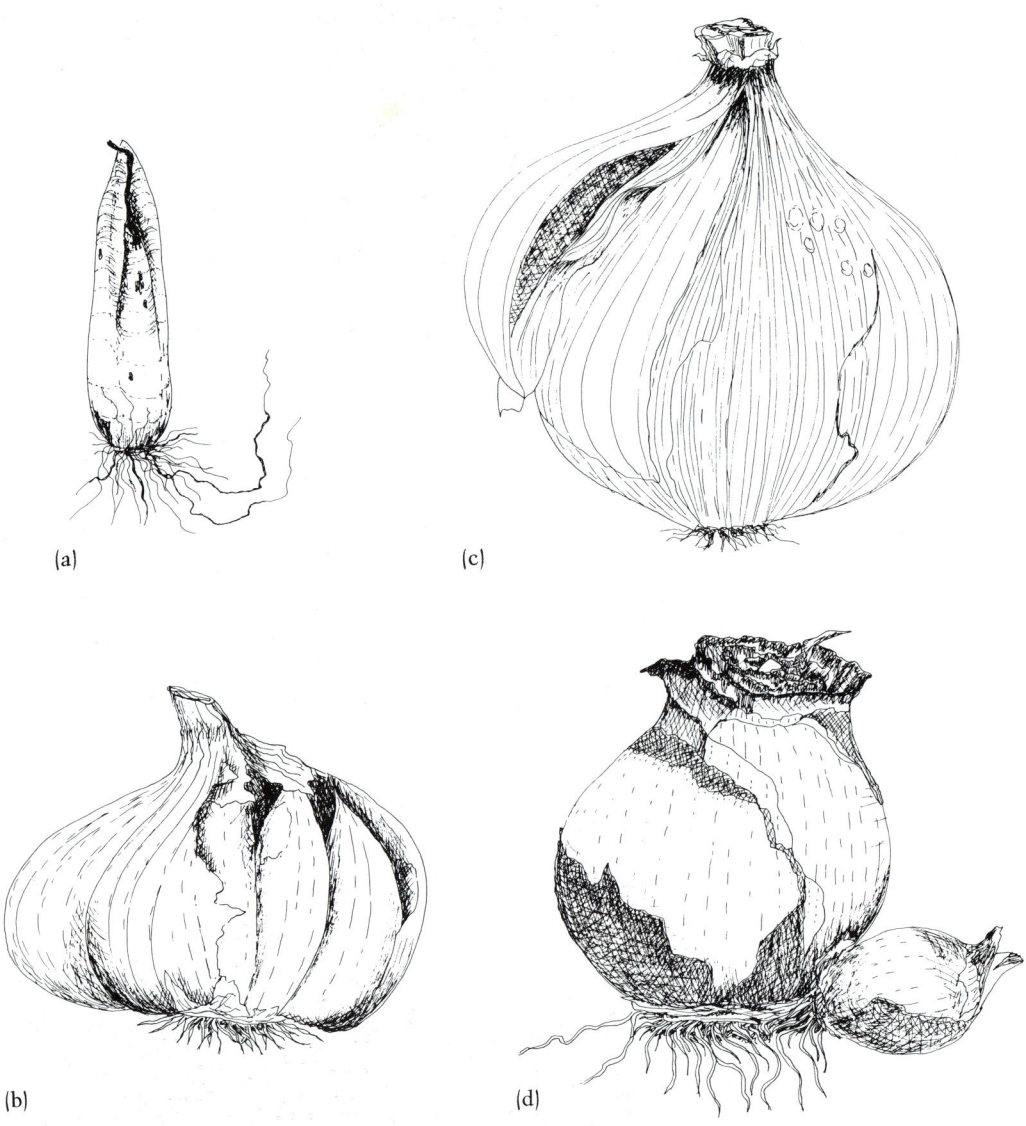

Fig. 5.2.5 A selection of bulbs; (a) *Erythronium dens-canis*, the dog's tooth violet; (b) *Allium sativum* (garlic); (c) *Allium cepa* (onion); (d) *Hyacinthus orientalis* cultivar (hyacinth).

In some cases, however, it appears that crystals act in part by enhancing the penetration of toxins through the stratum corneum. These include several alkaloids in daffodil bulbs (Gude *et al.* 1988), bromelin in pineapples (Polunin 1951) and an insoluble substance in *Dieffenbachia* (Kuballa *et al.* 1981).

CHEMICAL IRRITANTS 57

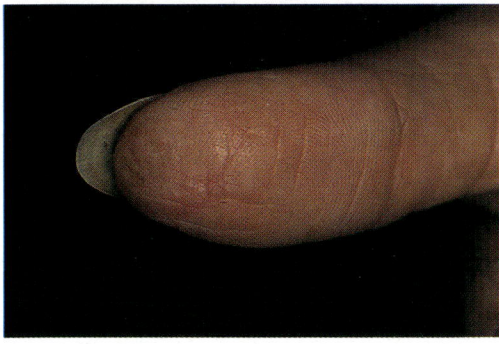

Fig. 5.2.6 Irritant fingertip dermatitis due to bulb handling.

5.2.2 Irritant sap or latex

Irritant substances in plants belong to several different chemical families, including alkaloids, glycosides, proteolytic enzymes, saponins, phenolic compounds and anthraquinones. Members of the buttercup family (Ranunculaceae) contain the unsaturated lactone, protoanemonin, formed after injury to the plant by the breakdown of the

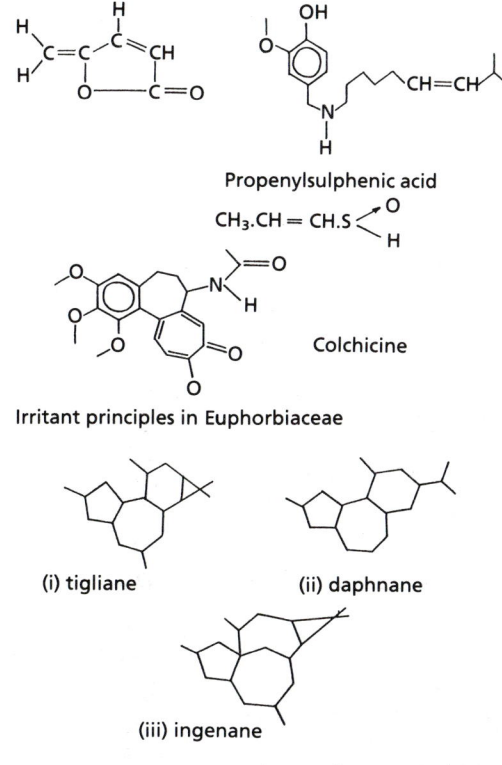

5.1 Some irritant principles in plants.

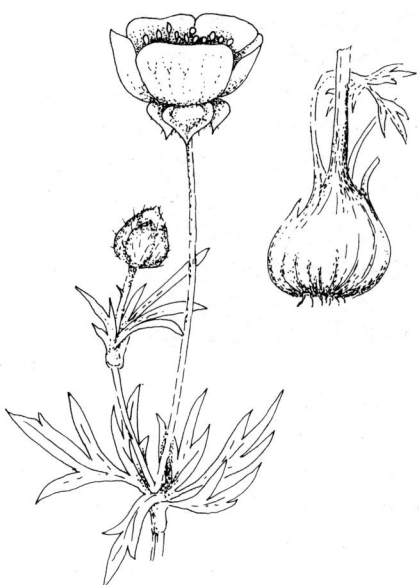

Fig. 5.2.7 *Ranunculus bulbosus*, the bulbous buttercup.

glycoside ranunculin. Protoanemonin (**5.I**) causes severe vesiculation and linear streaks after contact with field buttercups (*Ranunculus* spp.) (Fig. 5.2.7) and may lead to a false diagnosis of a phototoxic reaction (Woods 1962). However, hyperpigmentation is absent or mild and transient. Apart from *Ranunculus*, irritant members of the family include *Anemone* and *Clematis* (Fig. 5.2.8). A notable genus is *Pulsatilla*, which includes the European pasque flower (*P. vulgaris*) and the American prairie crocus (*P. patens*), a common species on dry prairies of Minnesota; the leaves in particular induce bullous irritant reactions (Vance 1982). Protoanemonin rapidly polymerizes to anemonin, which is non-irritant. Thus, only fresh plants cause irritant reactions (Shearer 1938). The irritant properties of Ranunculaceae have been used med-

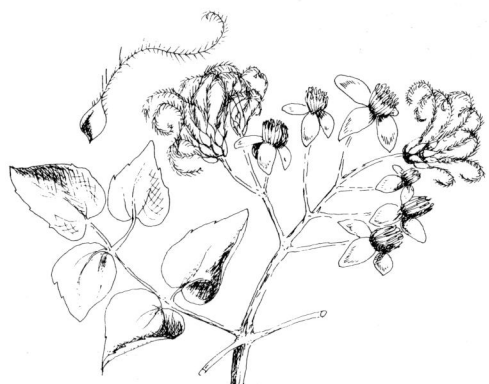

Fig. 5.2.8 *Clematis vitalba*, old man's beard.

icinally. An ointment made from the sap of celandine, *Ranunculus ficaria*, is applied as an astringent to haemorrhoids (Mitchell & Rook 1979) and the North American Indians have used Ranunculaceae as cold remedies and to revive unconscious people (Turner 1984).

The spicy taste of many Cruciferae (including mustard, horseradish, etc.) is due to irritant thiocyanates derived from glycosides; these are rarely allergenic (see pp. 128−9).

Similarly, capsaicin and related capsaicinoids contribute the pungency to chilli peppers (Lundblad *et al.* 1987). Capsaicin (**5.I**) induces erythema without blistering (Smith *et al.* 1970). The well-known lachrymatory properties of onion are due in part to propenylsulphenic acid (**5.I**). (Vohora *et al.* 1973). Colchicine (**5.I**) is a cytotoxic alkaloid derived from the 'autumn crocus' (pp. 256−7).

The spurge family (Euphorbiaceae) contains a large number of species with a highly irritant latex (Fig. 5.2.9). The family includes several common weeds, some popular ornamental house plants and border or rock garden perennials, some of which are detailed in Table 5.2.2. For a detailed discussion of irritant members of this family, the review by Webster (1986) is strongly recommended. *Euphorbia* is named after Euphorbus, who was the physician of King Juba of Numidia and who discovered the therapeutic properties of a species growing in the Atlas mountains. Several species have been used medicinally. Dioscorides mentioned the use of *E. characias* ssp. *wulfenii* as a purge, emetic and depilatory and to destroy 'hanging warts' (Huxley & Taylor 1977).

A few members of the family are grown as ornamental house plants. Fortunately, few of these are irritant, although *Codiaeum* and

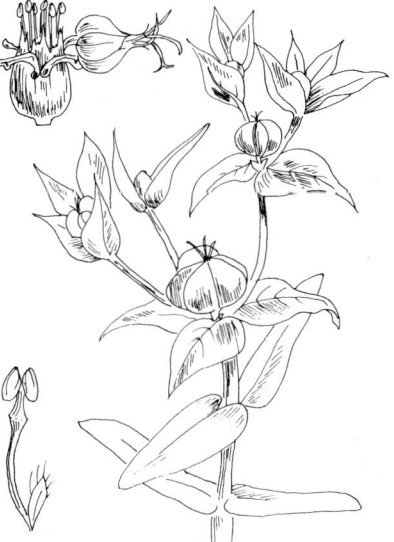

Fig. 5.2.9 *Euphorbia lathyrus*, mole plant or caper spurge. The seed capsules (which are explosive) resemble capers and contain an irritant latex.

Table 5.2.2 Irritant members of the spurge family (Euphorbiaceae).

WEEDS
Euphorbia spp., including:
E. *peplus* (petty spurge) (Fig. 5.2.10). A common annual weed in all temperate zones. Causes irritant contact dermatitis (Calnan 1975).
E. *helioscopia* (sun spurge). Causes severe keratoconjunctivitis (Mitchell & Rook 1979). Toxic to livestock (Schmidt & Evans 1980).
E. *lathyrus* (caper spurge, mole plant) (Fig. 5.2.9) European, planted in USA to keep away gophers. Fruits resemble caper buds but are explosive, yielding a poisonous sap. A troublesome weed in Australia (Francis & Southcott 1967).

ORNAMENTAL BORDER/ROCK GARDEN PLANTS
Euphorbia myrsinites. Attractive low-growing plants: bracts turn red in late summer. Mediterranean native, often grown as rock garden plant (Fig. 5.2.11). Irritant dermatitis reported in a child (Spoerke & Temple 1979).
E. *marginata* (snow on the mountain, Japanese edelweiss). Native to southern USA. Annual herb; upper leaves and bracts variegated white and green. A noxious weed in New South Wales and southern Australia (Francis & Southcott 1967). Once used to brand cattle in Texas. Irritant dermatitis developed in a child who was hit in the face (Pinedo et al. 1985) and in a flower arranger (Urushibata & Kase 1991).
Several other spp., e.g. E. *characias* and E. *griffithii*, are popular herbaceous plants.
Ricinus communis (castor oil plant). Sometimes grown as an ornamental annual. Allergenic (see p. 206).

HOUSE PLANTS
Euphorbia pulcherrima (poinsettia). Remarkably non-irritant but an allergen (see pp. 205–6).
Codiaeum variegatum v. *pictum* (florist's Croton) (Fig. 7.5.98). Probable sensitizer (see p. 205) (van Ketel 1979, Cleenewerck & Martin 1989).
Synadenium grantii (African milk bush). An increasingly popular foliage plant. Irritant dermatitis has been reported in a child (Spoerke et al. 1985).

OTHER SPECIES
Euphorbia tirucalli (naked lady, Indian tree spurge, pencil tree). See text.
Hippomane mancinella (Mancinella tree). See text.
Hura crepitans (sandbox tree). South America. Bat-pollinated. Explosive, irritant capsules.
Jatropha urens (see stinging plants p. 31).

Euphorbia pulcherrima are sensitizers. *Synadenium grantii* is an increasingly popular foliage plant which is irritant. Several succulent euphorbias are grown as ornamentals, notably *E. milii* var. *splendens*, the 'crown of thorns'. Fortunately, they appear relatively harmless. One succulent species, *E. tirucalli*, is, however, highly irritant and may cause blindness. This is occasionally grown in specialist collections and is widely cultivated as a burglar-proof hedge in parts of Africa and India. The plant is rich in hydrocarbons and attempts were made in Florida to cultivate it commercially as a 'green' source of gasoline (Webster 1986).

Perhaps the most formidable member of the Euphorbiaceae is the 'Manchineel tree' or 'beach apple' (*Hippomane mancinella*). At one

CHEMICAL IRRITANTS   61

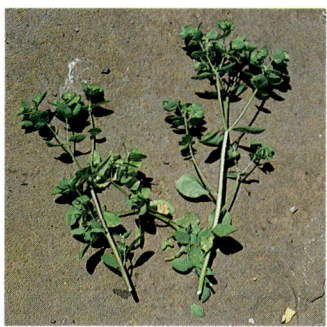

Fig. 5.2.10 *Euphorbia peplus*, the petty spurge. Note milky latex exuding from the bases of the broken stems.

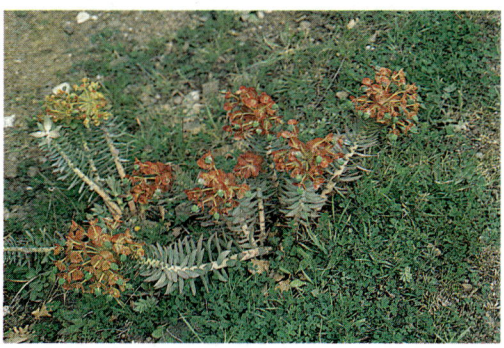

Fig. 5.2.11 *Euphorbia myrsinites* (photographed in Greece); the flower bracts often become reddish in the summer.

time, this species was common along beaches from Trinidad to south Florida; a rarer, and even more toxic, species (*H. horrida*) is endemic to the island of Hispaniola. Now *H. mancinella* is mostly restricted to areas of the Everglades National Park (Howard 1981). The Spanish explorer Oviedo, in 1555, wrote that 'the pestilent nature of this tree is such that it cannot be declared in a few words. If a man do but repose himself to sleep a little while under the shadow of the same, he has his head and eyes swollen when he rises, that the eyelids are joined with the cheeks. And if it chance one drop or more of dew of the said tree to fall into the eye, it utterly destroys the sight.' (Quoted in Allen 1943.) The tree grows up to 10 m with a spread of 6 m. The fruit resembles a small crab apple, with a pleasant odour. The whole plant exudes a milky latex when damaged. If the fruit is bitten, it causes severe oral pain, mucosal swelling and blistering; there may be dysphagia and later desquamation of the mucosa. In the unlikely event of swallowing the fruit, painful vomiting and bloody diarrhoea may follow (Earle 1938). Skin contact causes a severe, even blistering eruption, notably affecting hands, face and genitalia. Even the dried wood is toxic to cut and burn (Woods & Calnan 1976).

The active principles of the Euphorbiaceae are tigliane polyol (phorbol) esters (**5.I**). Some genera, including *Hippomane*, produce daphnane (tricyclic diterpenoid) and ingenane orthoesters, also found in members of the daphne family (Thymelaceae) (**5.I**) (Adolph & Hecker 1984).

References

Aaron T.H. & Muttitt E.L.G. (1964) Vesicant dermatitis due to prairie crocus. (*Anemone patens* L.). *Archives of Dermatology* **90**: 168–71.

Adolph W. & Hecker E. (1984) On the active principles of the spurge family. X. Skin irritants, cocarcinogens and cryptic carcinogens from the latex of the Manchineel tree. *Journal of Natural Products* **47**: 490–6.

Allen P.H. (1943) Poisonous and injurious plants of Panama. *American Journal of Tropical Medicine* **23** (suppl.): 1–76.

Arditti J.R. (1982) *Dieffenbachia*: uses, abuses and toxic constituents: a review. *Journal of Ethnopharmacology* **5**: 293–302.

Calnan C.D. (1975) Petty spurge (*Euphorbia peplus* L.). *Contact Dermatitis* **1**: 128–30.

Cheavin W.V.S. (1938) The crystals and crystoliths found in plant cells: part I. Crystals. *Microscope* **2**: 155–8.

Cleenewerck M.-B. & Martin P. (1989) Occupational contact dermatitis due to *Codiaeum variegatum* L., *Chrysanthemum indicum* L., *Chrysanthemum xhortorum* and *Frullania dilatata* L. In Frosch P.J., Dooms-Goossens A., Lachapelle J.M., Rycroft R.J.G. & Scheper R. (eds) *Current Topics in Contact Dermatitis*. Springer-Verlag, Berlin.

Earle K.V. (1938) Toxic effects of *Hippomane mancinella*. *Transactions of the Royal Society of Tropical Medicine and Hygiene* **32**: 363–70.

Ellis W., Barfort P. & Mastman G.J. (1973) Keratoconjunctivitis with corneal crystals caused by the *Dieffenbachia* plant. *American Journal of Ophthalmology* **76**: 143–7.

Franceschi V.R. & Herner H.T. (1980) Calcium oxalate crystals in plants. *Botanical Review* **46**: 361–426.

Francis D.F. & Southcott R.V. (1967) *Plants Harmful to Man in Australia*. Miscellaneous Bulletin No. 1. Botanic Gardens, Adelaide.

Gonçalo S., Sousa I., Moreno A. & Leitão A. (1986) Occupational dermatitis from *Salix vimminalis*. *Contact Dermatitis* **14**: 188–9.

Gude M., Hausen V., Heitsch H. & Konig W.A. (1988) An investigation of the irritant and allergic properties of daffodils (*Narcissus pseudonarcissus* L., Amaryllidaceae). A review of daffodil dermatitis. *Contact Dermatitis* **19**: 1–10.

Hjorth N. & Mitchell J.C. (1974) *Polygonum* dermatitis. *Contact Dermatitis Newsletter* **15**: 448.

Hjorth N. & Wilkinson D.S. (1968) Contact dermatitis. IV. Tulip fingers, hyacinth itch and lily rash. *British Journal of Dermatology* **80**: 696–8.

Howard R.A. (1981) Three experiences with the Manchineel (*Hippomane* spp., Euphorbiaceae). *Biotropica* **13**: 224–7.

Huxley A. & Taylor W. (1977) *Flowers of Greece and the Aegean*. Chabbo & Windus, London.

Kerner J., Mitchell J. & Maibach H.I. (1973) Irritant contact dermatitis from *Agave americana* L.: incorrect use of sap as 'hair restorer'. *Archives of Dermatology* **108**: 102–3.

Kuballa B., Lugnier A.H.M. & Anton R. (1981) Study of *Dieffenbachia*-induced edema in mouse and rat hindpaw: respective role of oxalate needles and trypsin-like protease. *Toxicology and Applied Pharmacology* **58**: 444–51.

Lampe K.L. & Fagerström R. (1968) *Plant Toxicology and Dermatitis*. Williams & Wilkins, Baltimore.

Lundblad L., Lundberg J.M., Anggård A. & Zetterström R. (1985) Capsaicin pretreatment inhibits the flare component of the cutaneous allergic reaction in man. *European Journal of Pharmacology* **113**: 461–2.

Merrick C., Fenney J., Clarke E.C., Hodnett T. & Fletcher G. (1991) A survey of skin problems in floristry. *Contact Dermatitis* **24**: 306.

Mitchell J. & Rook A. (1979) *Botanical Dermatology.* Greengrass, Vancouver.

O'Donovan W.J. (1942) Dermatosis bullosa striata pratensis. Agrimony dermatitis. *British Journal of Dermatology* **54**: 39–46.

Pinedo J.M., Saavedra V., Conzalez-de-Canales F. & Llamas P. (1985) Irritant dermatitis due to *Euphorbia marginata*. *Contact Dermatitis* **13**: 44.

Pohl R.W. (1961) Poisoning by *Dieffenbachia*. *JAMA* **177**: 812–13.

Polunin I. (1951) Pineapple dermatosis. *British Journal of Dermatology* **63**: 441–55.

Rycroft R.J.G., Lovell C.R., Harries P.G., Winter P. & Mallet A.I. (1987) Occupational irritant contact dermatitis from chicory. *Bollettino di Dermatologia Allergologica e Professionale* **2**: 77–82.

Sakai W.S., Shiroma S.S. & Nagao M.A. (1984) A study of raphide microstructure in relation to irritation. *Scanning Electron Microscopy* **II**: 979–86.

Schmidt R.J. & Evans F.J. (1980) Skin irritants of the sun spurge (*Euphorbia helioscopia* L.). *Contact Dermatitis* **6**: 204–10.

Shearer G.D. (1938) Some observations on the poisonous properties of buttercups. *British Veterinary Journal* **94**: 22–32.

Shelley W.B. & Arthur R.P. (1955) Studies on cowhage (*Mucuna pruriens*) and its pruritogenic proteinase, mucunase. *Archives of Dermatology* **72**: 399–406.

Smith J.G., Crounse R.G. & Spence D. (1970) The effects of capsaicin on human skin, liver and epidermal liposomes. *Journal of Investigative Dermatology* **54**: 170–3.

Snyder D.S., Hatfield G.M. & Lampe J.F. (1979) Examination of the itch response from the raphides of the fishtail palm, *Caryota mitis*. *Toxicology and Applied Pharmacology* **48**: 287–92.

Spoerke D.G. & Temple A.R. (1979) Dermatitis after exposure to a garden plant (*Euphorbia myrsinites*). *American Journal of Diseases of Childhood* **133**: 28–9.

Spoerke D.G., Montanio C.D. & Rumack B.H. (1985) Pediatric exposure to the houseplant *Synadenium grantii*. *Veterinary and Human Toxicology* **27**: 283–4.

Turner N.J. (1984) Counter irritant and other medicinal uses of plants in the Ranunculaceae by native peoples in British Columbia and neighboring areas. *Journal of Ethnopharmacology* **11**: 181–201.

Urushibata O. & Kase K. (1991) Irritant contact dermatitis from *Euphorbia marginata*. *Contact Dermatitis* **24**: 155–6.

Vance J.C. (1982) Toxic plants of Minnesota. Skin toxicity of the prairie crocus (*Anemone patens* L.). *Minnesota Medicine* **65**: 149–51.

Van der Werff P.J. (1959) Occupational diseases among workers in the bulb industries. (Preliminary report). *Acta Allergologica* **14**: 338–55.

Van Ketel W.G. (1979) Occupational contact dermatitis due to *Codiaeum variegatum* and possibly to *Aeschynanthus pulcher*. *Dermatosen in Beruf und Umwelt* **27**: 141–2.

Vohora S.B., Rizwan M. & Khan J.A. (1973) Medicinal uses of common Indian vegetables. *Planta Medica* **23**: 381–393.

Webster G.L. (1986) Irritant plants in the spurge family (Euphorbiaceae). *Clinics in Dermatology* **4**(2): 36–451.

Wong W.W. (1949) Keratoconjunctivitis due to crownflower. *Hawaiian Medical Journal* **8**: 339–41.

Woods B. (1962) Irritant plants. *Transactions of the St John's Hospital Dermatological Society* **48**: 75–82.

Woods B. & Calnan C.D. (1976) Toxic woods. *British Journal of Dermatology* **95** (suppl. 13): 1–97.

6 Phytophototoxic reactions

6.1 Introduction

The term 'phytophotodermatitis' was coined by Robert Klaber (1942) to describe a cutaneous reaction caused by sun exposure after contact with plants. In humans, the reactions are phototoxic, consisting of erythema with or without blistering followed by hyperpigmentation. This reaction is due to photosensitizing substances which are found in certain plant families. It can occur in any individual, if the degree of skin contamination and the dosage of irradiation are adequate. Allergic mechanisms are not involved. True photoallergic reactions to plants have not been proven to date, with the exception of one case of *Parthenium* dermatitis (see p. 173), although some plant constituents, such as psoralens, may photosensitize. Confusingly, individuals who are repeatedly exposed to volatile allergens (e.g. Compositae oleoresin or colophony) may subsequently become abnormally sensitive to light (persistent light reactivity); this is *not* a photoallergic reaction to the plant constituent and is discussed further on p. 148. This chapter discusses phototoxic reactions to plants and their products; a brief historical review is followed by an account of the mechanisms of phototoxicity, clinical features and details of the major plant genera which have been implicated.

6.1.1 Historical background

The ability of some plants to cause hyperpigmentation has been recognized since 1500 BC. In ancient Egypt, the juice of *Ammi majus* was rubbed on patches of vitiligo and the patient was encouraged to lie in the sunlight. *Angelica* leaves are used even today in Chinese herbal medicine for the same purpose. Observations on the use of plants in folk medicine, notably by El Mofty in Egypt, led to the development of photochemotherapy (PUVA) in vitiligo and psoriasis.

Several authors in the late 19th and early 20th centuries observed skin reactions from plants such as parsnips although the role of sunlight was not recognized. Oppenheim in 1932 described 'dermatosis bullosa striata pratensis', attributing the linear streaks and blisters to rubbing against meadow grass while sunbathing. Behçet *et al.* (1939), investigating phototoxic reactions to figs, found that the active wavelength of light lay in the 'near UV' spectrum. Klaber (1942) confirmed it to be between 320 and 400 mm. Kuske (1940) noted that a phototoxic potential was restricted to a few plant families and identified the photosensitizers as furocoumarins (psoralens).

Other chemical patterns emerged, reflecting different patterns of exposure to phototoxic substances. 'Berloque dermatitis' (see pp. 83–4), with its characteristic hyperpigmented lesions resembling pendants, was attributed to eau de cologne containing bergamot oil (Freund 1916). More recently, the use of powered string trimmers by scantily clad operators has led to an extensive macular hyperpigmented eruption ('strimmer rash') (Freeman et al. 1984, Oakley et al. 1986) (see p. 83).

Furocoumarins (psoralens) appear to be primarily responsible for phytophototoxic reactions in humans. Although other phototoxic substances, such as α-terthienyl, have been isolated in members of the daisy family (Compositae) (Arnason et al. 1981) they are probably not of clinical relevance. The role of other photoactive substances in animals has been well reviewed by Pathak (1986).

Geeldikkop ('yellow thick head') is a disorder of sheep which ingest plants such as *Tribulus terrestris* (puncture vine or debbeltje) in South Africa. Clinical features include photosensitivity, oedema, jaundice and blindness. It appears that these plants cause cholestasis, preventing the excretion of phylloerytherin, a porphyrin breakdown product of dietary chlorophyll. Increased tissue levels of phylloerythrin cause photosensitivity (Rimington & Quin 1937). Cholestasis is induced by icterogenic and rehmannic acid, which are also found in the grasses *Panicum laeisfolium* and *P. coloratum* as well as in *Lippia* species (Verbenaceae) (Rimington & Quin 1937).

Ingestion of several species of St John's Wort (*Hypericum* spp.) causes severe phototoxicity in animals without systemic ill effects (see Fig. 6.3.9). This is a direct toxic effect of hypericin (hexahydroxy-2,2-dimethylnaphthodianthrone) (Brockmann et al. 1957). Photosensitivity was recorded in the USA and Australia; the number of plants has been successfully reduced by 'biological control' using a beetle *Chrysolina gemellata* (Pathak 1986). The flowers of buckwheat (*Fagopyron* spp., Polygonaceae) contain pigments which are structurally similar to hypericin and which similarly cause photosensitivity in grazing animals in the USA (Blum 1964).

References

Arnason T., Chan G.F.Q. Wat C.K. et al. (1981) The role of oxygen in photosensitization with polyacetylene and thiophene derivatives. *Photochemistry and Photobiology* **33**: 821.
Behçet H., Ottenstein B., Lion K. et al. (1939) Les dermatites des figues. Recherches des influences cliniques, physiques et allergiques pouvant provoquer la dermatitie

des figues. *Annales Dermatologie et Syphiligraphie* **32**: 125.
Blum H.F. (1964) *Photodynamic Action and Diseases Caused by Light*. Hafner Publishing Co., New York.
Brockmann H., Kluge F. & Muxfeldt U. (1957) Totalsynthese des hypericins. *Chemische Berichte* **90**: 2302.
Freeman K., Hubbard H.C. & Warin A.P. (1984) Strimmer rash. *Contact Dermatitis* **10**: 117–18.
Freund E. (1916) Uber bisher noch nicht beschribene Kunstliche Hautverfarbungen. *Dermatologische Wochenschrift* **63**: 931.
Klaber R. (1942) Phyto-photo-dermatitis. *British Journal of Dermatology* **54**: 193–211.
Kuske H. (1940) Perkutane Photosensibilisierung durch pflanzliche Wirkstoffe. *Dermatologica* **82**: 273.
Oakley A.M.M., Ive F.A. & Harrison M.A. (1986) String trimmer's dermatitis. *Journal of the Society of Occupational Medicine* **36**: 143–4.
Oppenheim M. (1932) Dermatite bulleuse striée consécutive aux bains de soleil dans les pres (dermatitis bullosa striata pratensis). *Annales Dermatologie et Syphilographie* **3** (series 7): 1–7.
Pathak M.A. (1986) Phytophotodermatitis. *Clinics in Dermatology* **4**: 103–21.
Rimington C. & Quin J.I. (1937) Dikoor or geeldikkop on grassveld pastures. *Journal of the South African Veterinary Medical Association* **8**: 141.

6.2 The naturally occurring psoralens and other plant photosensitizers and their mode of action

B.E. JOHNSON

Phytophotodermatitis as customarily described appears to consist of a specific pattern of phototoxic skin reactions (Table 6.2.1) in which delayed erythema, blistering and hyperpigmentation are the major features. However, less obvious phototoxic reactions and photoallergy may also occur.

Table 6.2.1 The major reaction patterns of cutaneous phototoxicity.

Type	Skin reactions	Photosensitizers or diseases
1	Prickling or burning during exposure; immediate erythema; oedema/urticaria with higher doses; sometimes delayed erythema/hyperpigmentation	Coal tar, pitch, anthraquinone-based dyestuffs, benoxaprofen, amiodarone, chlorpromazine, erythropoietic protoporphyria
2	Exaggerated sunburn	Drugs such as chlorpromazine, chlorthiazides, quinine, demethylchlortetracycline
3	Late onset erythema; blisters with slightly higher doses; hyperpigmentation only with low exposures	Psoralens, phytophotodermatitis, berloque dermatitis
4	Increased skin fragility giving blisters with trauma	Nalidixic acid, frusemide, tetracycline, naproxen, amiodarone, porphyria cutanea tarda

6.2.1 Chemistry of the furocoumarins

Furocoumarins, (**6.I**) heterocyclic compounds produced in a biosynthetic process in which a furan ring becomes fused with the benz-a-pyrone coumarin, have been isolated from species of Umbelliferae,

6.I Molecular structures of the linear furocoumarin, Psoralen, demonstrating the numbering system commonly used, and of the angular furocoumarin, Angelicin.

Rutaceae, Moraceae and Leguminosae identified as having a role in classical phytophotodermatitis and it is evident that a number of these naturally occurring compounds are the phototoxic agents involved (Musajo & Rodighiero 1962, Pathak et al. 1962, Mitchell & Rook 1979). The nomenclature has varied (Scott et al. 1976) but is now simplified by using the conventional ring numbering system for the coumarin and prime numbers for the furan moiety as suggested by Spath (1937).

Only two forms of furano-coumarin condensation occur in nature. In the first, the furan ring is joined at its 3'2' bond to the 6,7 bond of the coumarin to produce linear furocoumarins known as psoralens. They appear to derive their name from the leguminous plant, *Psoralea corylifolia*, the Bavachee, seeds of which have been used for centuries in the Ayurvedic medicine treatment for vitiligo (Soine 1964).

Psoralen itself was isolated as the photoactive component of these seeds and characterized as a furocoumarin in 1933 (Jois et al. 1933). In the second form the furan ring is reversed with condensation at the coumarin 7,8 bond to produce angular furocoumarins known as angelicins related to the angelicin (isopsoralen) obtained from the umbellifer, *Angelica archangelica*.

6.2.2 Relative phototoxicity

Naturally occurring furocoumarins are limited in number, Soine (1964) listing some 19 psoralens and five angelicins as the major forms. The range is even more restricted in the Umbelliferae (Nielsen 1970). Moreover, not all furocoumarins are phototoxic. The phototoxic potential of those that are varies depending first on whether the molecule is linear (e.g. strongly positive psoralen) or angular (weakly phototoxic angelicin) and secondly on the substituent components of the molecule, all of which in the naturally occurring psoralens decrease the potential but, in the angelicins, may increase it.

8-MOP
8-methoxypsoralen

5-MOP
5-methoxypsoralen

6.II Molecular structures of the photosensitizing psoralens, Xanthotoxin (8-MOP) and Bergapten (5-MOP).

5-MOP (bergapten)
+++

Pimpinellin
++

Angelicin
+

Sphondin
+

Isobergapten
−

Isopimpinellin
−

6.III Molecular structures of the furocoumarins in Heracleum laciniatum (Kavli et al. 1983c). Cutaneous phototoxicity: +++ very phototoxic; ++ phototoxic; + minimally phototoxic; − non-phototoxic.

The severe acute reactions of phytophotodermatitis are associated with psoralen itself and its major derivatives 8-methoxypsoralen and 5-methoxypsoralen (**6.II**) and possibly with the angelicin derivative, pimpinellin (5,6-dimethoxyisopsoralen) (**6.III**).

6.2.3 Distribution of the phototoxic furocoumarins

The active component of bergamot oil from *Citrus bergamia*, the bergamot lime, was originally isolated in the 1830s and called bergapten (Fowlks 1959, Marzulli & Maibach 1970). It was characterized as 5-Methoxypsoralen (5-MOP) and identified as the major phototoxic component of the lime peel extract by Kuske (1938). 8-Methoxypsoralen (8-MOP) was first isolated as xanthotoxin from *Fagara xanthoxyloides* and was characterized by Thoms (1911) who recognized its similarity to bergapten. Fahmy and Abu Shady (1948), investigating the photoactive components of *Ammi majus*, used in the treatment of vitiligo, extracted 8-MOP, 5-MOP and imperatorin (8-isopentenyloxypsoralen) from these plants.

Large-scale surveys such as those of the Umbelliferae generally by Neilsen (1970) and of the *Heracleum* species by Mohlo et al. (1971) were concerned with taxonomy. There have been numerous, more restricted studies concerned with the isolation, characterization and quantification of the phototoxic furocoumarins from genera or individual species (e.g. Bourgaud et al. 1989). Some of these are summarized in Table 6.2.2. The furocoumarin content may vary with *geographical location*. For instance, 5-MOP, psoralen, isopimpinellin and angelicin were found in leaves of *Heracleum mantegazzianum*, the giant hogweed (Molho et al. 1971), but in specimens from the Tayside region of Scotland, 8-MOP is the major photosensitizing component of leaf (52 mg/100 g wet weight), stem (10 mg/100 g wet weight) and fruit (22 mg/100 g wet weight) (Gumar 1976).

Finally, the concentration of furocoumarins may increase in response to *fungal attack*. Fresh celery (*Apium graveolens*) contains 10–100 µg/g wet weight of psoralens in healthy plants (Beier et al. 1983, Berkeley et al. 1986, Ljunggren 1990) made up of psoralen, 8-MOP and 5-MOP (Seligman et al. 1987) but 320 µg/g in specimens infected with species of fungus such as *Sclerotina sclerotium* (Wu et al. 1972). Harvesters and canners are particularly at risk when handling diseased celery (see p. 87). The development of disease-resistant cultivars of celery has led to an increased natural furocoumarin content in these plants and similar increased exposure to phototoxic compounds may occur with other vegetables such as parsnips.

The figures for psoralen content become of more than academic interest when it is shown that, after 1 h under occlusion, as little as

Table 6.2.2 Distribution of some naturally occurring phototoxic furocoumarins.

Family	Genus	Species	Common name(s)	Psoralen	8-Methoxypsoralen (8-MOP, ammoidin, methoxsalen, xanthotoxin)	5-Methoxypsoralen (5-MOP, bergapten, heraclin, majudin)
Umbelliferae (Apiaceae)	Ammi	majus	Queen Anne's lace		+	+
	Heracleum	laciniatum	Tromsø palm			+ 7–9
		sphondylium	Cow parsnip		+	+
		mantegazzianum	Giant Russian hogweed		+	+
		hypoleucum				+
	Cymopterus	watsonii	Spring parsley		+ 50–350	+ 30–100
	Pastinaca	sativa	Parsnip		+ 28–350	+ 24–302
		opaca			+ 155	+ 220
		urens			+ 220	+ 260
	Apium	graveolens	Celery	+	+	+
Rutaceae	Citrus	bergamia	Bergamot lime			+
	Dictamnus	albus (fraxinella)	Burning bush Gas plant		+	+
	Fagaria	xanthoxyloides			+	
Moraceae	Ficus	carica	Fig		+ 65	+ 35

Table 6.2.2 *Continued*

8-Isopentenyl-oxypsoralen (imperatorin)	5-Methoxy-8-isopentenyl-oxypsoralen (phellopterin)	6-Methoxyisopsoralen (sphondin)	5-Methoxyisopsoralen (isobergapten)	Angelicin (isopsoralen)	5,6-Dimethoxypsoralen (pimpinellin)	5,8-Dimethoxypsoralen (isopimpinellin)	References and notes (values given are in mg/100 g dried plant material, unless otherwise stated)
+							(Fahmy & Abu Shady 1948)
		+ 8–10		+ 4–5	+ 6–8		5-MOP and pimpinellin major phototoxic compounds, especially in roots and leaves (Kavli *et al.* 1983a, 1983b, 1984); see **6.III**
+	+						(Weimark & Nilsson 1980) (Beyrich 1968)
+	+			+	+	+	(Beyrich 1968)
	+	+	+		+	+	(Beyrich 1968)
							(Williams 1970)
+ 16–485						+ 44–135	In roots, stem, leaf and fruits (Beyrich 1965, 1966)
+ 315	+ 25					+ 95	(Beyrich 1965)
+ 330	+ 45					+ 125	(Beyrich 1965)
							10–100 g psoralens/g wet weight in healthy plants (Beier *et al.* 1983; Berkeley *et al.* 1986; Llunggren 1990), 320 g/g in specimens infected with *Sclerotina* (Wu *et al.* 1972)
							(Kuske 1938)
							(Moller 1978)
							(Thoms 1911)
							In leaves (Rodighiero & Antonello 1959); absent from ripened fruit (Zaynoun *et al.* 1984)

Table 6.2.3 Phototoxic compounds in *Ficus carica*, the fig plant (Zaynoun et al. 1984).

	Psoralen			Bergapten		
	Leaf sap (mg/dl)	Stem sap (mg/dl)	Leaf (mg/100 g)	Leaf sap (mg/dl)	Stem sap (mg/dl)	Leaf (mg/100 g)
April	150–209	54–55	60	19–62	1–24	29
October	46–65	6–16	4–24	30–45	1–9	1–8

1 µg of 8-MOP per square centimetre of skin surface is sufficient to produce blistering after exposure to only 2.4 J/cm^2 of artificial UVA, equivalent to approximately 10 min exposure to summer sunlight in the UK. Ljunggren (1990) reported an unusual case which might be included as phytophotodermatitis, his patient having ingested large quantities of celery soup before using a UVA sunbed.

Similar excesses with parsnips containing 40–50 µg/g wet weight of psoralens (Ivie *et al.* 1981) could lead to the same result, the standard oral dose of 8-MOP for PUVA treatment being 40 mg per 70 kg body weight.

6.2.4 Mechanisms of phototoxicity

Photosensitization is a process in which reactions to normally ineffective radiation are induced in a system by the introduction of a specific radiation absorbing component, the photosensitizer (Blum 1964, Lamola 1974, Spikes 1977, Johnson 1984, Kochevar 1987). In biological systems the process is generally considered in terms of harmless doses of UVA (315–400 nm) or visible radiation being absorbed by a 'foreign' molecular species present at non-damaging concentrations, reactions resulting from the involvement of cell and tissue constituents in the dissipation of the absorbed energy.

Where oxygen is involved in the reaction, the term photodynamic action is used and radical species of photosensitizer, substrate and oxygen may all be formed (Type I) or excited singlet state oxygen may be produced (Type II). Early studies of psoralen photochemistry established the possibility of radical production by exposure to UVA (Pathak *et al.* 1961) but the photosensitized killing of bacteria with 8-MOP is independent of oxygen (Oginsky *et al.* 1959) unlike that with toluidine blue (Matthews 1963). Other tests for psoralen-induced oxygen-dependent photosensitization such as photodynamic haemolysis and the oxidation of serum proteins were negative (Musajo & Rodighiero 1962). The mechanisms for photosensitization by the major furocoumarins involved in phytophotodermatitis appeared to differ from those for other common photosensitizers and evidence for a photosensitized interaction between psoralens and DNA was first presented by Musajo et al. (1965). Now it is clear that the major pathway for psoralen photosensitization in biological systems is a UVA-induced covalent binding of the psoralen molecule into nuclear DNA (6.IV) producing

6.IV Mechanisms of 8-MOP photoadduct formation with thymine molecules in DNA.

monofunctional photoadducts and bifunctional, interstrand cross-links with pyrimidine bases in the DNA (Musajo & Rodighiero 1972, Pathak et al. 1974, Scott et al. 1976, Song & Tapley 1979, Gasparro 1988, Averbeck 1989). Monoadducts are formed by cycloaddition at the 3,4 double bond of the coumarin or the 4'5' bond of the furan and it is the 4'5' product which, when exposed to UVA, gives rise to cross-links. Substitution at either of these points or an inappropriate stereochemistry, as in the angular compounds, makes cross-linking impossible. While monoadducts may produce mutations and cell death, these effects are greatly increased by cross-link formation. The skin reactions obtained by psoralen monoadduct formation alone, produced by wave-lengths around 400 nm, if perceptible at all, are very mild (Gange 1989). It would appear that for practical purposes, in terms of psoralen concentration and UVA exposure, it is cross-linking of DNA, mainly in the epidermis, which results in the severe skin damage of phytophotodermatitis. An exception to this rule would appear to be presented by pimpinellin (5,6-dimethoxyisopsoralen), an angular compound which is approximately half as active as bergapten but does produce phototoxic bullae in skin (Kavli *et al.* 1983a).

The cutaneous reactions of classical phytophotodermatitis are so specific and differ so markedly from the reaction pattern associated with photodynamic action that it is difficult to accept that they might be mediated through this oxygen-dependent mechanism. Although there is unequivocal photochemical evidence for the possibility of alternative, oxygen-dependent or -independent pathways for furocoumarin-induced photosensitization, involving lipid or protein rather than DNA (Mizuno *et al.* 1974, Midden 1988), many furocoumarins which perform well in this respect photosensitize the skin less well and oxygen deprivation does not block the cutaneous photosensitization obtained with 8-MOP (Auletta *et al.* 1986, Wolf *et al.* 1988). Even so, if delayed hyperpigmentation alone, the mechanism for which is not known, is taken as a part of phytophotodermatitis, the equally efficient action of oxypseudanin with that of 8-MOP as described by Kuske (1938) would appear to involve an alternative pathway. Similarly, the furochromone, khellin, does not elicit the classical reactions of phytophotodermatitis but does photosensitize the skin to produce hyperpigmentation (Abdel-Fattah *et al.* 1982, Ortel *et al.* 1986) (**6.V**).

Khellin
(furanochrome)

6.V Molecular structure of the furochromone, Khellin.

Plant substances which photosensitize in model systems through photodynamic action have been isolated mainly from the daisy family, Compositae, and are identified as polyacetylenes such as phenylheptatriene or the thiophene, α-terthienyl (Towers *et al.* 1977, Towers 1980, Wat *et al.* 1980) (**6.VI**). α-terthienyl may also photosensitize through an oxygen-independent pathway *in vitro* (Kagan *et al.* 1980). However, cutaneous photosensitization induced by α-terthienyl is the typical photodynamic Type I reaction pattern, pitch smarts and their sequelae (Chan *et al.* 1977, Towers *et al.* 1979) (see Table 6.2.1). Although there is some association between chemical constituents of the Compositae and the abnormal photosensitivity

6.VI Molecular structures of potentially phototoxic compounds in the Compositae.

seen in photosensitivity dermatitis (Addo *et al.* 1985), this type of response after accidental contact with plants has not been reported and it is evident that either the phototoxic compounds do not come in contact with the skin in high enough concentration or they do not penetrate the stratum corneum.

6.2.5 Photoallergic reactions

A rare example of atypical phytophotodermatitis may be produced through contact with furocoumarin containing plants (Ljunggren 1977). This is a delayed hypersensitivity response as in contact allergic dermatitis but is produced as a photoallergic reaction. It also occurred after repeated photopatch tests with extracts from *Heracleum laciniatum* (Tromso palm) and was due more to the poorly phototoxic sphondin and isobergapten constituents rather than the phototoxic bergapten and pimpinellin (Kavli *et al.* 1982). None the less, repeated phototoxic insult with 8-MOP has also given rise to this type of response (Plewig *et al.* 1978) and this may well be the result of an alternative protein pathway of furocoumarin photosensitization.

References

Abdel-Fattah A., Aboul-Enein M.N., Wassel G. *et al.* (1982) An approach to the treatment of vitiligo by khellin. *Dermatologica* **165**: 136–40.

Addo H.A., Sharma S.C., Ferguson J., Johnson B.E. & Frain-Bell W. (1985) A study of Compositae plant extract reactions in photosensitivity dermatitis. *Photodermatology* **2**: 68–79.

Auletta M., Gange R.W., Tan O.T. & Matzinger E. (1986) Effect of cutaneous hypoxia upon erythema and pigment responses to UVA, UVB and PUVA (8-MOP + UVA) in human skin. *Journal of Investigative Dermatology* **86**: 649–52.

Averbeck D. (1989) Recent advances in psoralen phototoxicity mechanism. *Photochemistry and Photobiology* **50**: 859–82.

Beier R.C., Ivie G.W., Oertli E.H. & Holt D.L. (1983) HPLC analysis of linear furocoumarins (psoralens) in healthy celery (*Apium graveolens*). *Food and Chemical Toxicology* **21**: 163–5.

Berkeley S.F., Hightower A.W., Beier R.C. *et al.* (1986) Dermatitis in grocery workers associated with high natural concentrations of furocoumarins in celery. *Annals of Internal Medicine* **105**: 351–5.

Beyrich T. (1965) Die Furocoumarin von *Pastinaca urens* Req. *Pharmazie* **20**: 655–6.

Beyrich T. (1966) Die Furocoumarin von *Pastinaca sativa* L. *Pharmazie* **21**: 365–72.

Beyrich T. (1968) Vergleichende Untersuchung uber das Vorkommen an Furocoumarinen in einigen Arten der Gattung Heracleum. *Pharmazie* **23**: 336–9.

Blum H.F. (1964) *Photodynamic Action and Diseases Caused by Light.* Hafner Publishing Company, New York.

Bourgaud F., Allard N., Guckert A. & Forlot P. (1989) Natural sources of furocoumarins (psoralens). In Fitzpatrick T.B., Forlot P., Pathak M.A. & Urbach F. (eds) *Psoralens: Past, Present and Future of Photochemoprotection and Other Biological Activities.* John Libey Eurotext, Paris, pp. 219–30.

Chan G.F.Q., Prihoda M., Towers G.H.N. & Mitchell J.C. (1977) Phototoxicity evoked by alpha-terthienyl. *Contact Dermatitis* **3**: 215–16.

Fahmy J.R. & Abu-Shady H. (1948) The isolation and properties of ammoidin, ammidin and majudin, and their effect in the treatment of leukodermia. *Quarterly Journal of Pharmacy and Pharmacology* **21**: 499–503.

Fowlks W.L. (1959) The chemistry of the psoralens. *Journal of Investigative Dermatology* **32**: 249–54.

Gange R.W. (1989) 8-MOP photosensitization in human skin: split irradiation studies. In Fitzpatrick T.B., Forlot P., Pathak M.A. & Urbach F. (eds) *Psoralens: Past, Present and Future of Photochemoprotection and Other Biological Activities.* John Libbey Eurotcxt, Paris, pp. 117–23.

Gasparro F.P. (1988) Psoralen DNA interactions: thermodynamics and photochemistry. In Gasparro F.P. (ed.) *Psoralen DNA photobiology, Vol. II.* CRC Press, Boca Raton, Florida, pp. 5–36.

Gumar A.W.S. (1976) *A quantitative study of phytophotodermatitis.* Thesis, University of Dundee.

Ivie G.W., Holt D.L. & Ivey M.C. (1981) Natural toxicants in human foods: psoralens in raw and cooked parsnip root. *Science* **213**: 909–10.

Johnson B.E. (1984) Light sensitivity associated with drugs and chemicals. In Jarrett A. (ed.) *The Physiology and Pathophysiology of the Skin.* Academic Press, New York, pp. 2541–606.

Jois H.S., Manjunath B.L. & Rao S.V. (1933) Chemical examination of the seeds of *Psoralea corylifolia* (Linn). *Journal Indian Chemical Society* **10**: 41–6.

Kagan J., Gabriel R. & Reed S.A. (1980) Alpha-terthienyl, a non-photodynamic phototoxic compound. *Photochemistry and Photobiology* **31**: 465–9.

Kavli G., Volden G. & Raa J. (1982) Accidental induction of photocontact allergy to *Heracleum laciniatum. Acta Dermato-Venereologica* **62**: 435–8.

Kavli G., Raa J., Johnson B.E., Volden G. & Haugsbo S. (1983a) Furocoumarins of *Heracleum laciniatum,* isolation, phototoxicity, absorption and action spectra studies. *Contact Dermatitis* **9**: 257–62.

Kavli G., Krokan H., Midelfart K., Volden G. & Raa J. (1983b) Extraction, separation, quantification and evaluation of the phototoxic potency of furocoumarins in different parts of *Heracleum laciniatum. Photobiochemistry and Photobiophysics* **5**: 159–68.

Kavli G., Midelfart K., Raa J. & Volden G. (1983c) Phototoxicity from furocoumarins (psoralens) of *Heracleum laciniatum* in a patient with vitiligo. Action spectrum studies on bergapten, pimpinellin, angelicin and sphondin. *Contact dermatitis* **9**: 364–6.

Kavli G., Krokan H., Myrnes B. & Volden G. (1984) High pressure liquid chromatographic separation of furocoumarins from *Heracleum laciniatum. Photodermatology* **1**: 85–6.

Kochevar I.E. (1987) Mechanisms of drug photosensitization. *Photochemistry and Photobiology* **45**: 891–5.

Kuske H. (1938) Experimentelle untersuchungen zur photosensibilisierung der haut durch pflanzliche wirkstoffe. *Archives fur Dermatologie und Syphilis* **178**: 112–23.

Lamola A.A. (1974) Fundamental aspects of spectroscopy and photochemistry of organic compounds; electronic energy transfer in biologic systems; and photosensitization. In Fitzpatrick T.B. (ed.) *Sunlight and Man*. University of Tokyo Press, Tokyo, pp. 17–55.

Ljunggren B. (1977) Psoralen photoallergy caused by plant contact. *Contact Dermatitis* **3**: 85–90.

Ljunggren B. (1990) Severe phototoxic burn following celery ingestion. *Archives of Dermatology* **126**: 1334–6.

Marzulli F.N. & Maibach H.I. (1970) Perfume phototoxicity. *Journal of the Society of Cosmetic Chemists* **21**: 695–715.

Matthews M.M. (1963) Comparative studies of lethal photosensitization of *Sarcina lutea* by 8-methoxypsoralen and by toluidine blue. *Journal of Bacteriology* **85**: 322–31.

Midden W.R. (1988) Chemical mechanisms of the bioeffects of furocoumarins: the role of reactions with proteins, lipids and other cellular constituents. In Gasparro F.P. (ed.) *Psoralen DNA Photobiology*. Vol. II. CRC Press, Boca Raton, Florida, pp. 1–49.

Mitchell J.C. & Rook A. (1979) *Botanical Dermatology*. Greengrass, Vancouver.

Mizuno N., Tsuneishi S., Matsuhashi S. *et al.* (1974) Some aspects on the action mechanism of 8-methoxypsoralen photosensitization. In Fitzpatrick T.B. (ed.) *Sunlight and Man*. University of Tokyo Press, Tokyo, pp. 389–409.

Mohlo D., Jossang P., Jarreau M.-C. & Carbonnier J. (1971) Derives furannocoumariniques du genre *Heracleum* et plus specialement de *Heracleum sprengelianum* Wight & Arn. et *Heracleum ceylanicum* Gardn. ex C.B. Clarke étude phylogenique. In Heywood V.H. (ed.) *The Biology and Chemistry of the Umbelliferae*. Academic Press, London, pp. 337–60.

Moller H. (1978) Phototoxicity of *Dictamnus alba*. *Contact Dermatitis* **4**: 264–9.

Musajo L. & Rodighiero G. (1962) The skin photosensitizing furocoumarins. *Experientia* **18**: 153–62.

Musajo L. & Rodighiero G. (1972) Mode of Photosensitizing action of furocoumarins. In Giese A. (ed.) *Photophysiology, Vol. VII*. Academic Press, London, pp. 115–47.

Musajo L., Rodighiero G., Colombo G., Torlone V. & Dall'Acqua F. (1965) Photosensitizing furocoumarins: interaction with DNA and photoinactivation of DNA containing viruses. *Experientia* **23**: 22–4.

Nielsen B.E. (1970) *Coumarins of umbelliferous plants*. Thesis, The Royal Danish School of Pharmacy, Copenhagen.

Oginski E.L., Green G.S., Griffith D.G. & Fowlks W.L. (1959) Lethal photosensitization of bacteria with 8-methoxypsoralen to long wavelength ultraviolet radiation. *Journal of Bacteriology* **78**: 821–33.

Ortel B., Tanew A. & Honigsmann H. (1986) *Current Problems in Dermatology* **15**: 265–71.

Pathak M.A., Allen B., Ingram D.I.E. & Fellman J.H. (1961) Photosensitization and the effect of ultraviolet radiation on the production of unpaired electrons in the presence of furocoumarins (psoralens). *Biochimica et Biophysica Acta* **54**: 506–15.

Pathak M.A., Daniels F., Jr. & Fitzpatrick T.B. (1962) The presently known distribution of furocoumarins (psoralens) in plants. *Journal of Investigative Dermatology* **39**: 225–39.

Pathak M.A., Kramer D.M. & Fitzpatrick T.B. (1974) Photobiology and Photochemistry of furocoumarins (psoralens). In Fitzpatrick T.B. (ed.) *Sunlight and Man*. University of Tokyo Press, Tokyo, pp. 335–68.

Plewig G., Hofman C. & Braun-Falco O. (1978) Photoallergic dermatitis from 8-methoxypsoralen. *Archives of Dermatological Research* **261**: 201–11.

Rodighiero G. & Antonello C. (1959) Recerche sul contenuto in psoralene e bergaptene delle foglie di *Ficus carica*. *Il Farmaco* **14**: 679–85.

Scott B.R., Pathak M.A. & Mohn G.R. (1976) Molecular and genetic basis of furocoumarin reactions. *Mutation Research* **39**: 29–74.

Seligman P.J., Mathias T., O'Malley M.A. *et al.* (1987) Phytophotodermatitis from celery among grocery store workers. *Archives of Dermatology* **123**: 1478–82.

Soine T.O. (1964) Naturally occurring coumarins and related physiological activities. *Journal of Pharmaceutical Sciences* **53**: 231–64.

Song P.S. & Tapley J.J., Jr. (1979) Photochemistry and photobiology of psoralens. *Photochemistry and Photobiology* **29**: 1177–97.

Spath E. (1937) Die naturlichen Cumarine. *Berichte der Deutschen Chemischen Gesellschaft* **70A**: 83–117.

Spikes J.D. (1977) Photosensitization. In Smith K.C. (ed.) *The Science of Photobiology*. Plenum, New York, pp. 87–110.

Thoms H. (1911) Uber die Konstitution des Xanthotoxins und seine Beziehungen zum Bergapten. *Berichte der Deutschen Chemischen Gesellschaft* **44**: 3325–32.

Towers G.H.N. (1980) Photosensitizers from plants and their photodynamic action. *Progress in Phytochemistry* **6**: 183–202.

Towers G.H.N., Wat C.-K., Graham E.A. *et al.* (1977) Ultraviolet-mediated antibiotic activity of species of Compositae caused by polyacetylenic compounds. *Lloydia* **40**: 487–98.

Towers G.H.N., Arnason T., Wat C.-K. *et al.* (1979) Phototoxic polyacetylenes and their thiophene derivatives (effects on human skin). *Contact Dermatitis* **5**: 140–4.

Wat C.-K., MacRae W.D., Yamamoto E., Towers G.H.N. & Lam J. (1980) Phototoxic effects of naturally occurring polyacetylenes and alpha-terthienyl on human erythrocytes. *Photochemistry and Photobiology* **32**: 167–72.

Weimarck G. & Nilsson E. (1980) Phototoxicity in *Heracleum sphondylium*. *Planta Medica* **38**: 97–111.

Williams M.C. (1970) Xanthotoxin and bergapten in spring parsley. *Weed Science* **18**: 479–80.

Wolf C., Steiner A. & Honigsmann H. (1988) Do oral carotenoids protect human skin against ultraviolet erythema, psoralen phototoxicity and ultraviolet-induced DNA damage? *Journal of Investigative Dermatology* **90**: 55–7.

Wu C.M., Koehler P.E. & Ayres J.C. (1972) Isolation and identification of xanthotoxin (8-methoxypsoralen) and bergapten (5-methoxypsoralen) from celery infected with *Sclerotina sclerotium*. *Applied Microbiology* **23**: 852–6.

Zaynoun S.T., Aftimos B.G., Abi Ali L. *et al.* (1984) *Ficus carica*: isolation and quantification of the photoactive components. *Contact Dermatitis* **11**: 21–5.

6.3 Clinical features

The characteristic eruption is composed of linear dusky red lesions, often bullous and associated with brown hyperpigmentation (Figs 6.3.1–6.3.4). Most cases present in mid to late summer, when the level of

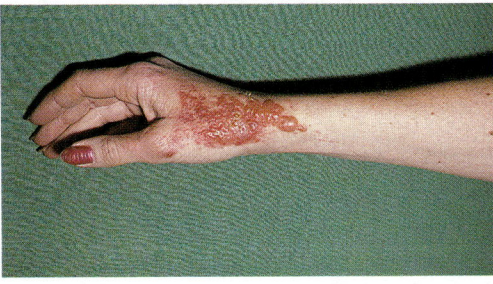

Fig. 6.3.1 Phototoxic reaction from handling rue. (Courtesy of Dr J. Adams.)

CLINICAL FEATURES

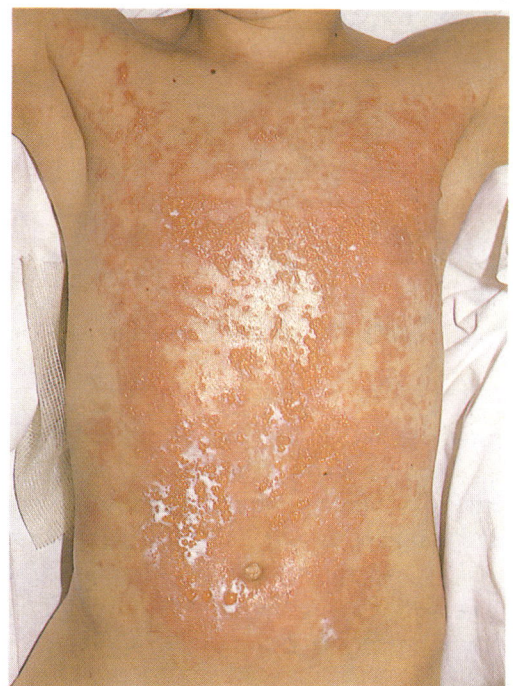

Fig. 6.3.2 Florid bullous eruption in a boy who retrieved a ball from a bed of rue on a sunny day, wearing only a pair of shorts. Note precise localization of eruption to areas of plant contact and light exposure.

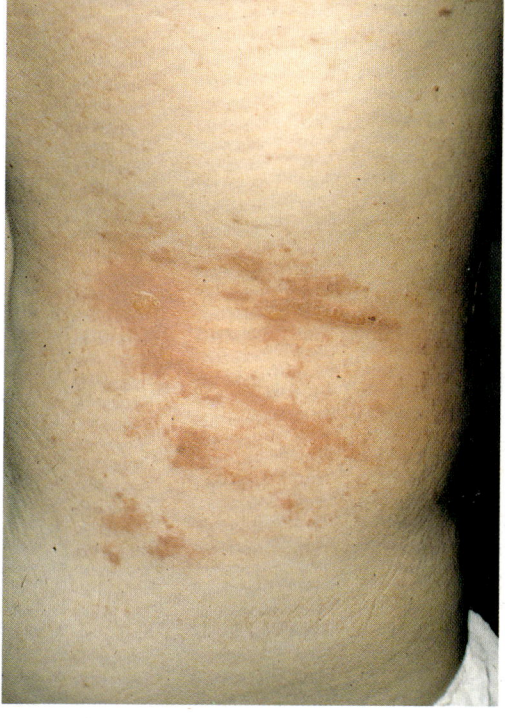

Fig. 6.3.3 Streaky hyperpigmentation. This may persist for several weeks or months after a phototoxic reaction. (Courtesy of Dr J. Adams.)

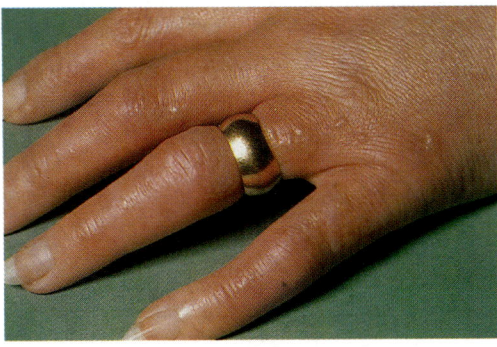

Fig. 6.3.4 Phototoxic reaction after handling a fig grown as a pot plant. (Courtesy of Dr J. Cook.)

psoralens is highest in the offending plants and the skin is unprotected by clothing. In the USA, the eruption can be misdiagnosed as poison ivy dermatitis; however, a phototoxic reaction is confined to the sites of contact and sun exposure, it is painful rather than pruritic and it is often followed by hyperpigmentation. Allergic contact dermatitis (e.g. poison ivy) is pruritic; the eruption will often continue to evolve after presentation and pigmentary change is rare (Sommer & Jillson 1967).

Table 6.3.1 Phototoxic reactions — 'at risk' activities.

Gardening
Brushing against rue plants or *Dictamnus* (especially USA)
Working amongst celery, parsnip or parsley
Clearing weeds with string trimmer
Pruning or harvesting figs

Canning and processing vegetables
e.g. celery

Rambling/jogging
Through fields and river banks
Rolling in the hay

Medication
Application of 'tan promoters' or perfumes containing bergamot oil (berloque dermatitis)
Excessive UV exposure after taking or applying psoralens for PUVA
Application of rue as an insect repellent

Play
Making peashooters with *Heracleum mantegazzianum*
Playing amongst rue bushes or Umbelliferae
Fighting with parsnips/celery, etc. (Fig. 6.3.6)

Ingestion
Ingestion of excessive psoralens (e.g. celery) especially before using sunbed
Ingestion of *Chlorella* (Japan)
Wearing 'leis' (garlands) of *Pelea anisata* (in Hawaii)

Phytophotodermatitis is especially common in children playing out of doors in the summer holidays when psoralens are most abundant in wild and garden plants. The resultant linear streaks have led to a misdiagnosis of battering (Campbell *et al.* 1982), in this case due to wild parsnip (*Pastinaca sativa*). In Europe, brushing against rue plants is probably the commonest cause of phototoxic reactions. The typical streak-like pattern also follows the application of rue to the skin as an insect repellent (Fig. 6.3.5) followed by sun exposure. It is also seen in individuals who are working among parsley, parsnip or celery plants in the summer. In the USA, *Dictamnus albus* (the burning bush or gas plant) (see Fig. 6.4.7) is more popular and may cause a similar eruption.

The pattern of the eruption is exactly related to areas of contact with the plant or plant product, followed by exposure to sunlight or an artificial UVA light source. The distribution may be bizarre, and can cause clinical confusion. After the giant Russian hogweed (*Heracleum mantegazzianum*) was introduced to Kew Gardens, the plant escaped from cultivation and naturalized itself on river banks and in damp areas. Apart from typical linear lesions seen in fishermen and bathers, the hollow stems were used by children as peashooters and trumpets causing striking perioral blisters (Drever & Hunter 1970). Similar re-

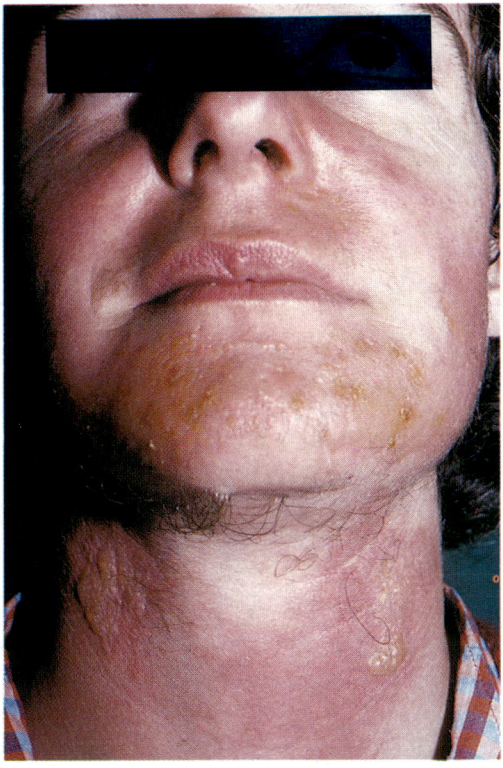

Fig. 6.3.5 Phototoxic reaction to rue used as an insect repellent. (Courtesy of Dr J. Adams.)

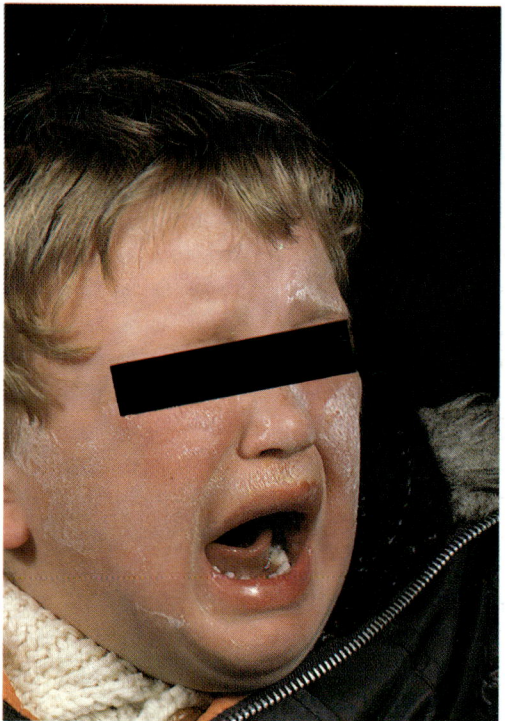

Fig 6.3.6 Diffuse phototoxic reaction on the face after playing 'Worzel Gummidge', in which the subject was hit on the face with a parsnip. He subsequently attended a football match in the afternoon. (Courtesy of Dr J. Ellis.)

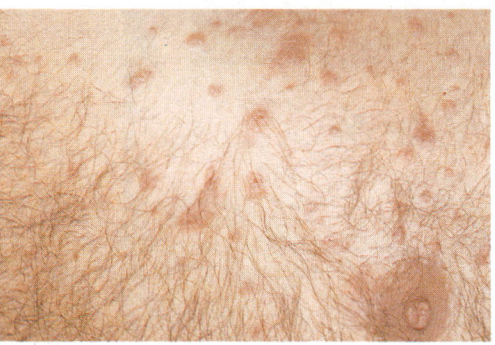

Fig. 6.3.7 'Strimmer rash'. A typical macular erythematous or bullous eruption on light-exposed areas, later becoming hyperpigmented. Because of the guttate appearance, a plant origin may not be suspected. (Courtesy of Dr N. Reynolds.)

actions have been reported to the Tromsø palm, *H. laciniatum* (Kavli et al. 1983). The stems of several Umbelliferae, including giant hogweed and cow parsnip as well as parsnip roots, are used in 'mock battles' (Fig. 6.3.6). The fruit capsules of *Pelea anisata*, the mokihana (Rutaceae), have been reported to cause bullous lesions in those who string or wear leis (garlands) in Hawaii, particularly for the celebration of Kamehameha Day in early June (Elpern & Mitchell 1984). Several psoralens have been isolated from this species (Yoke Marchant *et al.* 1985). Laboratory workers handling psoralens develop bullous lesions following spillage (e.g. Ena *et al.* 1991). Individuals with vitiligo may induce bullous reactions after self-treatment with topical psoralens and sunlight.

Modern power tools provide an ideal mechanism for delivery of plant sap to the skin of the operator. The string trimmer (e.g. 'Strimmer'®) is usually a petrol-driven device with a nylon cord revolving at about 10 000 revolutions/min. It acts as a modern labour-saving equivalent to a scythe, trimming scrubby areas of rank weeds (including several members of the Umbelliferae) and coarse grasses. Unfortunately, in so doing it delivers a 'buckshot spray' to the skin (Oakley et al. 1986). Although the manufacturers recommend protective clothing and goggles, this advice is frequently ignored in sunny weather. The resultant eruption, 'strimmer dermatitis' (Freeman et al. 1984) or 'string-trimmer's dermatitis' (Oakley et al. 1986) is composed of bright red irregular macules and papules on the anterior chest wall and arms, developing 12–24 h after exposure (Fig. 6.3.7). Some lesions may blister but always the lesions resolve leaving macular areas of hyperpigmentation which can sometimes resemble a lichenoid eruption or pityriasis lichenoides. Histology reveals a dermal capillaritis with a pericapillary lymphocytic infiltrate (Reynolds et al. 1990, 1991). The most commonly implicated species are the cow parsnip, *Heracleum sphondylium*, and cow parsley, *Anthriscus sylvestris* (Freeman et al. 1984, Oakley et al. 1986), although *H. mantegazzianum* has also caused the eruption in two cases (Reynolds et al. 1990, 1991).

Breloque (berlock) dermatitis (Fig. 6.3.8) (syn. photodermatitis pigmentaria or dermite pigmentée en forme de coulée) takes its name from the German word berlock or breloque (French), meaning a trinket or charm. The term was coined by Rosenthal in 1925 to describe pendant-like streaks of pigmentation on the neck, face, arms or trunk. Although he suspected that they were due to droplets of a fluid, he was unaware that Freund in 1916 had described pigmented macules due to sun exposure after the application of cologne water. The phototoxic ingredient proved to be bergamot oil, derived from the rind of fresh fruit of *Citrus bergamia* and several cases were reported in the 1950s and 1960s following increased use of perfumes containing bergamot oil and the passion for sunbathing (Harber et al. 1964). Since the introduction of artificial oil of bergamot and the reduced use of the natural product in perfumes, 'berloque' dermatitis has become rarer (Pathak 1986) (see Chapter 2, section 2.2).

Patients receiving PUVA therapy typically ingest psoralens (e.g. 8-methoxypsoralen 0.6 mg/kg body weight) 1–2 h before exposure to UVA. Toxic reactions may occur due to overdosage or if the patient receives accidental exposure to an additional UVA source (e.g. natural sunlight or strip lighting). Phototoxicity due to ingestion of naturally occurring psoralens appears to be rare in man, although recognized in

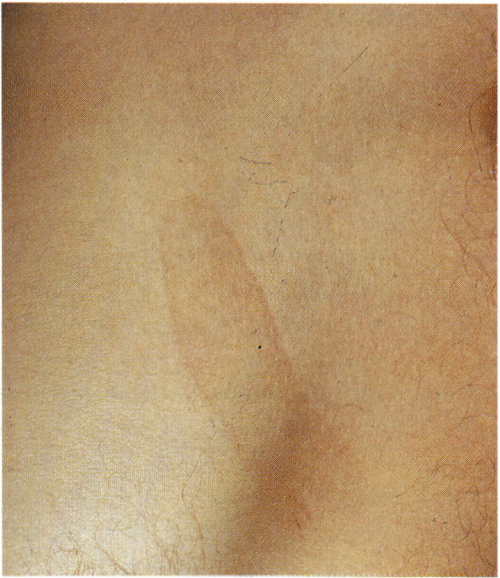

Fig. 6.3.8 Breloque (berlock) dermatitis. (Courtesy of Dr R.S.-H. Tan.)

grazing animals (Fig. 6.3.9 and see p. 65). Pathak (1986) describes an unsuccessful attempt to reproduce it in two fair-skinned 'volunteers' who ate 20 stalks of celery, 25 dried figs and 250 g of parsley before exposing their backs to the midday sun. The gastrointestinal effects of this experiment are not recorded! The advent of improved fungus-resistant cultivars of vegetables such as celery, which contain greater amounts of psoralens, and the vogue for UVA sunbeds may lead to an increased prevalence, as in a recent description of a severe reaction in an individual who consumed vast amounts of celery soup before using a sunbed (Llunggren 1990). In Japan, phototoxicity has been reported in five patients who ingested a preparation containing an alga (*Chlorella* species) as a 'natural health food' (Jitsukawa *et al.* 1984). The photosensitizer appears to be pheophorbide A, a chlorophyll derivative.

Phototoxic reactions are entirely preventable. Operatives working amongst phototoxic plants or using string trimmers should wear pro-

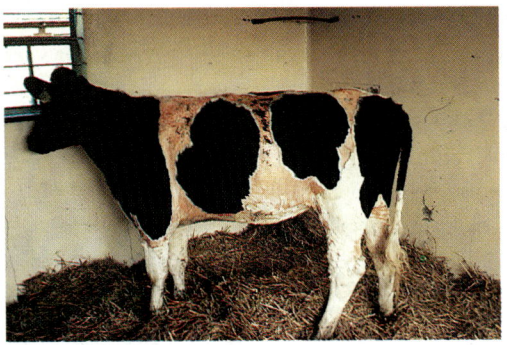

Fig. 6.3.9 Hepatogenous phototoxicity due to St John's wort (*Hypericum perforatum*) in a Friesian heifer. (Courtesy of Dr S. Shaw.)

tective clothing and avoid sun exposure. Rue in particular should not be planted near play areas. Many sunscreens, except those based on titanium dioxide, offer poor protection against UVA and should not be relied on. Artificial tanning promoters, e.g. those containing bergamot oil, are now out of favour. Treatment for an acute reaction is symptomatic. Severely affected individuals may need hospital admission, wet compresses and paraffin gauze dressings, together with potent analgesia. Steroids may be helpful if the eruption is oedematous. Hyperpigmentation may persist for several months and is best untreated. Depigmenting preparations containing hydroquinone are rarely necessary and run the risk of producing excessive hypopigmentation. Areas affected by phototoxic reactions may remain hypersensitive to UV light for several months or years, and sun protection is advisable.

References

Campbell A.N., Cooper C.E. & Dahl M.G.C. (1982) 'Non-accidental injury' and wild parsnips. *British Medical Journal* **284**: 708.
Drever J.C., Hunter J.A.A. (1970) Giant hogweed dermatitis. *Scottish Medical Journal* **15**: 315–19.
Elpern D.J. & Mitchell J.C. (1984) Phytophotodermatitis from mokihana fruits (*Pelea anisata* H. Mann, fam. Rutaceae) in Hawaiian lei. *Contact Dermatitis* **10**: 224–6.
Ena P., Cerri R., Dessi G., Manconi P.M. & Atzei A.D. (1991) Phototoxicity due to *Cachrys libanotis*. *Contact Dermatitis* **24**: 1–5.
Freeman K., Hubbard S.H.C. & Warin A.P. (1984) Strimmer rash. *Contact Dermatitis* **10**: 117–18.
Freund E. (1916) Uber bisher noch nicht beschriebene Kunstliche Hautverfarbungen. *Dermatologische Wochenschrift* **63**: 931.
Harber L.C., Harris H., Leider M. et al. (1964) Berloque dermatitis, a technique for its deliberate reproduction. *Archives of Dermatology* **90**: 572–6.
Jitsukawa K., Suizu R. & Hidano A. (1984) Chlorella photosensitization. New phytophotodermatosis. *International Journal of Dermatology* **23**: 263–8.
Kavli G., Volden G., Midelfari K. et al. (1983) *In vivo* and *in vitro* phototoxicity of different parts of *Heracleum laciniatum*. *Contact Dermatitis* **9**: 269–73.
Ljunggren B. (1990) Severe phototoxic burn following celery ingestion. *Archives of Dermatology* **126**: 1334–6.
Oakley A.M.M., Ive F.A. & Harrison M.A. (1986) String trimmer's dermatitis. *Journal of the Society of Occupational Medicine* **36**: 143–4.
Pathak M.A. (1986) Phytophotodermatitis. *Clinics in Dermatology* **4**: 103–21.
Reynolds N.J., Matthews C.N.A. & Burton J.L. (1990) Strimmer dermatitis (poster summary). *British Journal of Dermatology* **123**, Suppl 37: 63.
Reynolds N.J., Burton J.L., Bradfield J.W.B. & Matthews C.N.A. (1991) Weed wacker dermatitis (letter). *Archives of Dermatology* **127**: 1419–20.
Rosenthal O. (1925) Breloque dermatitis: Berliner Dermatologische Gesellschaft. *Dermatologische Zeitschrift* **42**: 295.
Sommer R.G., Carpenter G. & Jillson O.F. (1967) Phytophotodermatitis (solar dermatitis from plants). Gas plant and wild parsnip. *New England Journal of Medicine* **276**: 1484–6.
Yoke Marchant Y., Turjman M., Flynn T., Balza F., Mitchell J.C. & Towers G.H.N. (1985) Identification of psoralen, 8-methoxypsoralen, isopimpinellin and 5,7 dimethoxycoumarin in *Pelea anisata* H. Mann. *Contact Dermatitis* **12**: 196–9.

6.4 Plants which cause phototoxic reactions

Numerous plants have been implicated and the major ones are listed in Table 6.4.1. Several species have been shown to be rich in psoralens and are therefore potentially phototoxic, although there are no well-documented clinical examples. These species are shown in brackets in the table. Other species have been blamed in the past; however, many of these are primary irritants which can produce bullous reactions; these include *Ranunculus* species (buttercups), *Brassica nigra* (mustard), and some Compositae, notably *Anthemis cotula*, the stinking mayweed, and *Achillea millefolium* (yarrow). Bindweed (*Convolvulus arvensis*) and beggars' ticks (*Agrimonia eupatoria*) were incriminated (Klaber 1942, O'Donovan 1942) but there is little evidence of their ability to photosensitize (Van Dijk & Berrens 1964). The two major plant families are Umbelliferae and Rutaceae. Figs (Moraceae) are another important cause.

Umbelliferae

Most members of this large family are native to western Asia, although many of the relatively small number of species in western Europe are common weeds. All the species of dermatological importance are similar in floral structure and precise identification can be confusing! The basic structure of an umbellifer is outlined in Fig. 6.4.1. As the name implies, the numerous small flowers are held in an umbel (a cluster of flowers on stalks of roughly equal length arising from a single point). Generally the flowerhead is made up of many small umbels, a 'compound umbel'. The fruits are distinctive, each being small, oblong or cylindrical. The stems are hollow and leafy and the flower heads are sheathed at the base by one or more leaf-like bracts. The common species of roadsides, fields and river banks are *Anthriscus sylvestris* (Fig. 6.4.2), a

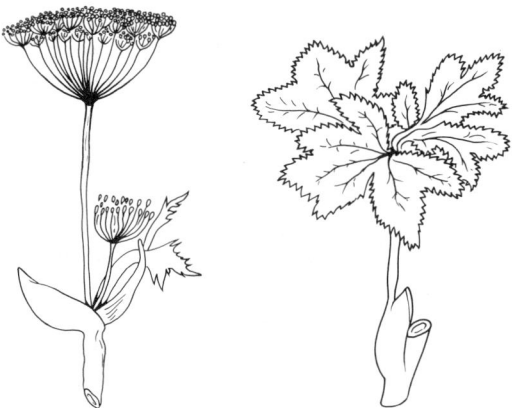

Fig. 6.4.1 *Peucedanum ostruthium* (masterwort), a typical member of the Umbelliferae. Note the characteristic compound-branched umbel (flowerhead).

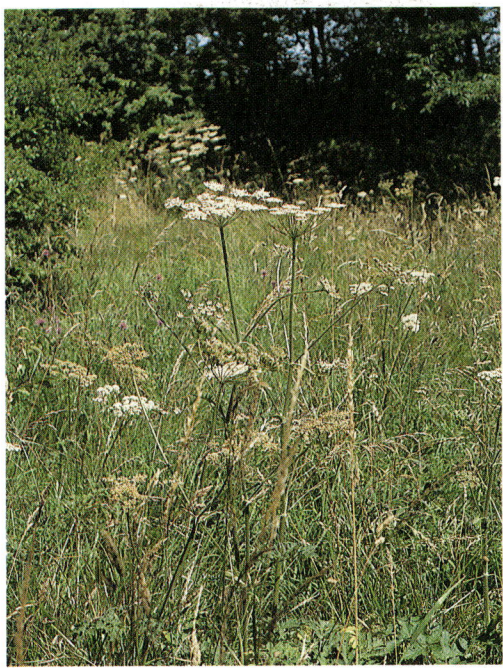

Fig. 6.4.2 *Anthriscus sylvestris* (cow parsley).

weed of cultivation probably originating from central Europe, *Daucus carota*, the wild carrot (often naturalized on waste ground), and *Heracleum sphondylium*, the cow parsnip or hogweed. All have white flowers. They are likely causes of 'strimmer rash'. Other species are listed in Table 6.4.1.

Heracleum mantegazzianum is an impressive plant (Fig. 6.4.3) resembling a much magnified version of our native hogweed (*Heracleum sphondylium*), but reaches a height of 3–4 m. Unlike *H. sphondylium*, the stems are red-spotted. Originally native to the Caucasus, it has become naturalized throughout all northern temperate areas, and causes severe phototoxic reactions in Europe and North America (Drever & Hunter 1970, Camm *et al*. 1976). It is particularly found on river banks and in moist places. Attempts to reduce the plant population by cutting down may aid water-borne dispersal of the seed heads (Editorial 1970).

Several important vegetables are members of the Umbelliferae. These include parsley, parsnip, carrot and celery (Figs 6.4.4, 6.4.5). Dermatitis due to celery, *Apium graveolens*, has been recognized since 1926 (Legrain & Berthe 1926). Workers gathering celery for canning are particularly at risk (Henry 1933) (see p. 69). More recently, Birmingham *et al*. (1961) have shown that celery infected with the filamentous fungus species *Sclerotinia sclerotiorum* and other fungus species is rich in psoralens (see p. 69). It appears that the psoralens are 'phyto-

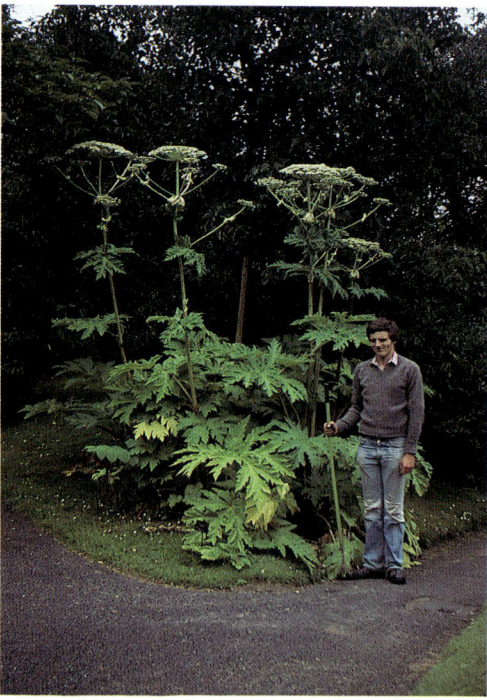

Fig. 6.4.3 *Heracleum mantegazzianum* (giant Russian hogweed). (Courtesy of Dr D. Gledhill.)

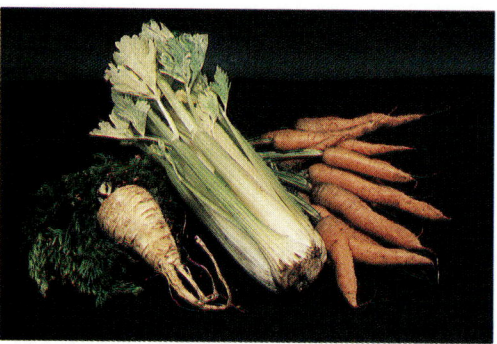

Fig. 6.4.4 Important members of the Umbelliferae (carrot, celery and parsnip).

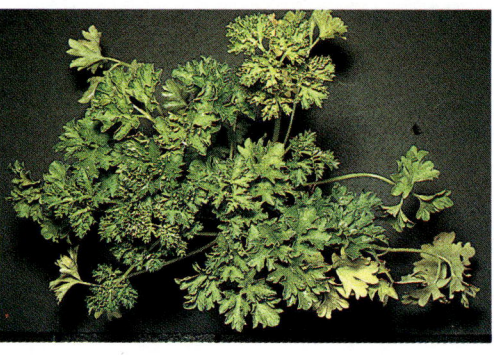

Fig. 6.4.5 *Petroselinum crispum* (parsley).

Table 6.4.1 Phototoxic plants. [ ] denotes that the species contains psoralens but phototoxic reactions have not been confirmed in humans.

Family	Botanical name	Common name	Distribution/comments
Umbelliferae (Apiaceae)	*Ammi majus*	Bishop's weed, Queen Anne's lace	Mediterranean. Occasionally grown as an ornamental in Britain and rarely naturalized on waste grounds. Greyish leaves; delicate lacy flower
	[*Anethum graveolens*]	Dill	West Asia. Garden herb
	Angelica archangelica	Angelica	Europe and Asia. Naturalized on river banks in UK. Candied leaf stalks used in confectionery. Hollow green stems. Greenish flowers on tall stems in late summer
	Angelica sylvestris	Wild angelica	Northern hemisphere, including UK. Common in moist places. Hollow purplish stems. Leaf stalks inflated, leaves oval, with saw-tooth notches at edges. Flowers pink and white in late summer
	Anthriscus sylvestris	Cow parsley, wild chervil	Europe and northwest Asia. Hairy stems with numerous white lace-like flowers. Oblong smooth fruit. Very common in fields and rough ground in UK except north Scotland. Flowers April–June. An important cause of 'strimmer dermatitis'
	Anthriscus cerefolium	Garden chervil	Similar but more slender. Shorter stems, only hairy above the nodes. Rarely naturalized in UK but an important garden herb
	Apium graveolens	Celery	Europe and Asia. In western Europe, found in wet places, especially near coasts. Most reactions due to garden forms (see text)
	Cachrys libanotis (Syn. *Hippomarathrum libanotis*)	—	Mediterranean. Common in meadows in west Sardinia (Ena *et al*. 1991)
	[*Cuminum cyminum*]	Cumin	Mediterranean and Asia. Cumin oil, previously used in perfumery, may be phototoxic
	Daucus carota	Carrot	Wild species common in northern temperate zones, near sea and on calcareous soil. Lance-shaped leaf lobes. Umbels of white flowers become concave in fruit. Stems have irritant hairs
	Foeniculum vulgare	Fennel	Euro-Mediterranean area including southern Britain on waste ground and near coasts. A common garden herb. Tall (1 m) stems with fine fern-like leaves. Plant dark green or bronze. Small yellow flowers. Whole plant has strong aniseed smell when crushed

Continued on p. 90

Table 6.4.1 Continued

Family	Botanical name	Common name	Distribution/comments
	Heracleum sphondylium	European cow parsnip, hogweed, cow parsley	Europe, including Britain. Common on roadsides, hedgerows. An important cause of 'strimmer dermatitis'. Large, coarse, oval leaves, irregularly cut at margins. Large umbels of white flowers; the petals of the outer flowers are enlarged. Mid–late summer
	Heracleum mantegazzianum	Giant Russian hogweed, wild rhubarb	Caucasus; introduced as an ornamental to Kew Gardens. Now naturalized by rivers in Europe (including UK). A massive plant, up to 4 m, with hollow red-spotted stems, oval leaves like *H. sphondylium* but up to 1 m in length. Flower heads up to 0.5 m diameter. An important cause of phototoxic reactions (see text)
	Other spp. of *Heracleum* contain psoralens and have been implicated in phototoxic reactions. These include *H. dulce*, *giganteum*, *laciniatum* (the Tromso palm), *lanatum* (USA & Japan), and *persicum*		
	Levisticum officinale	Lovage	May cause phototoxic reactions when harvested (Ashwood-Smith *et al.* 1992)
	[*Libanotis buchtormensis*] (Seseli)		West Asia
	[*Ligusticum acutilobum*]		West Europe. Related to the herb lovage (*Levisticum*)
	Pastinaca sativa	Parsnip	Europe (including south & west Britain and Ireland), Asia. The cultivated parsnip is a selection of this species which has hollow stems, oval lobed leaves and yellow flowers. Both wild and cultivated forms cause phototoxic reactions (see text). Other species contain psoralens
	Petroselinum crispum	Parsley	Europe; naturalized on limestone in UK. A common herb. See text
	Peucedanum ostruthium	Masterwort	Europe, Asia, naturalized in north and west Britain in moist meadows. Hollow stems, broad jagged leaves
	Peucedanum galbanum	Blister bush	South Africa, especially Table Mountain where it flowers in midsummer (January–March). A potent cause of phototoxicity
	Psoralens are found in other *Peucedanum* species		
	[*Phellopteris littoralis*] (*Cymopterus*)		USA

PLANTS WHICH CAUSE PHOTOTOXIC REACTIONS

Family	Species	Common name	Description/Distribution
	[*Pimpinella* spp.]	Burnet saxifrage	Europe, Asia. A few species in North and South America
	[*Prangos* spp.]		Mediterranean, west Asia
Rutaceae	*Citrus*		All species originally native to Far East but many are widely cultivated in warm temperate zones. Phototoxic reactions may follow accidental spillage of juice or deliberately rubbing essential oils (e.g. bergamot) to the skin to induce hyperpigmentation (see text)
	aurantifolia	Lime	
	aurantium	Bitter orange	
	aurantium v. *bergamia*	Bergamot	
	limetta	Sweet lemon	
	limon	Lemon	
	medica v. *limonum*	(Source of oil of ledro)	
	paradisi	Grapefruit	
	sinensis	Sweet orange	
	Dictamnus albus (*D. fraxinella*)	Burning bush, gas plant Creosote plant	Mediterranean region, Asia. Cultivated as an ornamental border plant, especially in USA. Aromatic, up to 1 m high, leaves divided into up to 10 oval, leathery, finely toothed leaflets. Pink or white purple-marked flowers in long spikes. Upper four petals held erect, the lower petal points backwards. See text
	Phlebalium argentuem	Blister plant	West Australia, cultivated in California. Low-growing shrub to 1 m, silvery leaves and white, occasionally yellow, flowers
	[*Ptelea* spp.]	Hop tree	Southern USA, Mexico
	Pelea anisata	Mokihana	Hawaii; fruits used in garlands (leis). See text
	Ruta graveolens	Rue	Mediterranean, on rocky hillsides. A very popular garden plant. A low-growing, pungent shrublet with grey leaves deeply cut into oval segments and yellow flowers in midsummer
	Ruta chalepensis	Fringed rue	Similar, but leaf segments wedge-like. Flowers yellow, green-tinged, petals fringed. See text
	[*Skimmia laureola*]	Skimmia	East Asian shrubs; some are popular in cultivation
	[*Thamnosa montana*]	Turpentine broom	Southern USA and southwest Arabia. Occasionally cultivated. Aromatic shrub
Moraceae	*Ficus carica*	Fig	Asia; naturalized in Mediterranean and cultivated in north Europe. See text
Leguminosae	*Psoralea corylifolia*	Bavchi, scurf pea	Tropical and sub-tropical areas. Used therapeutically for vitiligo for 3½ millenia. See text

alexins', i.e. substances which are produced by the plant in response to fungal attack (Beier & Oertli 1983).

Rutaceae

This family has numerous members in the tropics and southern hemisphere and a few genera in southern Europe. Most species are shrubs or small trees, the flowers have four or five sepals and petals and the fruit is fleshy. The family includes *Citrus* species (including orange, lemon, etc., see Table 6.4.1). *C. aurantifolia*, the Persian lime, was reported as a major cause of phototoxic reactions in southeast USA, notably Florida (Sams 1941). More recently, an outbreak of phototoxic reactions was reported from Maryland in children making pomander balls with limes (Israel 1985). Limes are a major cause of phototoxic reactions in Nigeria (Olumide 1985).

Ruta graveolens, garden rue (Fig. 6.4.6), is a widely grown sub-shrub native to Mediterranean areas (Table 6.4.1). The cultivar 'Jackman's Blue' is popular. Both Discorides and Culpeper are enthusiastic about the therapeutic properties of rue. According to Culpeper, it 'takes away wheals and pimples', it 'cures the morphew, and takes away all sorts of

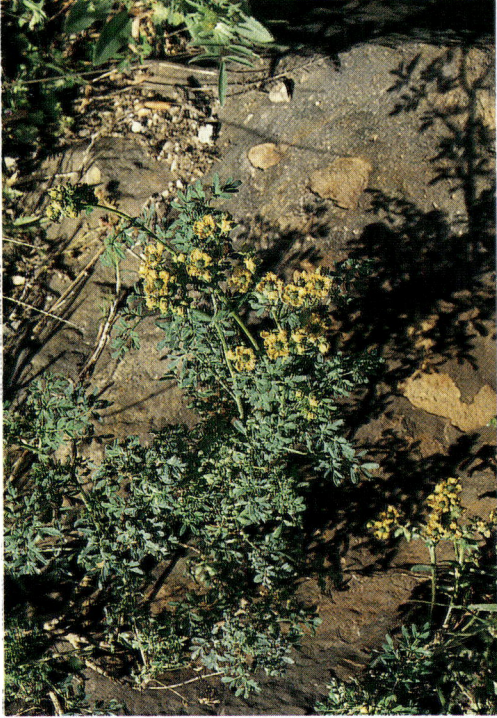

Fig. 6.4.6 *Ruta graveolens* (rue); note greyish lobed leaves and four-petalled flowers.

warts' and an ointment 'made of the juice thereof...cures St Anthony's fire, and all running sores in the head and the stinking ulcers of the nose, or other parts'. It is still used to ward off fleas and other biting insects. Rue is probably the commonest cause of phototoxicity acquired in the English garden (e.g. Gawkrodger & Savin 1983) and reactions can be severe, as shown in Figs 6.3.1, 6.3.2, 6.3.5.

Ruta corsica is a rarer species, endemic to Corsican and Sardinian mountains, and which can also cause phototoxicity (Ena & Camarda 1990). *Ruta* species contain bergapten, xanthotoxin and angelicins (Dall'acqua *et al.*, quoted in Ena & Camarda 1990).

Dictamnus albus (*D. fraxinella*), the gas plant, may be the burning bush (Fig. 6.4.7) encountered by the prophet Moses (*Exodus* Chapter 3). On a calm, hot day, the aromatic oil exuding from the plant can be briefly ignited without harming the plant. It is occasionally grown in Britain, but is a common yard plant in the USA and Canada (Sommer *et al.* 1967). Gardeners who prune the plant are at risk of phototoxicity which may be misdiagnosed as poison ivy dermatitis (Henderson & de Groseilliers 1984). The phototoxic substances, found in highest concentrations in the seed pods, include 8-methoxypsoralen and 5-methoxypsoralen (Moller 1978) (see Table 6.2.2).

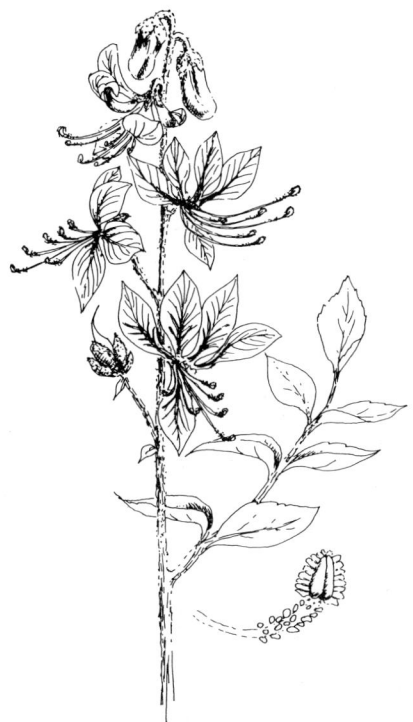

Fig. 6.4.7 *Dictamnus albus* (*fraxinella*), the 'burning bush'.

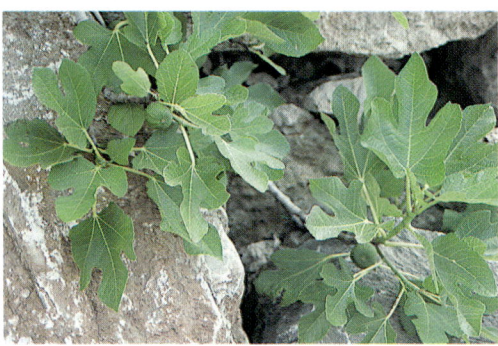

Fig. 6.4.8 *Ficus carica* (fig) bearing immature green fruit.

Moraceae (mulberry family)

Ficus carica, the fig tree (Fig. 6.4.8), is probably native to the Middle East, although it has been cultivated widely in Europe since ancient times. It is more widely mentioned as a food plant in the Bible than any other and the milky juice is used to destroy warts and to cure skin infections (Huxley & Taylor 1977). According to Culpeper, 'an ointment made of the juice and hog's grease, is an excellent remedy for the biting of mad dogs, or other venomous beasts, as most are'. Furthermore, 'if you tie a bull, be he ever so mad, to a fig tree, he will quickly become tame and gentle'.

Dioscorides in AD 50 noted that vitiligo would repigment if 'cataplasmed with ye leaves or ye boughes of ye Black Figge' (Mitchell & Rook 1979). Bullous dermatitis from the sap has been recognized since 1899 and is partly irritant in origin. In the Middle East and Mediterranean areas, fig dermatitis is common in the summer months (Berlin 1930). The psoralens are found chiefly in the leaves and unripe fruit (Zaynoun *et al.* 1984) (see Table 6.2.2). Phototoxic reactions to fig tree are seen in warmer summers in Britain.

References

Ashwood-Smith M.J., Ceska O., Yeoman A. & Kenny P.G.W. (1992) Photosensitivity from harvesting lavage (Levisticum officinale). *Contact Dermatitis* **26**: 356–7.

Beier R.C. & Oertli E.H. (1983) Psoralen and other linear furocoumarins as phytoalexins in celery. *Phytochemistry* **22**: 2595.

Berlin C. (1930) Feigenbaumdermatitis. *Dermatologische Wochenschrift* **90**: 733–6.

Birmingham D.J., Key M.M., Tublich G.E. *et al.* (1961) Phototoxic bullae among celery harvesters. *Archives of Dermatology* **83**: 73–7.

Camm E., Buck H.W.L. & Mitchell J.C. (1976) Phytophotodermatitis from *Heracleum mantegazzianum*. *Contact Dermatitis* **2**: 68.

Drever J.C. & Hunter J.A.A. (1970) Giant hogweed dermatitis. *Scottish Medical Journal* **15**: 315–19.

Editorial (1970) The giant hogweed. *Lancet* **ii**: 32.

Ena P. & Camarda I. (1990) Phytophotodermatitis from *Ruta corsica*. *Contact Dermatitis* **22**: 63.

Gawkrodger D.J. & Savin J.A. (1983) Phytophotodermatitis due to common rue (*Ruta graveolens*). *Contact Dermatitis* **9**: 224.

Henderson J.A. & Groseilliers J.P. (1984) Gas plant Dictamnus albus phytophotodermatitis simulating poison ivy. *Canadian Medical Association Journal* **130**: 889–91.

Henry S.A. (1933) Celery itch: dermatitis due to celery in vegetable canning. *British Journal of Dermatology* **45**: 301–9.

Huxley A. & Taylor W. (1977) *Flowers of Greece and the Aegean*. Chatto & Windus, London.

Israel E. (1985) Outbreak of phototoxic dermatitis from limes — Maryland. *MMWR Communicable Disease Center Surveillance Summary* **34**: 462.

Klaber R. (1942) Phyto-photo-dermatitis. *British Journal of Dermatology and Syphilology* **54**: 193–211.

Legrain M.M. & Berthe R. (1926) Dermite professionelle des mains et des avant-bras chez un remasseur de celeris. *Bulletin de la Societé Française de Dermatologie et Syphiligraphie* **33**: 662.

Mitchell J. & Rook A. (1979) *Botanical Dermatology*. Greengrass, Vancouver.

Moller H. (1978) Phototoxicity of *Dictamnus alba*. *Contact Dermatitis* **4**: 264–9.

O'Donovan W.J. (1942) Dermatitis bullosa striata pratensis. Agrimony dermatitis. *British Journal of Dermatology and Syphilology* **54**: 39–46.

Olumide Y.M. (1985) Contact dermatitis in Nigeria. *Contact Dermatitis* **12**: 241–6.

Sams W.M. (1941) Photodynamic action of lime oil (*Citrus aurantifolia*). *Archives of Dermatology and Syphilology* **44**: 571–87.

Sommer R.G., Carpenter G. & Jillson O.F. (1967) Phytophotodermatitis (solar dermatitis from plants): gas plant and wild parsnip. *New England Journal of Medicine* **276**: 1484–6.

Van Dijk E. & Berrens L. (1964) Milestones in dermatology: phytophotodermatitis. *Excerpta Medica* **18**: 371–3.

Zaynoun S.T., Aftimos B.G., Abi Abi L., Tevekjian K.K., Khalidid U. & Kurban A.K. (1984) *Ficus carica*: isolation and quantification of the photoactive components. *Contact Dermatitis* **11**: 21–5.

7 Allergic contact dermatitis due to plants

7.1 Mechanisms of allergic contact dermatitis

Allergic contact dermatitis is a specific immunological response to an external substance. In contrast to immunologically mediated contact urticaria, it is a manifestation of delayed (cell-mediated) immunity, analogous to tuberculin hypersensitivity. An allergic reaction can only occur in an individual who is already sensitized to the antigen and classically the reaction is restricted to sites of exposure (e.g. jean stud dermatitis in a nickel-sensitive patient). Some allergens, such as phosphorus sesquisulphide in match heads, are capable of spreading in the skin and produce a more diffuse response. Allergic contact dermatitis shows clinical and histological features of eczema. Initially, the lesions are papulovesicular, associated with a variable degree of erythema, oedema and crusting. Later, the skin thickens with scaling and lichenification. Early histological features occur within minutes to hours of exposure to the allergen and include a perivascular lymphocytic infiltrate. Subsequently, there is intercellular oedema in the epidermis leading to fluid-filled spaces which coalesce, forming vesicles (spongiosis). Basophils and eosinophils congregate in the upper dermis and there is endothelial damage to small blood vessels, with fibrin deposition and luminal narrowing. If antigenic stimulation continues, the process enters a more chronic phase and acanthosis and hyperkeratosis predominate (Dvorak *et al.* 1976).

A detailed discussion of the mechanisms of allergic contact dermatitis is outside the scope of this book and the reader is referred to the excellent review by Polak (1980). In brief, the exogenous substance (hapten) is typically of low molecular weight (500–1000 Da), enabling it to penetrate the epidermis. It forms conjugates with carrier problems in the skin (e.g. keratins), or in the case of some metals, binds directly to dermal collagen bundles. The antigenic complex is then recognized by a specific clone of lymphocytes (antigen recognition). These cells migrate from the skin via lymphatics to regional lymph nodes where they proliferate and differentiate. The resultant sensitized effector and memory cells are disseminated via blood vessels throughout the body (propagation phase). When the sensitized individual next encounters the allergen, an eczematous response develops at the site of contact, mediated by these cells (elicitation phase). In addition, further stimulation of memory cells also takes place (booster effect), explaining the increasingly severe response often observed on repeated exposure to the allergen. In some individuals, frequent re-exposure to small doses of the allergen may induce immunological tolerance and it is possible to induce oral hyposensitization to some allergens, notably poison ivy (Chapter 7.4).

Allergic sensitization requires intact, afferent and efferent limbs of the cellular immune system. Antigen presentation by epidermal Langerhans (macrophage-like) cells, and their interaction with lymphocytes and monocytes, appears to be essential for the induction of allergic contact dermatitis.

It is difficult to predict which chemicals are likely to cause delayed hypersensitivity in humans, although sensitization tests in guinea pigs will give a 'sensitizing index'. Most natural haptens are highly reactive and electron deficient ('electrophilic'). They react with electron-rich ('nucleophilic') groups on the surface of carrier proteins to form the conjugated antigen. Some naturally occurring substances such as the urushiols of poison ivy and poison oak (*Toxicodendron* spp.) are not electrophilic in their own right, but are oxidized to electrophilic orthoquinones. The allergens in plants belong to a variety of different chemical groups, some of which are illustrated (see **7.1**). The major allergen in each species of sensitizing plant (if known) is recorded in the test. For a more detailed discussion of the chemistry of allergic contact dermatitis the reader is referred to Dupuis and Benezra (1982).

Unfortunately, there is at present no reliable *in vitro* test which can confirm or refute a clinical diagnosis of allergic contact dermatitis. Techniques such as lymphocyte transformation and migration inhibition of macrophages give only indirect information. Despite its drawbacks, and the inconvenience to the patient, patch testing is essential in the investigation of suspected contact allergy.

7.2 Patch testing with plants and plant allergens

Patch testing should only be undertaken in a specialist dermatology department with expertize in the procedures and the interpretation of results. For further information on patch testing in general, the authoritative text by Cronin (1980) is strongly recommended. Plant material and extracts may give false negative or irritant false positive results. There is also a significant risk of active sensitization which is greater if unprocessed plant material is used and if the patch testing technique is not performed correctly. This can have devastating consequences to a professional horticulturist or florist. It is undesirable, although commonplace, to patch test the patient to a wide range of plants or a large 'routine' battery of plant extracts, many of which may share similar allergens. Multiple positive reactions are difficult to interpret and may reflect the 'angry back syndrome' (Mitchell 1975). It is essential to take a careful history, followed by patch testing with a selection of the most likely suspect plants, together with appropriate patch test batteries; in some individuals it may be necessary to perform further patch tests after an interval of a few weeks.

To obtain the maximum amount of information at minimal risk to the patient, it would be ideal to use a series of purified allergens at concentrations high enough to elicit a positive reaction but not high enough to sensitize or cause irritancy. Sadly, although many allergens have been identified in recent years, very few are available commercially and it is usually necessary to use the patient's own plant material, followed where appropriate by preparing an extract from it (Chapter 7.3).

Patch testing with standard batteries can often give useful, if sometimes indirect, information. Some examples are given in Table 7.2.1. Previously, a commercially prepared series of plant oleoresins (Hollister–Stier®) was used but it is now discontinued. The sesquiterpene lactone mix (see p. 149) appears to be a useful screening test for Compositae (daisy family) dermatitis, it should become available commercially by mid 1992. A simple feverfew (*Tanacetum parthenium*)

Table 7.2.1 Possible indicators of plant allergens in commercial series.

Allergen	Some plants with similar, or identical, allergens
Balsam of Peru 25% pet.	Conifers, cinnamon, citrus peel, *Styrax* (tinct. benz. co.), vanilla, ginger
Fragrance mix 16% Components:	
Cinnamyl alcohols	? Cinnamon
Cinnamaldehyde (eaxh 2%)	Cinnamon bark
Eugenol	Cloves, cinnamon
Amylcinnamaldehyde	Jasmine (*Jasminium*)
Hydroxycitronellal	? *Eucalyptus*, *Citronella*, cardamom
Geraniol	? *Pelargonium* ('geranium'), ? lavender, *Citronella*
Isoeugenol	? Cloves
Oak moss absolute	Lichens
Usnic acid/atranorin	Lichens
Colophony 20% pet. (also turpentine peroxides 0.3%, abietic acid 10%, etc.)	Conifers, *Eucalyptus*
Alantolactone (helanin 0.1% pet. may sensitize)	Compositae, liverwort (*Frullania* spp.), sweet bay (*Laurus*)
Primin	The purified major allergen in *Primula obconica* (?other spp.) may rarely give false negatives

extract appears to be a useful screen for chrysanthemum sensitivity (p. 162–3).

7.2.1 Identification of plants (see also Chapter 3)

Plant testing is valueless unless each plant is correctly identified. Several useful and inexpensive books are available and some are listed on p. 27. A common name is inadequate for identification; many plants have several vernacular names and the same name can be shared by two unrelated plant species (e.g. 'autumn crocus' may refer to true *Crocus*, a non-toxic member of the iris family, or *Colchicum*, a highly toxic cormous plant, the source of colchicine). Trade (lumber) names for woods are notoriously unreliable. The full botanical name is essential for a case report. Sometimes even varietal names are important. For example, a chrysanthemum grower may be able to grow some cultivars of chrysanthemums (X *Dendranthema*) and not others; it will be necessary to patch test all the cultivars grown by the patient. The same applies to growers of tulips and, to a lesser extent, narcissi.

Ask the patient to bring samples of all suspected plants, ideally fresh, but air-dried material is often acceptable. Where possible, the specimen should include leaves, stem and flowers and in some cases the root or bulbs (if any). Each plant should be packed separately; a jumble of plant leaves in a polythene bag will lead to contamination and confusing results. Reserve representative samples of the material for extraction and for precise identification, if required.

If you (and the patient) are unable to identify a plant found to give a positive patch test, the material should be sent to a department of botany or botanical garden for identification. It will help the taxonomist if you can give details of the habitat and a general description of the plant. If the material is to be sent by post, place fresh material in an inflated, sealed polythene bag without additional water and send it in a 'jiffy' bag or box lined with 'bubble' packaging. A squashed, festering mess of decaying plant in a polythene bag will not gladden the eye of the recipient! Alternatively plant material can be pressed between two paper towels and sandwiched between pieces of cardboard. It is reasonable to expect to be charged a fee for plant identification. Sometimes a 'garden visit' is necessary. This can provide useful information and not infrequently a valuable source of cuttings and seedlings for the horticulturally inclined dermatologist!

Before patch testing, ensure that the plant is not a recognized irritant (see Chapter 5). If there is a strong clinical suspicion that the plant is additionally causing an allergic reaction, make an extract (see p. 104) before proceeding with patch testing.

If the history and examination suggest phototoxicity, the plants should be compared with those in Chapter 6, section 6.4. It is pointless to patch test the patient (often a child) in such a case. If an unfamiliar plant is suspected of phototoxicity, photopatch tests may be appropriate in a control individual (ideally the investigator).

Where possible, avoid patch testing an individual with active dermatitis. False negative reactions are probable if the patient is taking systemic corticosteroids. It is useful to patch test using all portions of a suspected plant, i.e. leaf, flower head, stalk, individual petals and pollen. Inevitably, there will be much routine screening of innocuous material. The Finn chambers® are now in general use in patch testing clinics. An oblong sliver of leaf or petal can be placed across the aluminium disc, adhering to the surrounding adhesive tape. If the plant material is bulky or possesses hairs or spines, it can be lightly bruised or mashed with a little water and applied to the test chamber to reduce mechanical irritancy. Known chemically irritant plants should be avoided if at all possible (Chapter 5). Bulbs in particular may cause irritant reactions and in general a leaf of the bulbous plant is preferable or, in the case of garlic, a prepared extract (see p. 219). In the case of woods, avoid testing sawdust 'as is' where possible; a 10% suspension in petrolatum is preferable and controls should be tested for irritancy. It has been shown that irritants in general may augment the response to contact allergens by a non-specific mechanism (McLelland *et al.* 1991) although the practical implications of this finding are not yet clear.

Remember that false negative reactions can occur. Different specimens of the same species may vary in the concentration of allergens and the concentrations can vary even in an individual plant depending on season, degree of watering and general health of the plant. Usually a mature specimen is more allergenic than an immature one, although the reverse may be true (e.g. asparagus).

Apparent cross-reactions may occur between botanically unrelated plants which contain similar or identical allergenic substances. The sesquiterpene lactones are classical examples occurring in members of the daisy family (Compositae), sweet bay (*Laurus nobilis*), some members of the magnolia family (Magnoliaceae) and some liverworts (*Frullania* species). True cross-sensitization also occurs, e.g. between the long-chain monophenol gingkolic acid in *Gingko biloba* and urushiols in *Toxicodendron* species.

If a positive patch test is obtained with plant material the allergens should be extracted for further testing. The techniques for extraction of oleoresins are discussed in Chapter 7.3. Before further patch testing it is important to test differing dilutions for irritancy in 10–20 control subjects. Remember that an inappropriately high concentration of an oleoresin may cause active sensitization.

Photopatch testing is rarely of value in investigation of allergic contact dermatitis due to plants. There is only one well-documented case of photocontact allergy to *Parthenium hysterophorus* in India (see p. 173). Repeated exposure to volatile plant allergens, notably sesquiterpene lactones, sometimes leads to a syndrome of 'persistent light reactivity', a form of non-specific photosensitivity. Some patch test reactions are enhanced by irradiation of the test site ('photo-aggravation') although this does not necessarily imply that there is a component of photosensitivity.

In the following account, the important species known or reputed to cause allergic reactions are described and in most cases illustrated. The plant families are named and listed in the order used by the Royal Botanical Gardens, Kew. Thus closely related families will be found close to each other in the text.

References

Cronin E. (1980) *Contact Dermatitis*. Churchill Livingstone, Edinburgh.
Dupuis G. & Benezra C. (1982) *Allergic Contact Dermatitis to Simple Chemicals: A Molecular Approach*. Marcel Dekker, New York.
Dvorak H.F., Mihm C.M.J. & Dvorak A.M. (1976) Morphology of delayed-type hypersensitivity reactions in man. *Journal of Investigative Dermatology* **67**: 391–401.
McLelland J., Shuster S. & Matthews J.N.S. (1991) 'Irritants' increase the response to an allergen in allergic contact dermatitis. *Archives of Dermatology* **127**: 1016–19.
Mitchell J.C. (1975) The angry back syndrome: eczema creates eczema. *Contact Dermatitis* **1**: 193–4.
Polak L. (1980) Immunological aspects of contact sensitivity. An experimental study. In *Monographs in Allergy*, Vol. 15. Karger, Basel.

7.3 Preparation of plant extracts

M.G. ROWAN

Allergic responses to plant materials are due to their chemical constituents, usually compounds of the type known as secondary metabolites. These are low or medium molecular weight organic compounds of diverse chemical types synthesized via a wide variety of biosynthetic pathways. These compounds, which in many cases have no known function in the plant, are sporadically distributed across the plant kingdom, though in many instances related plant species contain the same or similar secondary metabolites. Occasionally, botanically unrelated plants such as cultivated chrysanthemums and the liverwort genus *Frullania*, may contain structurally similar allergens. Conversely, chemical variation may exist within a single species, some varieties possessing a particular chemical and others not. Where the actual allergenic chemical is known the knowledge of its distribution in the plant kingdom allows prediction of possible cross-reactions in patients. Conversely, a knowledge of a patient's cross-reaction pattern may yield clues as to the chemical nature of the allergen.

The purpose of preparing solvent extracts of possible plant allergens for testing is to isolate chemically elicited responses from those due to physical features of the plant such as spines, hairs and raphides. A minority of plant allergens have been chemically characterized and for those detailed isolation procedures have been published. Some recent examples include the isolation of falcarinol, the allergen of ivy and related species (Hansen & Boll 1986), and of the β-glucosidic ester of taraxinic acid from dandelion (Hansel *et al.* 1980). However, these procedures in which the emphasis is to obtain sufficient pure compound for chemical characterization lie outside the scope of this chapter.

Where a specific type of antigen is suspected particular extraction methods may be appropriate. Thus Hausen (1977) recommends a very brief (60 sec) diethyl ether wash of whole, fresh plant material for the extraction of sesquiterpene lactones from Compositae. This method exploits the fact that the sesquiterpene lactones occur in glandular structures on the surface of the plant, and minimizes the co-extraction of other plant constituents such as pigments. An alternative method of extracting parthenolide uses water as the extraction solvent, exploiting the appreciable water solubility of this compound (Hausen 1991).

An extraction procedure for the unknown allergens present in the majority of allergenic plants clearly requires to be as general and flexible as possible and for comparative purposes it is desirable to prepare the same type of extract, even where the allergen is known. Such an approach was proposed by Shelmire as long ago as 1940. He used a 24 h diethyl ether extract of dried plant material to investigate the allergenic properties of a wide range of wild and cultivated plants in Texas (Shelmire 1940).

7.3.1 Possible sources of error

In attempting to devise a suitable general procedure a consideration of the chemical nature of known natural allergens is important. A selection of chemical types is illustrated below and ranges from non-polar hydrocarbons such as limonene through moderately polar quinones and lactones to polar polyphenols (**7.I**). Such a range requires an extraction technique of very wide applicability and a few compounds may defeat even the most general methods. Such limitations must be borne in mind when interpreting patch test results using plant extracts. When in doubt different approaches to extraction should be tried.

Failure of the extraction process may lead to false negative results but, in addition, precautions must be taken to avoid false positives. Reagent grade solvents are frequently contaminated with various ma-

Limonene (citrus species)
α-methylene-γ-butyrolactone (tulip)
Primin (primula obconica)
Coronopilin (various compositae)
β-glucosyl taraxinate (dandelion)
Falcarinol (ivy)
Usnic acid (lichens)
Urushiols ('poison ivy')

7.1

terials such as plasticizers from plastic tubing, paint and grease from joints and taps. Extraction techniques involve the maceration of plant material with relatively large volumes of solvent, followed by removal of the solvent from the extract by distillation under reduced pressure. This inevitably results in the concentration of the contaminants in the extract. Clearly, such contaminants may themselves be allergenic or irritant and may interfere with the tests. In our laboratories, solvents are routinely re-distilled prior to phytochemical work but this requires specialized facilities. An alternative approach might be to use the purer high pressure liquid chromatography (HPLC) grade solvents and prepare suitable solvent controls for patch testing.

A further problem arises with diethyl ether and chloroform. Both these solvents are slightly unstable on storage, yielding peroxides and phosgene respectively. Peroxides in ether are an explosion hazard, and are also likely to react with unsaturated groups in the extractives. This may generate allergenic or irritant compounds from innocuous plant constituents. Before use, and especially before re-distillation, diethyl ether should be shaken with ferrous sulphate to remove peroxides.

Phosgene reacts with hydroxy groups and again may either generate or destroy allergens. Chloroform is supplied with added stabilizer to prevent phosgene build up but this will be removed if the solvent is re-distilled. Thus re-distilled chloroform should have about 2% ethanol added.

7.3.2 Preparation of plant material

At all stages in the collection and handling of the plant material it is important to avoid cross-contamination with other species. Samples collected in bulk for the preparation of standards should be rigorously cleaned of stray weeds whilst patients should be advised to collect, or ask their relatives to collect, suspect specimens from their own environment in separate bags.

Dried plant material is usually preferred for extraction. It is usually sufficient to air-dry the material for about 2 weeks, turning frequently to avoid the development of mould. If necessary the material may be dried more rapidly in an oven at about 60°C. Many secondary metabolites are quite stable under the conditions of drying and even volatile constituents such as terpenes may well be retained if the specialized glands and structures which contain them are not damaged. During slow drying many plant enzymes remain active and, for instance, many glycosides may be hydrolysed. This is not necessarily a disadvantage since, for example, the tulip allergen α-methylene-γ-butyrolactone occurs in the living plant as the weakly allergenic tuliposide A.

7.3.3 Extraction procedure

A general extraction procedure which we have used to prepare a series of standard suspensions in soft paraffin for patch testing is outlined below (Lovell & Rowan 1991). It is important to note that most of the organic solvents used in plant extraction are flammable and toxic. They are subject to the Control of Substances Hazardous to Health (COSHH) regulations and appropriate advice must be sought before embarking on extractions.

Coarsely powdered plant material is macerated with a sufficient volume of a mixture of chloroform and methanol (3:1) to form a mobile suspension and allowed to stand at room temperature overnight. The mixture is filtered and the residue extracted with a further batch of chloroform:methanol (3:1). The two filtrates are combined, then evaporated to dryness by distillation under reduced pressure at a temperature not exceeding 40°C. At this point the extractive is weighed and resuspended in a known volume of diethyl ether to give a reasonably homogeneous, pipettable suspension. Yellow soft paraffin (100 g) is melted at 65°C in a fume cupboard and a volume of the ether suspension equivalent to 1 g of plant extract is added dropwise with vigorous stirring. At this temperature the diethyl ether is rapidly evaporated to yield a fairly homogeneous 1% suspension of the plant extract in the paraffin. This suspension is poured into small screw-topped vials and cooled rapidly under a stream of water to maintain homogeneity. This method is particularly suitable for involatile compounds of moderate polarity such as the sesquiterpene lactones. For more polar compounds the method may be modified to use pure methanol for extraction or pure methanol followed by the normal chloroform : methanol mixture. Volatile compounds such as terpenes may be lost, at least in part, during the removal of the chloroform : methanol. If such compounds are suspected of being the allergenic constituents, the plant material may be extracted with dichloromethane and this extract added directly to the melted soft paraffin. The volatile dichloromethane evaporates whilst the non-polar terpenes dissolve in the soft paraffin. However, with this method it is less easy to control the content of extract in the soft paraffin mixture. Alternatively, volatile components may be isolated independently of other constituents by steam distillation, and the oil blended directly with the soft paraffin without the need to use a solvent.

When extracts are being prepared for use as part of a battery of standards for patch testing it is desirable to start with a relatively large amount of plant material to enable the use of a single standard over a long period of time. Dried plant material may be stored in the dark for a considerable period of time with relatively little loss of secondary metabolites. Alternatively the extractives may be stored in the dry state in an atmosphere of nitrogen at $-20°C$, and made up in yellow soft paraffin as required.

References

Hansel R., Kartarahardja M., Huang J.-T. & Bohlmann F. (1980) Sesquiterpenlacton--D-glucopyranoside sowie ein neues Eudesmanolid aus *Taraxacum officinale*. *Phytochemistry* **19**: 857–61.

Hansen L. & Boll P.M. (1986) Polyacetylenic falcarinol as the major allergen in *Schefflera arboricola*. *Phytochemistry* **25**: 529–30.

Hausen B.M. (1977) A simple method of extracting crude sesquiterpene lactones from Compositae plants for skin tests, chemical investigations and sensitising experiments in guinea pigs. *Contact Dermatitis* **3**: 58–60.

Hausen B.M. (1991) A simple method of isolating parthenolides from *Tanacetum* and other sensitising plants. *Contact Dermatitis* **24**: 153–5.

Lovell C.R. & Rowan M.G. (1991) Dandelion dermatitis. *Contact Dermatitis* **25**: 185–8.

Shelmire B. (1940) Contact dermatitis from vegetation. *Southern Medical Journal* **33**: 337–46.

7.4 Poison ivy and poison oak dermatitis

C. DANNAKER & H.I. MAIBACH

In this chapter we outline the physical and chemical characteristics of poison ivy and poison oak plants, as well as of related members of the plant family Anacardiaceae. The biological and physical findings resulting from allergic reactions to this plant are reviewed. Finally, we discuss measures to prevent allergic dermatitis, including personal protective measures, immunization, and chemical destruction of the plant.

No plant rivals the *Rhus* (*Toxicodendron*) genus in terms of the amount of disease produced. In North America, poison ivy and poison oak dermatitis are the most common causes of allergic skin reactions. In the USA 50% or more of the population may be allergic to these plants (Kligman 1958a). Millions of Americans annually suffer from poison oak or ivy dermatitis. Poison ivy and oak dermatitis knows no racial, age or sexual prejudices. Patch tests of recent emigrees to the USA from the Orient and South America gave positive results in many (Epstein 1984a). Sensitization of newborn infants to this plant family has been reported (Fisher 1986).

Allergic contact dermatitis to poison oak and ivy is a major cause of occupational disability amongst outdoor workers, especially in the western USA. Between 3000 and 5000 cases of poison oak dermatitis related to occupational exposure are reported annually in California and account for about 8% of the reported occupational diseases in the state (Occupational Disease in California 1983, San Francisco, California Dept of Industrial Relations, Division of Labor Statistics and Research, September 1985).

The plant family Anacardiaceae

The Anacardiaceae family includes the genus *Toxicodendron* (poison ivy, poison oak and poison sumac). There are many related cross-reacting species (mango, cashew, Japanese lacquer, Indian marking nut

Table 7.4.1 The Anacardiaceae family and cross-reacting plants.

Genus *Toxicodendron*	Related and cross-reacting cultivars
	African poison ivy — *Smodingium argutum*
Poison ivy	
T. radicans	Cashew — *Anacardium occidentale*
T. rydbergii	Ginkgo — *Ginkgo biloba*
	Grevillea, e.g. *G. robusta* Cunn
Poison oak	
T. diversilobum	Indian marking nut — *Semecarpus anacardium*
T. toxicarium	Japanese lacquer — *Rhus verniciflua*
Poison sumac	
T. vernix	Mango — *Mangifera indica*

and African poison ivy) (Table 7.4.1). Several unrelated genera such as *Ginkgo* and *Grevillea* all cross-react with *Toxicodendron* spp.

The taxonomy of poison oak and ivy is confusing. Some have recommended classifying *Rhus* as the genus, *Toxicodendron* as a subgenus. Most botanists consider the term 'Rhus' a misnomer and classify poison ivy as *Toxicodendron radicans* and poison oak as *Toxicodendron diversilobum*.

Confusion over classification of these weeds is due not to the misguided writings of humans but to the variable appearance of the genus (Kligman 1958a). American Boy Scouts learn the adage, 'leaves three, leave it be'. Although it is correct that in spring poison ivy and

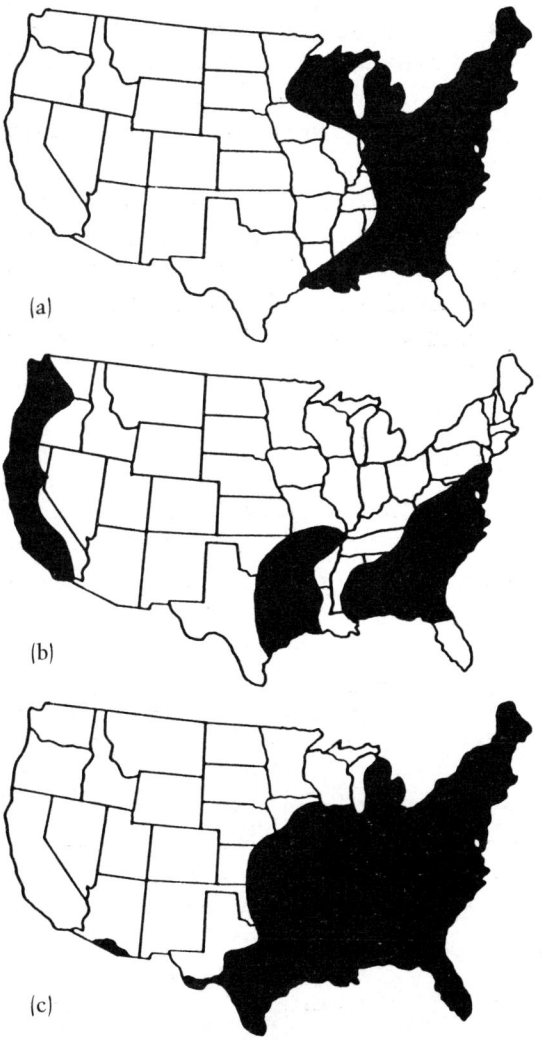

Fig. 7.4.1 Distribution of *Toxicodendron* species in USA; (a) poison ivy, (b) western and eastern poison oak, (c) poison sumac.

oak leaves appear in groups of three, clusters of five or more leaves can occur. The best defence against poison ivy and oak contact is to recognize the appearance of the plant in one's region (Epstein 1987). The distribution of *Toxicodendron* spp. in the USA is shown in Fig. 7.4.1.

7.4.1 Distribution and morphology

Poison oak and ivy typically grow along roads, hiking trails, or streams. When the plant structure is damaged such as by high winds or animal travel, the allergen responsible for allergic contact dermatitis may collect on the surface as a black sticky sap. This allergen is urushiol and is found within the stems, delicate canals and roots of the plant.

In spring and summer these plants form green ivy or oak-shaped leaves (Figs 7.4.2, 7.4.3). The leaves of poison ivy range from 3 cm to 15 cm long. Poison oak leaves are much shorter (3–7 cm). Poison ivy

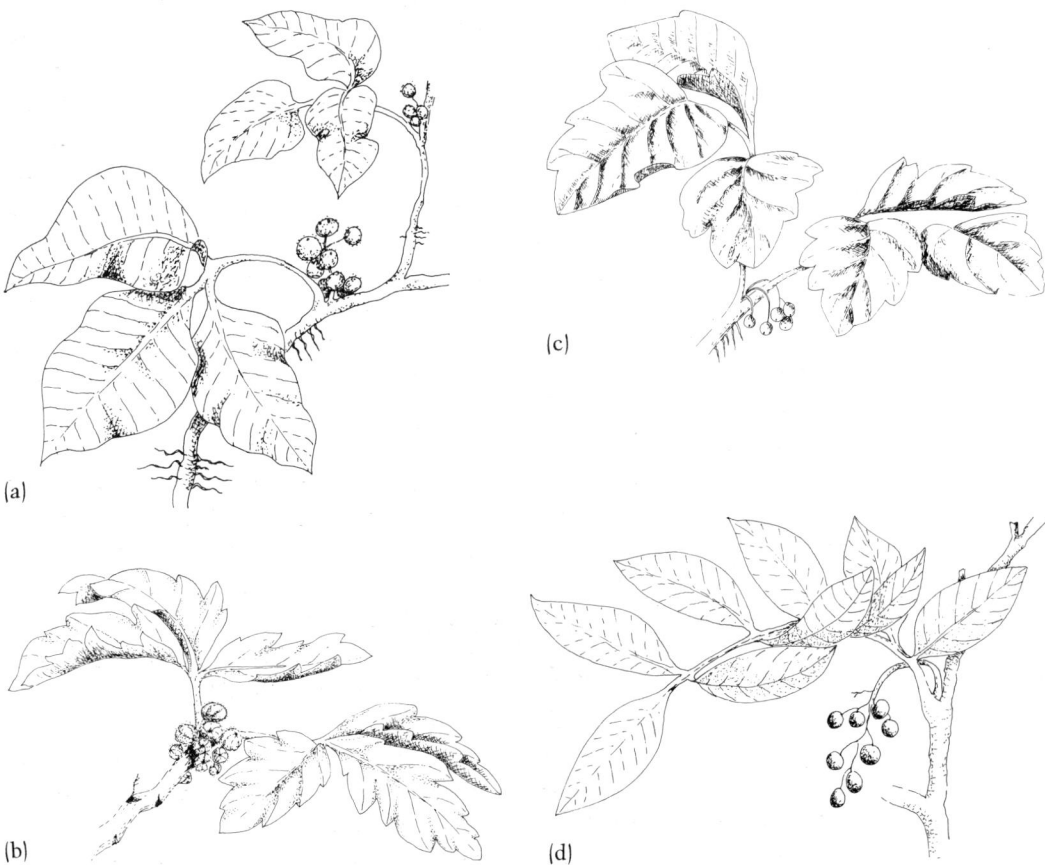

Fig. 7.4.2 Typical leaves of (a) poison ivy, (b) western poison oak, (c) eastern poison oak, (d) poison sumac.

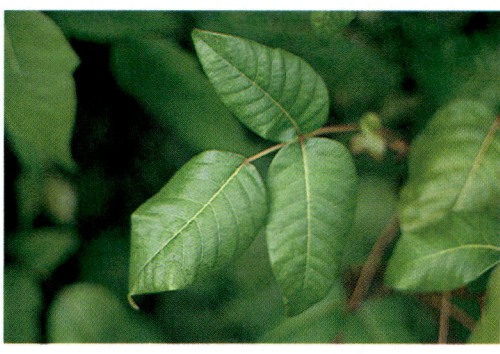

Fig. 7.4.3 *Toxicodendron radicans* (poison ivy) showing three-lobed leaves.

is scrambling and partial to climbing, whereas poison oak is more shrub-like, usually only 1–3 m high. Both may ascend trees but poison ivy is the more likely to climb to heights up to 40 m. It often clings to trees, telephone poles or houses. Poison oak usually remains as a small plant or it may form a bush or small tree.

These plants bloom with attractive white, waxy flowers followed by green berries that turn white in fall. In the fall the leaves turn attractive shades of red, yellow, violet or orange. Depending on water supply the plant may turn colour as early as spring. Novice hikers may unwittingly collect these poisonous leaves to adorn their homes. In winter the plant appears as dead vines. If these dry parts are burned, an airborne dermatitis can result due to retained allergen in the plant canals. Poison oak (*Toxicodendron diversilobum*) is native to the west coast of North America and grows at the edge of streams, thickets and wooded slopes. Poison ivy (*T. radicans*) is found in the eastern USA growing in rocky canyons and on wooded slopes. An eastern variety of poison oak exists (*T. toxicarium*) as well as poison ivy occurring in the midwestern USA (*T. rydbergii*).

Poison oak and ivy probably developed first in northern America. Oriental plants with cross-reacting sap allergens may be descendent relatives spread via a northern land bridge (Gillis 1975). Poison ivy, oak and sumac are indigenous to the USA, southern Canada and northern Mexico. Poison oak grows in the western USA and poison ivy in the east. In Texas, the two may intermingle and mixed cultivars have been observed (Epstein 1990). Poison sumac (*T. vernix*) grows in the southeastern USA. Swampy areas are its preferred habitat and it is prevalent in Florida.

Poison oak and ivy have been introduced to Europe and Japan. Due to their small numbers they are rarely a cause of allergic dermatitis. This weed has been used in Europe as an ornamental flower or a vine to strengthen dikes in the Netherlands and is found growing naturalized in France and Germany (Ippen 1983). Poison ivy dermatitis has been observed in the Japanese population (Epstein 1987).

Less is known concerning poison sumac (*T. vernix*). This plant grows as a shrub or small tree in swamps or peat bogs in the eastern USA. Exposure to this plant is much less common than to poison oak or ivy due to the isolated areas it inhabits. Fruit grows between the leaf and branch in poison sumac which enables distinction of this plant from benign sumac (*Rhus typhina*) where the fruit grows from the ends of branches (Fig. 7.4.2). Although it contains allergenic urushiols, these have not been as well characterized as in poison ivy and oak. The leaves are smooth-edged, oval and about 10 cm long. They number from seven to 13 per stem, usually in odd numbers. The leaves often angle up from the stem like rabbit ears.

Of greater importance to travellers allergic to poison ivy and oak are the shrubs, trees and other plants which contain chemicals that cross-react with the poison oak and ivy allergen, urushiol. These cross-reacting plants may be found in Central and South America, Japan, and South-East Asia.

7.4.2 Allergenicity

Contained in the oil of most members of the Anacardiaceae family is a substance called urushiol which is derived from the Japanese word for sap, kiurushi. Urushiol contains a mixture of pentadecylcatechols (PDCs). The base molecule of PDC has a completely saturated side chain at position 3 (**7.II**). Unsaturation of the side chain leads to

7.II Pentadecylcatechol skeleton.

greater allergenicity. Saturation of the carbon side chain as well as substitution of the catechol ring results in reduced allergenicity. This PDC, due to its complete side-chain saturation, is the least reactive urushiol. The location of the side chain at position 3 on the catechol ring increases antigenicity, whereas substitution at position 6 induces immunological tolerance (Baer *et al.* 1977).

Members of the Anacardiaceae family contain pyrocatechols with mixtures of C15 and C17 side chains containing one, two, three or no double bonds. For example, poison ivy contains mainly C15 side chains (3-*N*-pentadecylcatechols), poison oak the C17 (3-*N*-heptadecylcatechols), and poison sumac, C13. Other relatives belonging to the Anacardiaceae family contain similar chemicals which may cross-react with poison ivy/oak urushiol. Kligman (1958b) showed that ingestion of cashew nut shell oil (cardol and anacardic acids) may desensitize individuals allergic to poison ivy. Cardol is a resorcinol with a side chain similar to poison oak and ivy urushiol (5-pentadecadienylresorcinol). Dermatitis has been reported in poison ivy-sensitive individuals from ingestion of improperly shelled cashews contaminated with cashew oil (Marks et al. 1984).

The mechanism by which urushiol elicits allergic contact dermatitis probably begins with covalent binding of the PDCs to skin protein. In the presence of tissue oxygen with or without enzymes, a reactive quinone is created (Epstein 1990). Region specific nucleophilic attack takes place at the ring sites 4, 5 and 6 (Epstein 1987). Knowledge of the manner in which the reactive quinone is metabolized is helpful when attempting to design a good tolerogen. For example, epicutaneous application of the PDC analogue, 5-methyl-3-n-pentadecylcatechol in guinea pigs resulted in specific immune tolerance to poison ivy (Stampf et al. 1986). This was due to the methyl group located at the 5 position blocking nucleophilic attack which would have led to induction of effector cells and allergic contact dermatitis.

7.4.3 Cross-reacting plants

Urushiol-containing and cross-reacting plants may be found worldwide. They probably represent a common cause of dermatitis in urushiol-sensitive individuals which may be difficult to recognize.

Mango (*Mangifera indica* L.)

The mango is a delicious fruit found in eastern Asia, Burma and regions of India. It has been widely cultivated throughout the world, in particularly Hawaii, Florida, Mexico and Central America.

The mango tree is large, 15–30 m high, and bears a speckled or streaked greenish to yellow-red ovoid fruit. The leaves, stems and skin of the fruit contain urushiol and other long-chain phenols such as cardol which is chemically similar to urushiol (Fisher 1977). Other allergens such as B-pinene and limonene are also present (Benezra et al. 1985).

Allergic contact dermatitis occurs from eating the fruit with the peel intact. So-called mango poisoning may result in a vesicular eruption which is either confined to the lips and face or may be generalized. Climbing a mango tree can result in allergic dermatitis due to the content of urushiol in the leaves and bark of the tree. Symptoms of wheezing have also been reported, presumably due to immediate type hypersensitivity (Kahn 1942). The fruit needs simply to be peeled prior to eating to avoid contact with urushiol.

Cashew nut tree (*Anacardium occidentale* L.)

This small tree is native to the tropical Americas but is harvested now in most tropical countries. The cashew nut shell but not the kernel contains a brown oily juice. This juice possesses the contact allergen. Roasting the shell of the nut liberates irritating vapours. Modified cashew nut oil has industrial uses such as in ink, adhesives and resin manufacture.

Dermatitis has resulted from sensitized children handling and playing with the nuts (Orris 1958). Improperly shelled cashew nuts caused an outbreak of perioral and more generalized dermatitis in Pennsylvania (Marks *et al.* 1984). In India, cashew nut dermatitis may affect thousands of workers (Behl & Captain 1979). Roasting the nut shell must be complete for the allergen to be inactivated (Ratner & Spencer 1974). The allergens found in the cashew shell include cardanol, cardol and anacardic acid which are a monophenol, diphenol (resorcinol) and salicylic acid, respectively (Benezra *et al.* 1985).

Japanese lacquer tree (*Toxicodendron verniciflua* Stokes)

This tree is indigenous to Japan and China (Fig. 7.4.4). From its bark is derived a thick viscous sap used for varnishing furniture, floors, tea pots, rifle stocks, canes, wooden toilet seats and ornaments. Once applied, the lacquer may retain its allergenicity for hundreds and perhaps thousands of years (Toyama 1918).

The Japanese lacquer tree contains urushiols which differ from poison ivy by the positions of the double bonds on the 15-carbon side chain at positions 8, 11 and 13 instead of 8, 11 and 14 positions in poison ivy. Patients allergic to poison ivy usually cross-react to Japanese lacquer tree urushiol (Fig. 7.4.5) (Howell 1959).

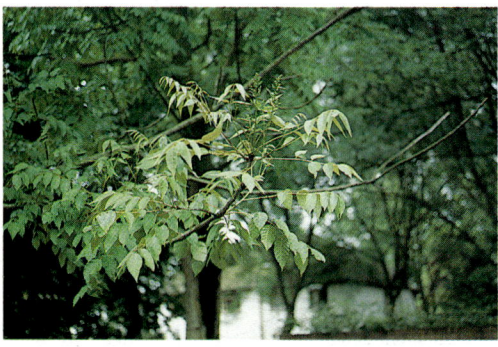

Fig. 7.4.4 Japanese lacquer tree planted in Oxfordshire. (Courtesy of Dr S. Powell.)

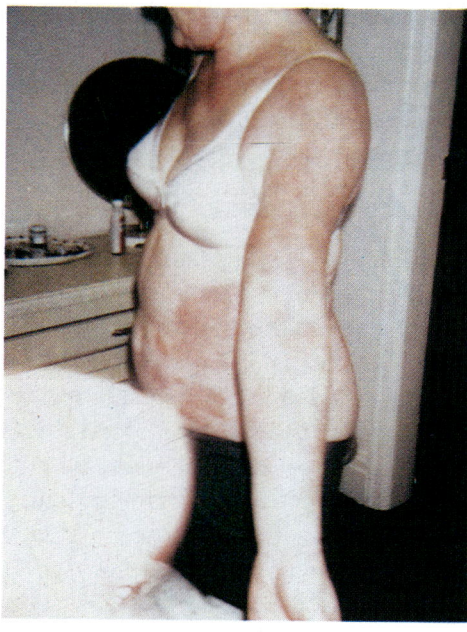

Fig. 7.4.5 Widespread dermatitis from Japanese lacquer tree. A patch test with material from the tree was positive. (Courtesy of Dr S. Powell.)

Marking nut tree (Bhilawa) (*Semecarpus anacardium* L.)

This tree bears a nut and is indigenous to India. The black juice of this nut is used to mark laundry in India and Malaya. Indian laundry workers called dhobies develop 'dhobie mark dermatitis' from the oil of this nut. Dhobie mark dermatitis affected English officers and servicemen stationed in India during World War II and who wore marked garments (Livinghood *et al.* 1943).

The marking nut liquid contains a pentadecylcatechol which is capable of cross-reacting with poison ivy/oak urushiol (Howell 1959).

Rengas tree (*Semecarpus* sp.)

The wood from the Rengas tree found in Malaysia is used for furniture and contains a sap which may cross-react with poison ivy (Epstein 1990).

African poison ivy (*Smodingium argutum* E. Mey)

This native of South Africa grows as both a shrub and a small tree. Allergic dermatitis is said to occur frequently. Contact has taken place from plants growing in South African gardens or school yards. Clinically, this dermatitis closely resembles its North American counterpart. It affects the uncovered parts with a streaky vesicular dermatitis corresponding to points of contact with the venomous leaves.

The leaves of this plant are thin and deeply notched. Like the American variety, the leaves are often trifoliate.

The sap of this plant is chemically similar to poison ivy (*Toxicodendron radicans* L.) (Findlay *et al.* 1974).

Miscellaneous cross-reacting plants

The ginkgo tree (*Ginkgo biloba* L.) (see pp. 233–4) is a member of the Ginkgoaceae family and contains the allergen ginkgolic acid. Ginkgolic acid contains a C15 side chain which chemically resembles poison ivy and oak urushiols. Stomatitis and proctitis have resulted from eating ginkgo fruit. This fruit should be considered inedible.

Grevillea, a member of the Proteaceae family, contains a resorcinol. This plant is indigenous to east Australia. A cultivar of *Grevillea*, Robyn Gordon, has been reported to cross-react with poison ivy urushiol (Menz *et al.* 1986).

The Brazilian pepper tree (*Schinus terebinthifolius*), which is also known as Florida holly, is a relative of the Ginkgo tree and a potential cause of allergic dermatitis (Morton 1978).

7.4.3 Clinical features

Poison ivy and oak contain the potent allergen urushiol. Some sensitized individuals may react within hours of exposure with an extremely pruritic, vesicular dermatitis. The majority of sensitive individuals react within 2–4 days of exposure. The first sensitizing dose, however, may not result in dermatitis for up to 3 weeks following exposure. Exposure may occur not only to the plant itself but to contaminated fomites such as pets, shoes, clothing, automobile tyres being changed, golf balls, etc. (Goldstein 1968).

An intense, oedematous and vesicular dermatitis is typical (Fig. 7.4.6). Streaks of vesicles corresponding to points of plant leaf contact help to suggest poison ivy/oak as the provoking agent. If the resin is

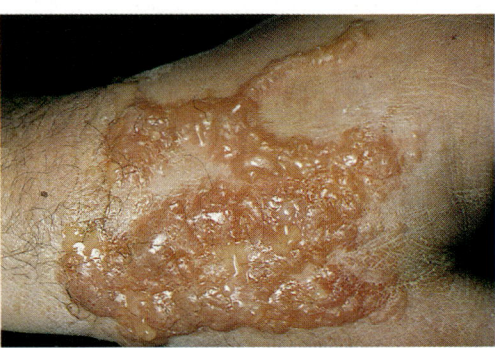

Fig. 7.4.6 Linear bullous lesions caused by poison ivy.

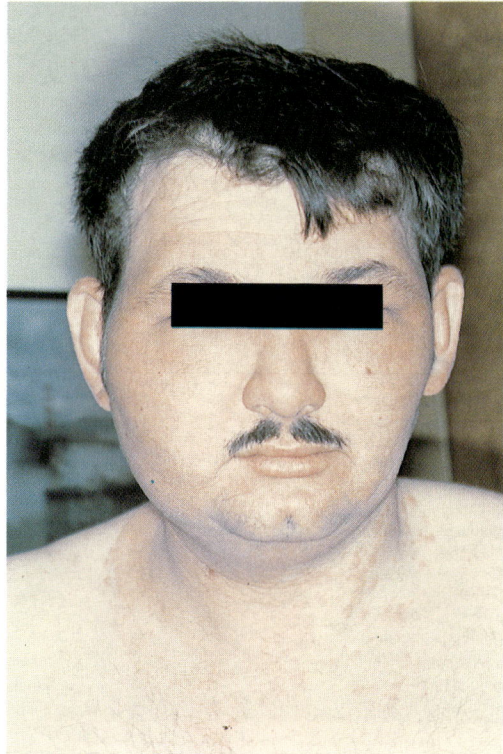

Fig. 7.4.7 Oedematous dermatitis of head and neck caused by poison oak. (Courtesy of Dr C. Dannaker.)

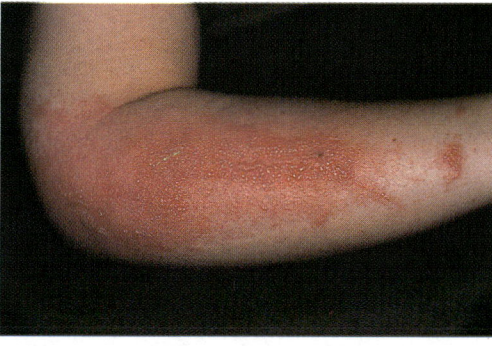

Fig. 7.4.8 Linear vesicular lesions from poison oak. (Courtesy of Dr J. Reeves.)

allowed to remain on the skin for a prolonged period or if exposure is extensive, confluent vesicles and bullae often result. If washing the resin off the skin is to be effective, this must occur within a few minutes of contact (Marks 1989).

The face and arms are often affected (Figs 7.4.7, 7.4.8). Secondary spread to the genitals is common (Fig. 7.4.9). Specks of black, oxidized urushiol may occur on contaminated clothing or skin. An airborne contact dermatitis may result from burning contaminated wood or brush.

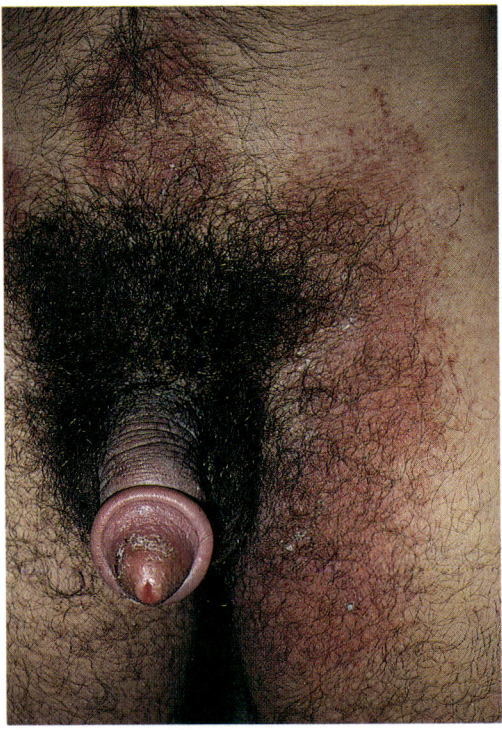

Fig. 7.4.9 Allergic dermatitis affecting the groin, caused by poison oak. (Courtesy of Dr J. Reeves.)

The vesicles cannot spread the allergic dermatitis but may become secondarily infected. The magnitude of exposure and the individual's immunological function may determine how soon following exposure dermatitis will develop. Thus, the impression that the dermatitis is spreading may occur as new lesions continue to develop in less heavily exposed areas, days after the initial outbreak of poison ivy/oak dermatitis. Intense pruritus is characteristic.

Untreated, the dermatitis usually lasts approximately 3 weeks, but in some instances may be protracted. Significant suffering from pruritus and eroded skin occurs. In dark-skinned individuals, severe blistering may result in permanent pigmentary post-inflammatory changes. Occasionally, urticaria, erythema multiforme and renal disease have followed allergic reactions to poison oak or ivy (Rytand *et al.* 1948, Devich *et al.* 1975, Pfaff 1987). Some authors consider much of the evidence for immune complex disease related to poison oak/ivy dermatitis to be circumstantial and suspect (Epstein 1984b).

7.4.4 Treatment and prevention

Removing urushiol resin as soon after exposure as possible is important. Waiting longer than 10 min will almost certainly result in elicitation of dermatitis in sensitized individuals. Bathing later than this may still help remove residual resin from the skin. Unfortunately, few quantified data are available on decontamination of skin and clothing. Contaminated clothing, camping gear, tools or pets must be washed with a mild detergent and water. Organic solvents such as isopropyl alcohol have also been used for cleansing skin or fomites.

Treatment of mild or localized dermatitis can include aluminium acetate compresses 1:40 (Domeboro) three to four times daily for 30 min and a strong topical corticosteroid cream such as fluocinonide or clobetasol propionate. Delicate areas such as the face and genitals must be treated with milder topical corticosteroids. Systemic antihistamines are often necessary to control severe itching.

When the allergic reaction is robust and medical contraindications do not exist, oral corticosteroids are the treatment of choice. Oral prednisone is usually started in a dose of 40–80 mg daily. Care should be taken not to discontinue treatment prematurely. Usually oral corticosteroids should be continued 10–14 or more days to avoid rebound of dermatitis. Intramuscular triamcinolone acetonide 40 mg will usually last for 3 weeks. Adrenal function returns to normal in 30–40 days. Usually, one injection is adequate to suppress a moderately severe bout of poison oak/ivy dermatitis.

7.4.5 Eradication

Physical means of plant destruction are inefficient and appropriate only for removal of a limited number of plants. Grubbing poison ivy/oak roots in early spring and late fall is often effective if the soil is moistened and the roots completely removed. Poison ivy can be pulled from tree trunks and the base of the root severed. Roots and stems should be buried and not burned. Smoke from their incineration is capable of causing allergic dermatitis in sensitized individuals. After 1 year of growth, seedling plants have an established root system and are resistant to destruction by ploughing (Crooks & Kligman 1976).

Poison oak/ivy remains quite resistant to destruction by herbicides once root growth is well established. Aminotriazole mixed with a triazine-type herbicide is effective against this weed when root growth is limited (Adams 1988). In the USA these pesticides are approved for non-food crops only. Other pesticides such as 2,4-dichlorophenoxyacetic acid, ammonium sulphamate and glyphosate are herbicides which have been used to eradicate poison ivy/oak. Often the roots are not destroyed by these herbicides and regrowth takes place the following season.

7.4.6 Barriers

Protective clothing is helpful in preventing skin contact with poison oak/ivy urushiol but care must be taken when removing contaminated apparel. Laundering is effective in removing urushiol from most clothing (Fisher 1977). Various clothing materials offer some ability to bind to urushiol. Unfortunately, Kevlar, a clothing material favoured by forestry workers, binds poorly to urushiol (Waali 1984).

Preventive creams claimed to prevent skin penetration of the poison ivy/oak allergen have been recommended. Most of these barrier creams have been found to be ineffective. They include sodium perborate, cottonseed oil, tyrosinase and chloroamide (Von Adelung 1913, Sizer & Prokesch 1945, Sulzberger et al. 1946, Waali 1984).

Several barrier preparations have shown promise in temporarily preventing percutaneous penetration of poison ivy/oak allergens. The polyamine salts of a linoleic acid dimer were shown to be 70% effective in preventing patch test reactions in sensitized patients to urushiol (Orchard et al. 1986). An organoclay compound (Ivy Block) may also prevent penetration by binding to urushiol (Epstein 1990). Stokoguard Outdoor Cream* successfully prevented poison ivy/oak dermatitis in a majority of sensitized patients in double-blind placebo-controlled testing when washed off within 8 h of urushiol exposure (Fisher 1990).

7.4.7   Hyposensitization

The feasibility of hyposensitization to urushiol has been reviewed in detail by Epstein (1984b). Although it is claimed the American Indians were able to hyposensitize themselves by chewing the leaves of *Toxicodendron* spp. a commercially effective preparation without significant side-effects has yet to be identified. The side-effects of pruritus ani, generalized eczematous eruptions, urticaria and vesicular rashes limit the usefulness of hyposensitization with purified urushiol (Epstein et al. 1982). Whether hyposensitization may result in immune complex nephritis is uncertain. Older reports of nephritis following hyposensitization have been reviewed and were felt to be inconclusive (Epstein 1984b). Although diacetylated urushiol produced tolerance and desensitization in guinea pigs (Watson et al. 1981), efficacy was found to be lacking in human trials (Marks et al. 1987). The search continues for analogues of urushiol which minimize side-effects and are capable of producing clinically relevant hyposensitization.

If a patient is willing to attempt desensitization therapy it should be realized that between 2 and 4 months of treatment are necessary to achieve desensitization and that maintenance therapy will be necessary† (Epstein 1990). Epstein's seminal work (1984b) concerning this subject

---

* Stokoguard Outdoor Cream available from Stockhausen — Skin Protection Division, PO Box 16025, Greensboro, North Carolina 27416, USA.
† Hollister-Stier, a division of Miles Inc., North 3525 Regal Spokane, Washington 99207 markets a poison ivy/oak hyposensitization kit.

should be reviewed before attempting this procedure. Very low concentrations of urushiol with a slow increase in dose over months are necessary to avoid severe side-effects. Due to widely varying sensitivity, a routine starting dose cannot be recommended. If successful, this method will result in *hypo*sensitization, not *de*sensitization to urushiol. Allergic skin reactions will tend to be less severe and resolve more quickly (Epstein 1984b). Immunization of unsensitized mentally disabled children with intramuscular purified urushiol resulted in partial tolerance to urushiol for up to 6 years (Epstein *et al.* 1981).

Firefighters usually suffer more bouts of poison ivy/oak dermatitis early in the season. Later, when poison ivy/oak contact is greater due to more extensive fires, outbreaks of allergic dermatitis appear to be reduced. This may represent a form of 'hardening' (Epstein 1990).

An effective and safe form of immunotherapy for prevention of poison ivy/oak dermatitis remains to be elucidated.

References

Adams R.M. (1988) Dermatitis caused by poison ivy and its relatives. *Current Concepts in Skin Disorders* **9**: 5–9.
Baer H., Hooton M.L., Dawson C.R. & Lerner D.I. (1977) The induction of immune tolerance in delayed contact sensitivity by the use of chemically related substances of low immunogenicity. *Journal of Investigative Dermatology* **69**: 215–18.
Behl P.N. & Captain R.M. (1979) *Skin-Irritant and Sensitizing Plants Found in India.* S. Chand, Ram Naga, New Delhi, pp. 28–29.
Benezra C., Ducombs G., Sell Y. & Foussereau J. (1985) *Plant Contact Dermatitis.* B.C. Decker, Philadelphia.
Crooks D.M. & Kligman D.L. (1976) *Poison Ivy, Poison Oak and Poison Sumac.* Farmers' Bulletin No. 1972. US Dept Agriculture, Government Printing Office, Washington DC.
Devich K.B., Lee J.C., Epstein W.L. *et al.* (1975) Renal lesions accompanying poison oak dermatitis. *Clinical Nephrology* **3**: 106–13.
Epstein W.L. (1984a) What factors determine unresponsiveness to poison oak/ivy? In Epstein E.E. (ed.) *Controversies in Dermatology.* WB Saunders, Philadelphia, pp. 424–7.
Epstein W.L. (1984b) Allergic contact dermatitis to poison oak and ivy. Feasibility of hyposensitization. *Dermatologic Clinics* **2**: 613–17.
Epstein W.L. (1987) The poison ivy picker of Pennypack Park: the continuing saga of poison ivy. *Journal of Investigative Dermatology* **88**: 7s–11s.
Epstein W.L. (1990) Poison oak and poison ivy dermatitis. In *Occupational Skin Disease*, 2nd edn. W.B. Saunders, Philadelphia.
Epstein W.L., Byers V.S. & Baer H. (1981) Induction of persistent tolerance to urushiol in humans. *Journal of Allergy and Clinical Immunology* **68**: 20–5.
Epstein W.L., Byers V.S. & Frankart W. (1982) Induction of antigen-specific hyposensitization to poison oak in sensitized adults. *Archives of Dermatology* **118**: 630–3.
Findlay G.H., Whiting D.A., Eggers S.H. & Ellis R.P. (1974) Smodingium (African 'poison ivy') dermatitis. *British Journal of Dermatology* **90**: 535–41.
Fisher A.A. (1977) The notorious poison ivy family of Anacardiaceae plants. *Cutis* **20**: 570.
Fisher A.A. (ed.) (1986) Poison sumac (Anacardiaceae) *Rhus* family. *Contact Dermatitis*, 3rd edn. Lea & Febiger, Philadelphia, pp. 405–17.

Fisher A.A. (1990) Efficiency of topical barrier creams in prevention of poison ivy dermatitis. *American Journal of Contact Dermatitis* **1**: 208.

Gillis W.T. (1975) Poison ivy and its kin. *Arnoldia* **35**: 93–123.

Goldstein N. (1968) The ubiquitous urushiols: contact dermatitis from mango, poison ivy, and other 'poison' plants. *Cutis* **4**: 679–85.

Howell J.B. (1959) Cross-sensitization in diverse poisonous members of the sumac family (Anacardiaceae). *Journal of Investigative Dermatology* **32**: 21–5.

Ippen H. (1983) Contact allergy to Anacardiaceae. A review and case reports of poison ivy allergy in central Europe. *Dermatosen in Beruf und Umwelt* **31**: 140–8.

Kahn I.S. (1942) Fruit sensitivity. *Southern Medical Journal* **35**: 858–9.

Kligman A. (1958a) Poison ivy (rhus) dermatitis. *Archives of Dermatology* **77**: 149–80.

Kligman A.M. (1958b) Cashew nut shell oil for hyposensitization against rhus dermatitis. *Archives of Dermatology* **78**: 359–63.

Livinghood C.S., Rogers A.M. & Fitz-Hugh T. (1943) Dhobie mark dermatitis. *JAMA* **123**: 23–6.

Marks J.G. (1989) Poison ivy and poison oak allergic contact dermatitis. In Maibach H.I. (ed.) *Immunology and Allergy Clinics of North America*. WB Saunders, Philadelphia, pp. 497–506.

Marks J.G., Demelfi T., McCarthy M.A. et al. (1984) Dermatitis from cashew nuts. *Journal of the American Academy of Dermatology* **10**: 627–31.

Marks J.G., Trautlein J.J., Epstein W.L. et al. (1987) Oral hyposensitization to poison ivy and poison oak. *Archives of Dermatology* **123**: 476–8.

Menz J., Rossi E.R., Taylor W.C. & Wall L. (1986) Contact dermatitis from *Grevillea* 'Robyn Gordon'. *Contact Dermatitis* **15**: 126–31.

Morton J.F. (1978) Brazilian pepper – its impact on people, animals and the environment. *Economic Botany* **32**: 353–9.

Orchard S.M., Fellman J.H. & Storrs F.J. (1986) Poison ivy/oak dermatitis. Use of linoleic acid dimer for topical prophylaxis. *Archives of Dermatology* **122**: 783–9.

Orris L. (1958) Cashew nut dermatitis. *New York Journal of Medicine* **58**: 2799–800.

Pfaff F. (1987) On the active principle of rhus toxicodendron and rhus venenata. *Journal of Experimental Medicine* **2**: 181–95.

Ratner J.H. & Spencer S.K. (1974) Cashew nut dermatitis: an example of internal-external contact-type hypersensitivity. *Archives of Dermatology* **1110**: 921–6.

Rytand D.A., Burnham D.K. & Cox A.J., Jr. (1948) Periarteritis nodosa following the dermatitis of poison oak and primrose. *Stanford Medical Bulletin* **6**: 319–23.

Shelmire B. (1946) Sodium perborate ointment and poison ivy dermatitis. *JAMA* **116**: 681–3.

Sizer I.W. & Prokesch C.E. (1945) The destruction by tyrosinase of the irritant principles of poison ivy and related toxicants. *Journal of Pharmacology and Experimental Therapeutics* **84**: 363–74.

Stampf J.-L., Benezra C., Byers V. et al. (1986) Induction of tolerance to poison ivy urushiol in the guinea pig by epicutaneous application of the structural analog 5-methyl-3-n-pentadecylcatechol. *Journal of Investigative Dermatology* **86**: 535–8.

Sulzberger M.B., Baer R.L. & Lanof A. (1946) Chloroamide containing ointments in prevention of experimental poison ivy dermatitis. *Journal of Investigative Dermatology* **7**: 145–6.

Toyama I. (1918) Rhus dermatitis. *Journal of Cutaneous Diseases* **36**: 157–65.

Von Adelung E. (1913) An experimental study of poison oak. *Archives of Internal Medicine* **11**: 148–64.

Waali E.E. (1984) *Testing Materials that Bond with Poison Oak/Ivy/Sumac*

Urushiol. Written report to USDA Forest Service Equipment Development Center, Missoula.

Watson E.S., Murphy J.C., Wirth P.W. *et al.* (1981) Immunologic studies of poisonous Anacardiaceae: I. Production of tolerance and desensitization to poison ivy and oak urushiols using esterified urushiol derivatives in guinea pigs. *Journal of Investigative Dermatology* **76**: 164–70.

7.5 Other plant families causing allergic contact dermatitis

The plant species which have been implicated in allergic reactions are described in the following pages. Amazingly, there is no internationally agreed system of classification of plant families. The following account follows the sequence recognized by the Royal Botanic Gardens, Kew, and adopted by many other botanic gardens. Most other classifications are similar, although it should be noted that Kew retain the term Compositae, rather than Asteraceae, for members of the daisy family.

The heading for each family is given in bold type, followed by the names of each genus (in capitals) and relevant species. Common names and geographical distribution are noted, where relevant, together with information on patch testing. Where patch testing vehicles are suggested, pet. = petrolatum and MEK = methylethylketone (butanone).

Algae

Common names: Seaweeds, slimes, blooms, etc.

Distribution: Worldwide, in damp places, fresh or salt water

The algae form a large, successful group of plants. Many are unicellular, forming the simplest form of plant life. Others are multicellular, forming long filamentous strands or branched fronds, as in many seaweeds (Fig. 7.5.1). Algae are usually classified according to their pigment (green, brown, red and blue-green) (Brightman 1966). Lichens (q.v.) are a symbiotic relationship between unicellular algae and fungi. Some unicellular algae are pathogenic to humans, notably *Prototheca* (Rippon 1982). Members of this genus may cause extensive cutaneous and subcutaneous infection in humans (Cox *et al.* 1974).

Many cutaneous reactions to algae are due to toxins. An example is seabather's itch, a papulovesicular eruption which may be caused by the blue-green alga, *Lyngbya majuscula* (Grauer & Arnold 1961); irritant toxins include lyngbyatoxin A (Cardellina *et al.* 1979) and debromoaplysiatoxin (Solomon & Stoughton 1978). A similar eruption caused by *Anabena* may have an allergic component; the blue pigment, phycocyanin, is the suspected sensitizer (Cohen & Reif 1953). 'Dogger bank itch', initially thought to be due to the alga *Fragillaria striatulata*, is in fact due to a marine animal *Alcyonidium gelatinosum*.

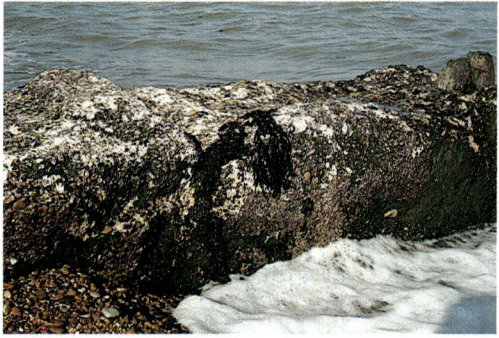

Fig. 7.5.1 Common seaweeds, *Pelvetia canaliculata* (channeled wrack) and *Cladophora rupestris* in a typical coastal habitat between tides, Felixstowe beach. (Courtesy of Dr R. Mallett.)

Atopics in the USA have a high incidence of prick test positivity using alga species (Bernstein & Safferman 1966); the significance is uncertain. *Chlorella*, ingested in Japan as an aphrodisiac, may cause phototoxic reactions (see p. 84). Brown algae (including many seaweeds) contain large amounts of iodine (430–2500 mg/kg dry weight). Van der Willigen *et al.* (1988) report contact dermatitis to Japanese sargassum in two eel fishermen. An eczematous eruption on the hands, arms, neck and face coincided with the fishing season (and maximum growth of the seaweed). Positive patch tests were obtained with water and saline extracts of the seaweed and also with 20% potassium iodide (Van der Willigen *et al.* 1988).

Bernstein I.L. & Safferman R.S. (1966) Sensitivity of skin and bronchial mucosa to green algae. *Journal of Allergy* **38**: 166–73.

Brightman F. (1966) *The Oxford Book of Flowerless Plants*. Oxford University Press, Oxford.

Cardellina J.H. *et al.* (1979) Seaweed dermatitis: structure of lyngbyatoxin A. *Science* **204** (4389): 193–5.

Cohen S.G. & Reif C.B. (1953) Cutaneous sensitisation to blue-green alga. *Journal of Allergy* **24**: 452–7.

Cox G.E., Wilson J.D. & Brown P. (1974) Protothecosis: a case of disseminated algal infection. *Lancet* **ii**: 379–82.

Grauer F.H. & Arnold H.L. (1961) Seaweed dermatitis. *Archives of Dermatology* **84**: 720–32.

Rippon J.W. (1982) *Medical Mycology*, 2nd edn. W.B. Saunders, Philadelphia, p. 651.

Solomon A.E. & Stoughton R.B. (1978) Dermatitis from purified sea algae toxin (debromoaplysiatoxine). *Archives of Dermatology* **114**: 1333–5.

Van der Willigen A.H., Habets J.M.W., Van Joost T., Stolz E. & Nienhuis P.H. (1988) Contact allergy to iodine in Japanese sargassum. *Contact Dermatitis* **18**: 250–2.

Lichens

Patch test:
Lichen as is (?)
Perfume mix 8% ⎫
Oak moss 2% ⎬ pet.
Atranorin 0.5% ⎭
D-usnic acid 1%
Evernic acid 1%   ⎫ pet.
Stitic acid 1%   ⎬ if
Fumarprotocetraric acid 1% ⎭ available

Lichens are dual organisms, composed of a symbiotic relationship between a fungus, which can only survive in the association, and which gives the plant its shape, and an alga, which is able to photosynthesize. This successful combination is able to produce a more elaborate and durable organism than either partner alone. Lichens are able to colonize inhospitable areas such as bare rock (Figs 7.5.2, 7.5.3), and as 'pioneer plants' can break down the rock surface; this, together with decaying material from the lichen, eventually forms soil conditions suitable for other plants. Many lichens are epiphytic (growing on trees), gaining nutrition from rain water running down tree trunks. Only a few species tolerate air polluted with sulphur dioxide and survive in towns. Lichens are variable in shape, either tubular, upright and branching, or flat and leaf-like or forming an amorphous greyish crust. Some of the lichens of dermatological interest are detailed in Table

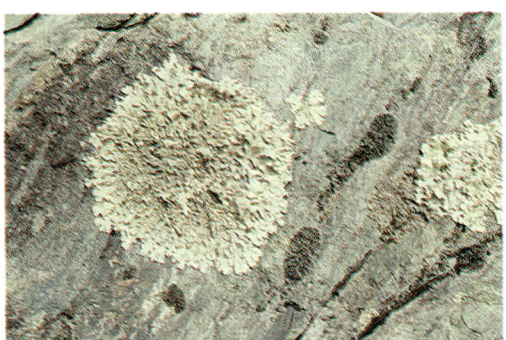

Fig. 7.5.2 *Parmelia* species. This genus of lichens is common on trees, rocks and walls. (Courtesy of Dr R. Champion.)

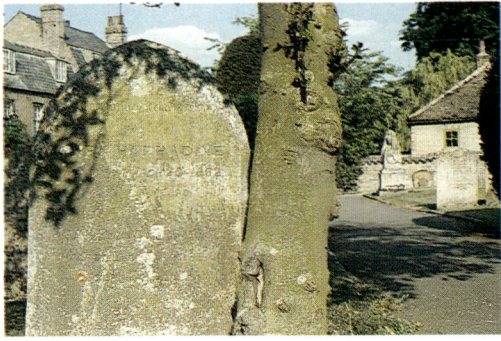

Fig. 7.5.3 *Lecanora conizaeoides* (a minute lichen) forming extensive greenish crusts on tree trunk and gravestone, Grantchester. (Courtesy of Dr R. Mallett.)

LICHENS

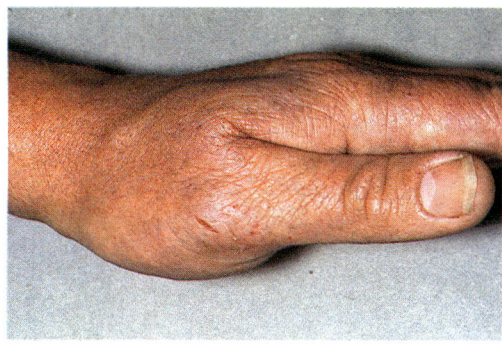

Fig. 7.5.4 Atopic dermatitis aggravated by lichen and grasses. (Courtesy of Drs R. Champion & R. Mallett.)

7.5.1. For excellent drawings and descriptions of lichens see Nicholson and Brightman (1966).

Eczematous eruptions (Fig. 7.5.4) on the face, hands and of the neck have been recognized in wood cutters and lumber workers since the early years of the century. However, Tenchio (1948) was the first to attribute it to the lichen *Parmelia caperata* growing on tree barks. Mitchell (1965) studying 'cedar poisoning' in lumber workers in British Colombia, found D-usnic acid (7.IIIa)

Usnic acid

7.IIIa

to be an antigen in the bark lichens. Champion (1971) also found D-usnic acid sensitivity in some, but not all, patients with lichen sensitivity. In a group of atopic individuals who developed exacerbation of eczema, as well as asthma and rhinitis, after exposure to lichens, three patients had positive patch tests with lichens, notably *Lecanora* spp. (Champion 1971). In addition to D-usnic acid (Mitchell 1966), the L-enantiomer (mirror image molecule) can also sensitize (Salo *et al.* 1981).

Several species are used in perfumery. *Evernia prunastri*, in particular, is a source of 'chypre'-like perfume (Guin & Jackson 1988). *Pseudevernia furfuracea* yields oak moss absolute. In perfume sensitivity due to oak moss the major sensitizer is atranorin (7.IIIb),

Atranorin

7.IIIb

followed by usnic, evernic and fumarprotocetraric acids (Goncalo *et al.* 1988). Dahlquist and Fregert (1980) obtained positive patch tests to atranorin in 1% of 760 'routine' patch test patients. *Usnea barbata* is also occasionally used in perfumery and may sensitize (Novak 1974). *Cladonia* spp. in particular are sometimes used in decoration, e.g. wreaths (Salo *et al.* 1981). Rarely, a photosensitive eruption may occur in conjunction with lichen sensitivity, perhaps reflecting 'persistent light reactivity'. In 16 patients sensitive to UVA and UVB, Thune and Solberg (1980) obtained positive patch tests with a mixture of eight lichen genera, namely *Cetraria*, *Cladonia*, *Hypogymnia*, *Parmelia*, *Physcia*, *Platismatia*, *Pseudevernia*, and *Umbilicaria*. Atranorin 1% was positive in seven patients (Thune & Solberg 1980).

Lichen sensitivity can be diagnosed by taking a careful clinical history and patch testing with perfume mix, oak moss and atranorin. Patch testing with lichens themselves may be misleading, as many lichens, especially *Parmelia*, grow together with liverwort species such as *Frullania*. The allergens in liverworts, sesquiterpene lactones, are structurally dissimilar from those found in lichens. However, in one recent study, Gonçalo *et al.* (1987) observed a high incidence of lichen sensitivity in patients with *Frullania* dermatitis; atranorin was *not* the main sensitizer. In general, it appears that lichens are weaker sensitizers than liverworts (Mitchell 1965).

Champion R.H. (1971) Atopic sensitivity to algae and lichens. *British Journal of Dermatology* **85**: 551–7.
Dahlquist I. & Fregert S. (1980) Contact allergy to atranorin in lichens and perfumes. *Contact Dermatitis* **6**: 111–19.
Gonçalo S. (1987) Contact sensitivity to lichens and Compositae in *Frullania* dermatitis. *Contact Dermatitis* **16**: 84–6.
Gonçalo S., Cabral F. & Gonçalo M. (1988) Contact sensitivity to oak moss. *Contact Dermatitis* **19**: 355–7.
Guin J.D. & Jackson D.B. (1988) Oak moss

Table 7.5.1 The lichens of dermatological importance (major allergenic species marked *).

Botanical name	Typical habitat	Description/comments
Cetraria spp.	Mostly heather and mountains in north	Broad, branched fronds. *C. islandica* brown, with stiff marginal spines. *C. nivalis* cream, with ridges and hollows and a crisped margin
* *Cladonia rangiferina*	Abundant in arctic/sub-arctic regions. In Britain, rare except Scottish and Welsh mountains. Heaths and moors	'Reindeer moss'. Much-branched, bluish grey. About 8 cm height. Stems turn yellow after touching with a drop of strong potassium hydroxide solution
* *Evernia prunastri* (see also *Pseudevernia*)	Common on trees/fences	'Mousse de Chêne'. Flattened, drooping, much-branched stems. Greenish grey, wrinkled upper surface; white on under surface
Hypogymnia physodes	Common on tree bark. Tolerates pollution. *Evm. elegans* common on twigs/old heather stems in moorland	Pale grey, upper surface smooth. Has an air space between upper and lower surfaces, giving it an inflated appearance. Cannot be detached from stone/bark without tearing. *Evm. elegans* has narrow lobes, turned up at the tips
Lecanora spp. (see Fig. 7.5.3)	Walls, tombstones. Tolerates pollution. Common in towns	Grey granular crusts, often chalky white at the margin
* *Parmelia* spp. (see Fig. 7.5.2)	Many spp. common on trees	Mostly grey or grey-green, forming large rosettes. Individual lobes, narrow, fan shaped at tips. *P. caperata*, uniquely, has yellow-green lobes
Physcia spp.	Chiefly rocks and walls	Relatively small rosettes; many species are covered with a white powder, notably at the tips of the lobes
Platismatia glauca	Common on fences, walls, trees, rocks	Broad lobes of thin texture, having a wavy crisped appearance. Upper surface grey, sometimes with bluish tinge; under surface brown, smooth, shining
* *Pseudevernia furfuracea* (= *Evernia*, *Parmelia furfuracea*)	Rocks, stone walls, fences, trees	'Oak moss'. Used in perfumery. Much-forked branches. Upper surface dark grey with numerous small, bristle-like projections. Under surface matt black or mottled grey and black
Umbilicaria spp.	Rocks, especially in mountain areas	Brownish grey, often 'pebbled' surface and lace-like holes at the edges. Some species hairy at margins. *U. pustulata* ('tripe de roche') edible, but unexciting!
* *Usnea*	Trees, often in dense shade	'Old man's beard' lichens. Long, often hanging stems, attached to tree by small disc-like holdfasts. Much branched, moss-like. Green/grey or red (*U. rubiginea*). Occasionally used in perfumery

photosensitivity in a ragweed-allergic patient. *Contact Dermatitis* **18**: 240–2.
Mitchell J.C. (1965) Allergy to lichens. *Archives of Dermatology* **92**: 142–6.
Mitchell J.C. (1966) Stereoisomeric specificity of usnic acid in delayed hypersensitivity. *Journal of Investigative Dermatology* **47**: 167–8.
Nicholson B.E. & Brightman F.M. (1966 revised 1979) *The Oxford Book of Flowerless Plants*. Oxford University Press, Oxford.
Novak M. (1974) Contact sensitisation to constituents of perfume composition in antiphlogistic ointment. *Ceskoslovensko Dermatologica* **49**: 375.
Salo H., Hannuksela M. & Hausen B.M. (1981) Lichen picker's dermatitis (*Cladonia alpestris* (L) Rab). *Contact Dermatitis* **7**: 9–13.
Tenchio F. (1948) Etiologie de l'eczema des bucherons. *Dermatologica* **97**: 72–7.
Thune P.O. & Solberg Y.J. (1980) Photosensitivity and allergy to aromatic lichen acids, Compositae oleoresins and other plant substances. *Contact Dermatitis* **6**: 81–7.

Jubulaceae (liverworts)

FRULLANIA spp.

Distribution: Worldwide, especially in temperate and sub-tropical forests
Patch test: Plant as is: Compositae (NB may sensitize)

The liverworts derive their common name from the resemblance of some species to the lobes of the liver. *Frullania*, however, belongs to a group of leafy liverworts; these are moss-like with regularly branching stems. Of the European species, *F. dilatata* is the commonest, forming red or dark green tufts on trees. *Frullania tamarisci* (Fig. 7.5.5) has a more glossy appearance and favours shady rocks, although sometimes found in beech forests. Forestry workers come into close contact with *Frullania* species and allergic contact dermatitis was first recorded by Le Coulant and Lopes in 1960. Since then there have been several reports in forestry workers throughout continental Europe (e.g. Fernandez de Corres 1984, Gonçalo *et al.* 1987). Mitchell (1981) reported 112 cases, due to *F. nisquallensis*, in forestry workers on the west coast of Vancouver Island, British Columbia. Benezra *et al.* (1985) illustrate *Frullania* dermatitis in a child who was playing on a woodpile.

Exposed areas of skin are typically affected, with an 'airborne' pattern on the face and vee of the neck, superficially resembling photosensitivity but involving 'shaded' areas such as the eyelids and nasolabial folds. The hands may become oedematous, with involvement of finger webs but often sparing of the palms. Le Coulant *et al.* (1966) described involvement of the male genitalia and intertriginous folds. Sometimes frank erythroderma may develop. The Canadian workers, working in cold wet conditions, wear rash-protective clothing and skin involvement is less extensive (Mitchell 1981). Photosensitivity does not appear to occur, although photoaggravation of allergic reactions has been reported (Bruley *et al.* 1986).

The allergens are sesquiterpene lactones (**7.IV**), and it is not surprising that cross-reactions are reported with botanically unrelated plants that contain similar allergens, e.g. *Laurus nobilis* (sweet bay) (Asakawa *et al.*

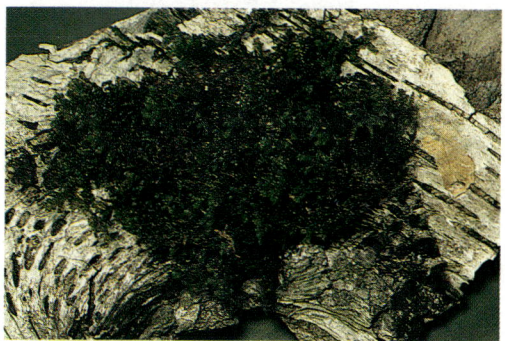

Fig. 7.5.5 *Frullania tamarisci*, Dartmoor. (Courtesy of Mr C. Parsons.)

(+)-frullanolide (in F. *dilatata*)
(−)-frullanolide (in F. *tamarisci*)
(+)-cis-β-cyclocostunolide

7.IV Allergens in *Frullania* spp.

1974), *Magnolia grandiflora* (Gonçalo 1987) and several Compositae (Mitchell et al. 1970, Mitchell 1981, Fernandez de Corres 1984). Enantiomers (mirror-image molecules) of frullanolide have been found in *F. dilatata* and *F. tamarasci*; cross-sensitivity does not occur (Barbier & Benezra 1982). Several other sesquiterpene lactones have been isolated from *Frullania* spp. (Asakawa et al. 1983). Several of Mitchell's patients also reacted to lichen acids (e.g. 75% to 1% usnic acid) Mitchell (1981) and Gonçalo (1987) found sensitivity to *Parmelia* species (lichens) in 27 of 48 *Frullania*-positive foresters. This probably represents separate sensitization to lichens (*Parmelia* and *Frullania* often grow together). *Frullania* may cause active sensitization (Mitchell 1981, Tomb 1992) and should not be used as a screening patch test, but only in individuals whose history suggests *Frullania* dermatitis.

Mildly affected individuals may be able to return to work. Le Coulant et al. (1966) report successful hyposensitization by continued application of the plants. Other workers have not observed 'hardening' (Mitchell 1981).

Asakawa Y., Benezra C., Foussereau J., Muller J.C. & Ourisson G. (1974) Cross-sensitisation between *Frullania* and *Laurus nobilis*. *Archives of Dermatology* **110**: 957.

Asakawa Y., Matsuda R., Toyota M. et al. (1983) Sesquiterpenes from *Chiloscyphus*, *Clasmatocolea* and *Frullania* species. *Phytochemistry* **22**: 961–4.

Barbier P. & Benezra C. (1982) Stereospecificity of allergic contact dermatitis (ACD) induced by two natural enantiomers, (+) and (−) − Frullanolides, in guinea pigs. *Naturwissenschaften* **69**: 296–7.

Benezra C., Ducombs G., Sell Y. & Foussereau J. (1985) *Plant Contact Dermatitis*. B.C. Decker, Toronto.

Bruley C., Beltzer-Garelly E., Kaufman P., Binet O. & Robin J. (1986) Allergy and photoallergy to *Frullania*. *Photodermatology* **1**: 49–50.

Fernandez de Corres L. (1984) Contact dermatitis from *Frullania*, Compositae, and other plants. *Contact Dermatitis* **11**: 74–9.

Gonçalo S. (1987) Contact sensitivity to lichens and Compositae in *Frullania* dermatitis. *Contact Dermatitis* **16**: 84–6.

Le Coulant P. & Lopes G. (1960) Role pathogene des muscinees — hepatiques dans les industries du bois. *Archives des Maladies Professionelles de Medicine du Travail et de Securite Sociale* **21**: 374–6.

Le Coulant P., Texier L., Maleville J., Geniaux M., Tamisier J.M. & Bancons F. (1966) L'allergie an *Frullania*: son role dans la dermite du bois de chene. *Bulletin de la Société Française de Dermatologie et Syphilologie* **73**, 440.

Mitchell J.C. (1981) Industrial aspects of 112 cases of allergic contact dermatitis from *Frullania* in British Columbia during a 10 year period. *Contact Dermatitis* **7**: 268–9.

Mitchell J.C., Fritig B., Singh B. & Towers G.H.N. (1970) Allergic contact dermatitis from *Frullania* and Compositae. The role of sesquiterpene lactones. *Journal of Investigative Dermatology* **54**: 233–9.

Tomb R.R. (1992) Patch testing with *Frullania* during a 10-year period: hazards and complications. *Contact Dermatitis* **26**: 220–3.

Magnoliaceae

This family includes *Magnolia* itself (Fig. 7.5.6), as well as the tulip tree (*Liriodendron*). Many species are cultivated as ornamentals and the heartwood of *L. tulipifera* is grown for timber in the USA, where it is native. Schulz and Hausen (1980) report allergic contact dermatitis in two woodworkers handling *L. tulipifera*; patch tests were positive to shavings and bark, negative in 10 controls. *Liriodendron tulipifera* contains potentially antigenic quinones and also sesquiterpene lactones (Doskotch et al. 1972, Schulz & Hausen 1980). These latter molecules are also found in several botanically unrelated genera, including members of the daisy family (Compositae), sweet bay (*Laurus nobilis*) and liverworts, e.g. *Frullania* spp. (Mitchell et al. 1970). Parthenolide, a sesquiterpene lactone found in feverfew, *Tanacetum parthenium* (Compositae), has also been isolated from *Magnolia grandiflora* (Wiedhopf et al. 1973) and the Asiatic tree, *Michelia champaca* (Govindachari et al. 1964).

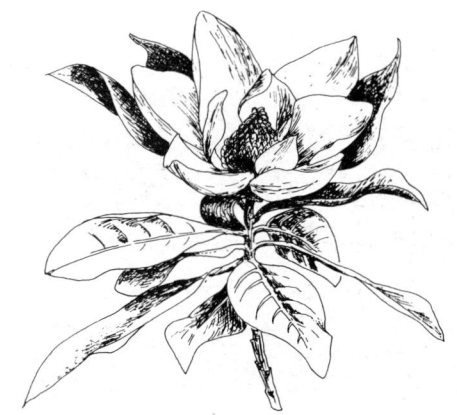

Fig. 7.5.6 *Magnolia grandiflora*.

Doskotch R.W., Hufford C.D. & El-Feraly T.S. (1972) Further studies on the sesquiterpene lactones tulipinolide and epitulipinolide from *Liriodendron tulipifera* L. *Journal of Organic Chemistry* **37**: 2740–4.

Govindachari T.R., Joshi B.S. & Kamat V.N. (1964) Revised structure of parthenolide. *Tetrahedron Letters* **52**: 3927–33.

Mitchell J.C., Fritig B., Singh B. & Towers G.H.N. (1970) Allergic contact dermatitis from *Fullania* and Compositae. The role of sesquiterpene lactones. *Journal of Investigative Dermatology* **54**: 233–9.

Schulz H.K. & Hausen B.M. (1980) Tulpenholz-Allergie (*Liriodendron tulipifera* L, Magnoliaceae). *Dermatosen in Beruf und Umwelt* **28**: 158–60.

Wiedhopf R.M., Young M., Bianchi E. & Cole J.R. (1973) Tumour inhibitory agent from *Magnolia grandiflora* (Magnoliaceae). *Journal of the Pharmaceutical Society* **62**: 345.

Illiciaceae

ILLICIUM verum

Common name: Star anise
Distribution: South China, Tonkin. The dry fruits are used in oriental cooking
Patch test: 0.5% star anise oil

Star anise, an important spice (Fig. 7.5.7), takes its name from the cluster of fruits of this tree which, together with *Pimpinella anisum* (see

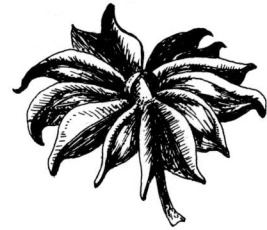

Fig. 7.5.7 Star anise pod.

p. 142), yield oil of anise (oleum anisi stellati). Contact dermatitis was reported by Greenberg and Lester (1954). The most likely sensitizer is anethole (**7.V**) which is also an irritant. Other potential sensitizers are the terpenoids, pinene, limonene and safrole. Rudzki and Grzywa (1976), testing with the oil, found 1–7% dilutions to be irritant and to produce active sensitization. A 0.5% dilution elicited positive patch tests in actively sensitized patients.

Greenberg L.A. & Lester D. (1954) *Handbook of Cosmetic Materials*. Interscience, New York.
Rudzki E. & Grzywa Z. (1976) Sensitising and irritating properties of star anise oil. *Contact Dermatitis* **2**: 305–8.

H₃CO–⟨benzene⟩–CH=CH–CH₃
Anethole
7.V

Annonaceae

This tropical family includes *Cananga odorata*, a tree native to Malaysia. The hanging sprays of greenish-yellow flowers have a fragrance redolent of hyacinths and are worn as garlands. Ylang ylang perfume was traditionally obtained by steam distillation of the flowers. It contains several allergens, including derivatives of geraniol and linalool. Rudzki *et al.* (1976) patch tested 200 subjects with 2% concentrations of 35 essential oils; four reacted to ylang ylang oil. Cananga oil (extracted from trees growing in Java) contains more sesquiterpenes and is an important sensitizer in Japan (Nakayama *et al.* 1974, quoted in Mitchell & Rook 1979). *Cananga odorata* is also a source of Macassar oil, which our Victorian forefathers applied liberally to their hair. The 'antimacassar' was later developed to protect chairs from greasy scalps.

Mitchell J. & Rook A. (1979) *Botanical Dermatology*. Greengrass, Vancouver.
Rudzki E., Grzywa Z. & Bruo S. (1976) Sensitivity to 35 essential oils. *Contact Dermatitis* **2**: 196–200.

Papaveraceae

The bleeding heart, *Dicentra spectabilis* (Fig. 7.5.8), is a beautiful and popular herbaceous perennial. It is listed as a cause of sensitization by Lampe and Fagerstrom (1968). Recurrent dermatitis of the hands, forearms and neck was attributed to this species by Harville (1933). Patch testing with an ether extract (diluted in alcohol) was positive, but no control data were recorded.

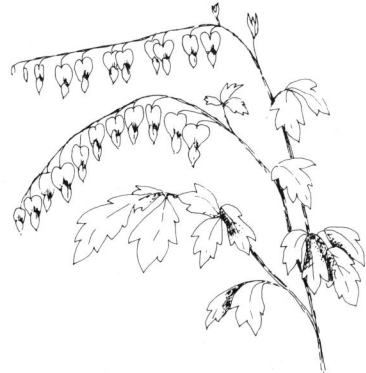

Fig. 7.5.8 *Dicentra spectabilis*, the 'bleeding heart'.

Harville C.H. (1933) Contact dermatitis to a common plant. *Journal of Allergy* **4**: 527–9.
Lampe K.F. & Fagerstrom R. (1968) *Plant Toxicity and Dermatitis. A Manual for Physicians*. Williams & Wilkins, Baltimore.

Brassicaceae (Cruciferae)

This large family includes several important vegetables, such as cabbage (*Brassica oleracea*), cauliflower (*B. oleracea* v. *botrytis*), radish (*Raphanus sativus*), horse radish (*Armoracia rusticana*), turnip (*Brassica campestris*) and mustard (*Brassica nigra*). Several species contain thioglucosides which are broken down enzymatically, in the presence of water, to isothiocyanates (mustard oils) (**7.VI**), which contribute the hot spicy flavour and are also potent irritants. Mustard oil plasters have been used as rubefacients. There are a few examples of allergic contact dermatitis to members of this family.

BRASSICA nigra

Brassica nigra (Fig. 7.5.9) (black mustard) is a common herb in central and southern Europe, naturalized in many temperate countries. In Britain, it is found particularly on the south-western coastline on cliffs, banks and riversides. It bears four-petalled yellow flowers in June–August and four-angled seed pods.

Contact urticaria and anaphylaxis has been reported in food handlers (Kavli & Moseng 1987) and a consumer (Panconesi *et al.* 1980). These latter authors also describe delayed

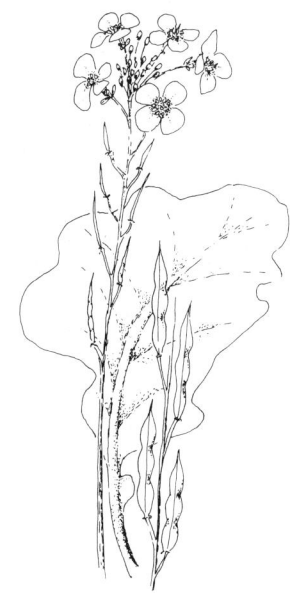

Fig. 7.5.9 *Brassica nigra*.

hypersensitivity. Dannaker and White (1987) reported contact dermatitis due to mustard powder in a salad maker. Patch tests were positive using 1% mustard powder in aqueous suspension. Patch tests were negative to thiurams and thioureas. The allergen appears to be allylisothiocyanate (**7.VI**). Allylisothiocyanate (synthetic oil of mustard) 0.1% is a useful non-irritant material for patch testing (Gaul 1964).

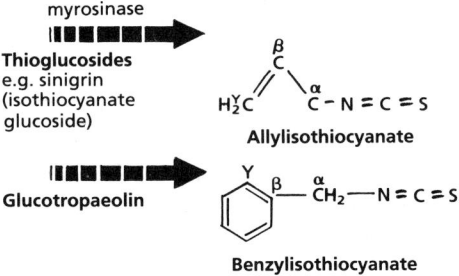

7.VI Mustard oils.

Dannaker C.J. & White I.R. (1987) Cutaneous allergy to mustard in a salad maker. *Contact Dermatitis* **16**: 212–14.
Gaul L.E. (1964) Contact dermatitis from synthetic oil of mustard. *Archives of Dermatology* **90**: 158.

Kavli G. & Moseng D. (1987) Contact urticaria from mustard in fish-stick production. *Contact Dermatitis* **17**: 153–5.

Panconesi E., Sertoli A., Fabbri P., Giorgini S. & Spallanzini P. (1980) Anaphylactic shock from mustard after ingestion of pizza. *Contact Dermatitis* **2**: 294–5.

BRASSICA oleracea v. botrytis (cauliflower)

A plant grower with hand eczema was patch test positive to cauliflower 'as is' and to 10% aqueous and ethanolic extracts; positive reactions were also obtained with several thiurams, including the fungicide tetramethylthiuramdisulphide (Van Ketel 1975, Van Ketel & Bruynzeel 1987).

Van Ketel W.G. (1975) A cauliflower allergy. *Contact Dermatitis* **1**: 324.

Van Ketel W.G. & Bruynzeel D.P. (1987) Contact dermatitis due to plants in Amsterdam. *Bolletino di Dermatologia Allergologica e Professionale* **2**: 132–8.

RAPHANUS sativus

Raphanus sativus (radish) (Fig. 7.5.10) is unknown in the wild. The leaves are irritant (Shelmire 1940) and a waitress who was chopping salads developed an acute vesiculo-bullous dermatitis of both palms attributed to radish. Patch tests were positive to the tuberous root and also to allylisothiocyanate 0.1% and benzyl isothiocyanate in petrolatum (Mitchell & Jordan 1974).

Mitchell J.C. & Jordan W.P. (1974) Allergic contact dermatitis from the radish, *Raphanus sativus*. *British Journal of Dermatology* **91**: 183–9.

Shelmire B. (1940) Contact dermatitis from vegetation. *Southern Medical Journal* **33**: 337–46.

Capparidaceae

CAPPARIS spinosa

Common name: Caper bush
Distribution: Mediterranean, extending throughout Asia. Common in walls and dry rocky areas, especially near the coast

This sprawling shrub has greyish oval leaves and showy white-pink flowers with several prominent stamens (Fig. 7.5.11). Capers, the pickled flower buds, are used widely,

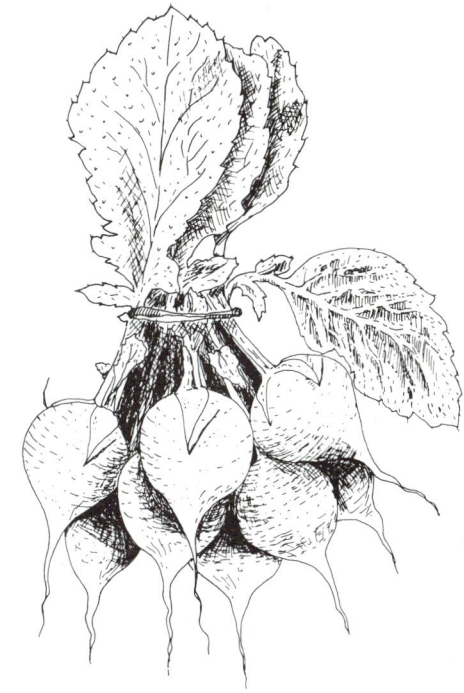

Fig. 7.5.10 *Raphanus sativus* (radish).

particularly as a condiment in 'fast foods', such as burgers. Several *Capparis* species are irritant, containing glucocapparin, a protein which is broken down to form isothiocyanates (Mitchell 1974). Vena *et al.* (1990) report allergic contact dermatitis in a middle-aged housewife who applied a compress of the minced leaves and fruits to an area of

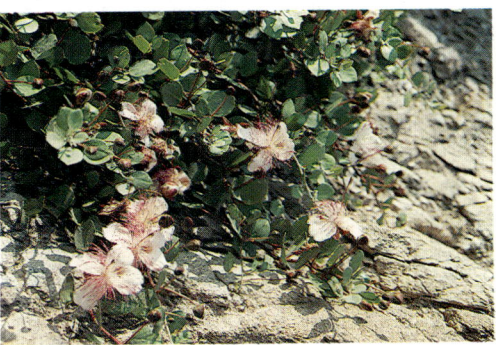

Fig. 7.5.11 *Capparis spinosa* (caper plant), photographed on the Mani peninsula, southern Greece.

epicondylitis, producing acute vesiculobullous dermatitis. On patch testing, the patient also cross-reacted to oil of mustard, which also contains isothiocyanates.

Mitchell J.C. (1974) Contact dermatitis from plants of the caper family (Capparidaceae). *British Journal of Dermatology* **91**: 13–20.
Vena G.A., Angelini G., Filotico R. & Foti C. (1990) Contact allergy to *Capparis spinosa* L (abstr.). *Contact Dermatitis* **23**: 261.

Cistaceae

CISTUS creticus

Common name: Rock rose
Distribution: Mediterranean region.
   Commonly grown in warmer gardens

The leaves of this beautiful sub-shrub (Fig. 7.5.12) exude an aromatic gum, ladanum, which was used extensively in medicinal plasters. Today, the gum is still collected in Crete by pulling a flail through the plants.

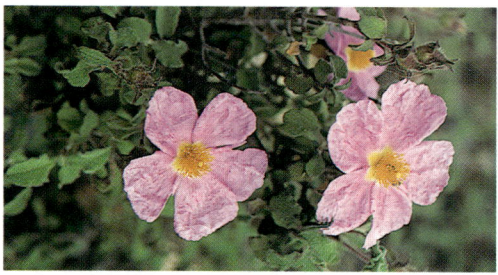

Fig. 7.5.12 *Cistus creticus*, photographed in Crete.

Many species and cultivars of *Cistus* are cultivated in sunny rock gardens and shrubberies, although they are susceptible to winter damp. English and Cronin (1988) report a positive open test to a leaf of *C. creticus* in a housewife with dermatitis (Fig. 7.5.13). Her skin improved when the plant was removed from her garden. It is perhaps surprising there are no other reports of allergic contact dermatitis to this genus.

English J.S. & Cronin E. (1988) Allergic contact dermatitis from *Cistus creticus. Contact Dermatitis* **18**: 123.

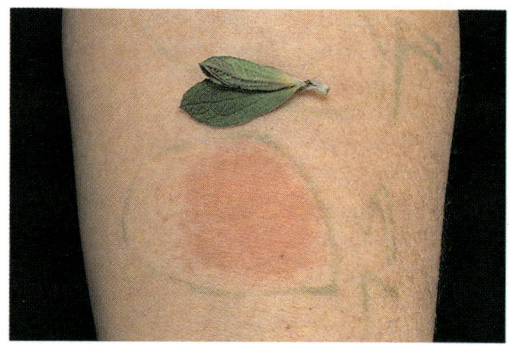

Fig. 7.5.13 Open patch test with *Cistus creticus* leaf. (Courtesy of Dr J. English.)

Caryophyllaceae

DIANTHUS caryophyllus

Common name: Carnation pink
Distribution: Europe. Numerous cultivars and hybrids
Patch test: Leaf and flower petal as is. Twenty per cent ether extract Eugenol 2% pet.

The carnation (Fig. 7.5.14) is a popular plant, grown in borders, rock gardens or greenhouses. It is also used frequently in floristry as the fragrant blooms are long-lasting. The plants are compact, with grey, needle-like leaves and showy, mostly double, flowers in pink, white or red shades. Despite its popularity, cutaneous reactions are rare. Shelmire (1940)

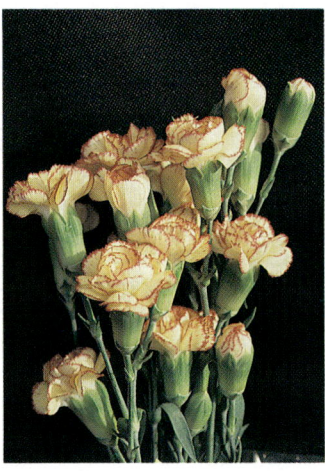

Fig. 7.5.14 Carnation.

describes it as a 'minor sensitizer' in housewives and florists. Van Grutten (1980) reports dermatitis in a flower seller who imported Italian carnations. A patch test with the leaf was positive. Cross-reaction may occur with Eugenol.

Shelmire B. (1940) Contact dermatitis from vegetation. *Southern Medical Journal* **33**: 337–46.
Van Grutten M. (1980) Carnation dermatitis in a flower seller. *Contact Dermatitis* **6**: 289.

Malvaceae

The mallow family includes many ornamental genera such as *Lavatera* and *Althea* (hollyhock), which are irritant. Cotton, derived from the capsules of *Gossypium* species, may cause severe anaphylactic reactions (see Chapter 4.3). *Hibiscus* contains many spectacular greenhouse and hardy shrubs and hardy annuals. Okra (gumbo) (Fig. 7.5.15) is the immature fruit of *H. esculentus*, widely grown in tropical America and in Japan. Positive patch tests to okra were obtained in a series of food handlers with fingertip dermatitis (Sinha *et al.* 1977). Okra is covered with sharp trichomes, and has an irritant mucilage, both of which may give false positive patch test reactions. In a recent questionnaire study of 50 okra farmers, 32 had cutaneous symptoms and signs, including pruritus, erythema in fingers, hands and arms, oedema and sometimes even bullae. Patch tests were positive in 9.8–30% using a homogenate of leaves and immature pods of different strains, diluted 20–40-fold in distilled water (positive in 3.8–9% of controls) (Matsushita *et al.* 1989). Immature pods contain a proteolytic enzyme, akin to mucunain and bromelin; this may also be the principle allergen (Manda *et al.* 1992). Dermatitis has also been reported to the allied species *H. cannabinus* (ambary plant) in operatives working on a collective farm. Positive patch tests were obtained using a 0.1–0.3% aqueous suspension of plant material (Karimov 1985).

Karimov A.M. (1985) Dermatitis caused by the ambary plant (*Hibiscus cannabinus*). *Vestnik Dermatologii i Venerologii* **11**: 63–4.
Manda F., Tadera K. & Aoyama K. (1992) Skin lesions due to okra (*Hibiscus esculentus* L.) proteolytic activity and allergenicity of okra. *Contact Dermatitis* **26**: 95–100.
Matsushita T., Aoyama K., Manda F., Ueda A., Yoshida M. & Okamura J. (1989) Occupational dermatoses in farmers growing okra (*Hibiscus esculentus* L). *Contact Dermatitis* **21**: 321–5.
Sinha S.M., Pasricha J.S., Sharma R.C. & Kandhari K.C. (1977) Vegetables responsible for contact dermatitis of the hands. *Archives of Dermatology* **113**: 776–9.

Linaceae

LINUM usitatissimum

Common names: Flax. Linseed oil plant
Distribution: Europe, often cultivated

Linseed oil is obtained by compressing the seeds of this attractive blue-flowered annual. The residual 'cake' is used to feed cattle. The seeds cause mechanical irritation, affecting longshore workers who unload the grain as well as operatives in oil extraction factories and paint factories. Dermatitis is reported from cigarette paper made from flax (Weber, quoted in Schwartz *et al.* 1957). Tye (1950) reported positive patch tests to the cooked, bleached flax fibre destined for cigarette paper manufacture. Linseed oil may be allergenic (Schwartz *et al.* 1957).

Schwartz L, Tulipan L. & Birmingham D.J. (1957) *Occupational Diseases of the Skin*, 3rd edn. Lea & Febiger, Philadelphia.
Tye M.J. (1950) Cigarette paper dermatitis. *Journal of Investigative Dermatology* **14**: 77–8.

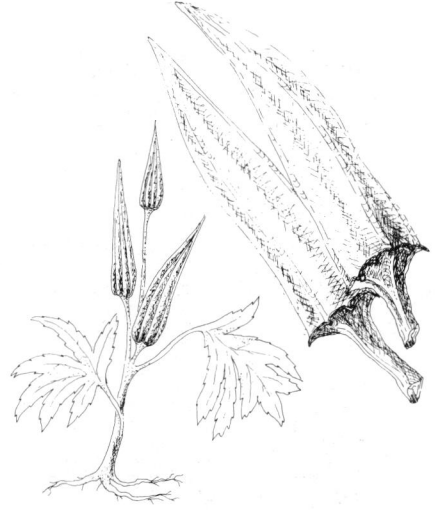

Fig. 7.5.15 Okra pod.

Zygophyllaceae

LARREA tridentata

Common name: Creosote bush
Distribution: Southwest USA (desert areas). South America

This globose, strongly aromatic, shrub has shiny 'polished' leaves, which are covered with a sticky secretion. Members of the genus are common in Argentina, particularly near the city of Mendoza, and in the western foothills of the Andes. The leaves and roots are used in herbal teas and in bath essences. Because of its resinous coating it burns readily and is ideal for starting bonfires and barbecues, the chief source of exposure. Allergic contact dermatitis was first reported by Smith (1937) and may be under-recognized in the USA (Shasky 1986). Leonforte (1986) reported six cases in Argentina. In common with other aromatic members of the family Zygophyllaceae, *Larrea* contains several potentially allergenic phenols, alkaloids and amines; these substances may protect the plant from attack by leaf-chewing insects (Leonforte 1986).

Leonforte J.F. (1986) Contact dermatitis from *Larrea* (creosote bush). *Journal of the American Academy of Dermatology* **14**: 202–7.
Shasky D.R. (1986) Contact dermatitis from *Larrea tridentata* (creosote bush). [Letter] *Journal of the American Academy of Dermatology* **15**: 302.
Smith L.M. (1937) Dermatitis caused by creosote bush. *Journal of Allergy* **8**: 187–8.

Geraniaceae

PELARGONIUM cvs.

Common name: Geranium
Distribution: Chiefly Southern Africa. Widely grown as ornamental pot/tub or bedding plants
Patch test: Leaf (as is) of patient's own plant. Geraniol 10%

Strictly speaking, *Geranium* (Fig. 7.5.16) is a genus of hardy herbaceous plants, including some British natives. However, the name is applied popularly to species and cultivars of the genus *Pelargonium*. Most species are sub-

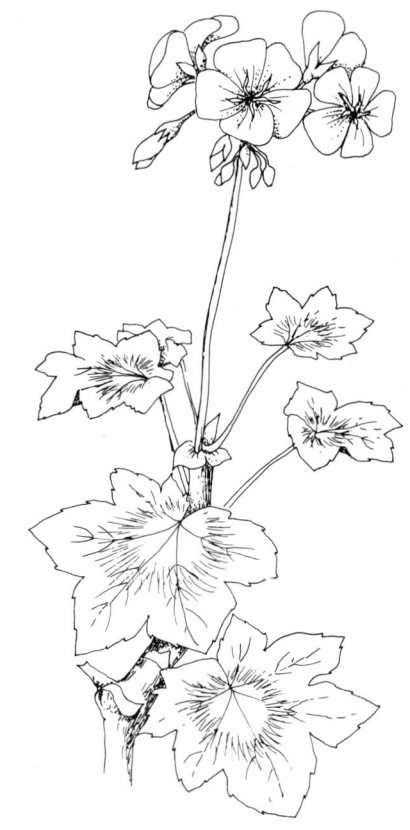

Fig. 7.5.16 *Pelargonium zonale* cultivar (geranium).

shrubs, although several are tuberous or succulent. This genus is based in Southern Africa, although a few members extend to Australia and the Middle East. Several cultivars are grown, notably forms of the zonal geranium (*P. zonale*) and ivy-leaved geranium (*P. peltatum*). Several species have aromatic leaves, including the rose geranium (*P. graveolens*). Cultivars of this species are grown on a large scale commercially on the island of Reunion as a source of geranium oil used in perfumery as a substitute for attar of roses (Van der Walt & Vorster 1988). Although geranium oil is irritant, Opdyke (1975) was unable to achieve sensitization using a maximization test. However, a few cases of allergic contact dermatitis have been reported. Anderson (1923) described vesicular hand dermatitis in a young man after removing dead leaves. Both zonal cultivars and forms of the rose geranium appear to sensitize (Rook 1961,

Hjorth 1969). Geranium oil may cause perfume dermatitis (Klarmann 1958).

Ointments containing geraniol (such as Blastoestimulina®) are reported to sensitize when used on chronic leg ulcers (Romaguera et al. 1986, Guerra et al. 1987).

The allergen may be geraniol. Cross-reactions occur with lemon-grass (*Citronella*) (Keil 1947).

Anderson J.W. (1923) Geranium dermatitis. *Archives of Dermatology and Syphilology* **7**: 510.
Guerra P., Aguilar A., Urbina F., Cristobal M.C. & Garcia-Perez A. (1987) Contact dermatitis to geraniol in a leg ulcer. *Contact Dermatitis* **16**: 298–9.
Hjorth N. (1969) Plant dermatitis. *Contact Dermatitis Newsletter* **6**: 126.
Keil H. (1947) Contact dermatitis due to oil of citronella. *Journal of Investigative Dermatology* **8**: 327–334.
Klarmann E.G. (1958) Perfume dermatitis. *Annals of Allergy* **16**: 425.
Opdyke D.L.T. (1975) Monographs on fragrance raw materials. *Food and Cosmetic Toxicology* **13**: 451.
Romaguera C., Grimalt F. & Vilaplana J. (1986) Geraniol dermatitis. *Contact Dermatitis* **14**: 185–6.
Rook A. (1961) Plant dermatitis — botanical aspects. *Transactions of the St John's Hospital Dermatological Society* **46**: 41–7.
Van der Walt J.J. & Vorster P.J. (1988) *Pelargoniums of Southern Africa*, Vol. 3. Annals of Kirstenbosch Botanic Gardens No. 16, p. 64.

Rutaceae

CITRUS spp.

Common names: C. aurantium — Seville orange; C. sinensis — orange; C. limon — lemon; C. deliciosa — mandarin; C. paradisi — grapefruit
Distribution: ?Asia. Widely cultivated in temperate zones
Patch test: Peel as is (irritant) or 5–10% dispersion in pet. citrus oil 5% pet.

Citrus fruit, notably lemon and *C. bergamia* (the source of bergamot oil) are important causes of phototoxic reactions (see Chapter 6). The peel is also irritant and may cause Type I hypersensitivity (Niinimäki 1987). Allergic contact dermatitis is unusual, although it has been described in food handlers (Schwartz 1938) and a bartender (Cardullo et al. 1989). Patch testing with orange peel and an ether extract yielded significant positive patch tests; there was some cross-reactivity with balsam of Peru (Hjorth 1961). Hjorth (1971) describes exacerbation of hand dermatitis in a patch test-positive patient who ate a jar of marmalade! Patch testing is difficult because citrus fruit peel is often waxed and dyed. Sensitization may be due to carnauba wax (Greenberg & Lester 1954) or dyes such as carotene and Citrus Red 3 dye (Mitchell 1972). Irritancy may preclude patch testing with peel (Schwartz 1938). Alternatively, false negative results may occur because the allergen located within the peel does not reach the skin. A homogenate dispersed in petrolatum may be preferable.

Citrus fruits contain psoralens, notably bergapten. Potential sensitizers include geraniol, citral (Cardullo et al. 1989) and a hydroperoxide derivative of D-limonene (Schwartz 1938) (**7.VII**). Limonene itself is probably not a sensitizer (Cardullo et al. 1989).

7.VII Allergens in citrus fruits.

Cardullo A.C., Ruszkowski A.M. & Deleo V.A. (1989) Allergic contact dermatitis resulting from sensitivity to citrus peel, geraniol and citral. *Journal of the American Academy of Dermatology*. **21**: 395–7.
Greenberg L.A. & Lester D. (1954) *Handbook of Cosmetic Materials*. Interscience, New York.
Hjorth N. (1961) *Eczematous Allergy to Balsams, Allied Perfumes and Flavouring Agents*. Munksgaard, Copenhagen.
Hjorth N. (1971) Allergy to balsams. *Spectrum* **8**: 97.
Mitchell J.C. (1972) Allergic contact dermatitis from a food dye presenting as 'sock dermatitis'. *Contact Dermatitis Newsletter* **11**: 247.

Niinimäki A. (1987) Scratch-chamber tests in food handler dermatitis. *Contact Dermatitis* **16**: 11–20.

Schwartz L. (1938) Cutaneous hazards in the citrus fruit industry. *Archives of Dermatology* **37**: 631–49.

Rutaceae

RUTA spp.

Common name: Rue
Distribution: Mediterranean, central Europe. *Ruta graveolens* widely grown as a herb

This genus of highly aromatic, low-growing shrubs is an important cause of phototoxic reactions (Chapter 6). In addition, Gonçalo *et al.* (1989) report allergic contact dermatitis to *R. chalepensis*, the fringed rue. This species is similar to the common rue, *R. graveolens*, but has leaves deeply cut into wedge-like segments; the petals are fringed, unlike those of *R. graveolens*, which are toothed (Huxley & Taylor 1977). In addition to psoralens, both species contain α-pinene, limonene and eucalyptol. In the patient described by Gonçalo *et al.* (1989) closed patch tests were positive with the plant and 'photoaggravation' (which may be non-specific) was demonstrated by UV-irradiation of the patch test site. Cross-reactivity was noted with lemon oil and turpentine.

Gonçalo S., Correia C., Couto J.S. & Gonçalo M. (1989) Contact and photocontact dermatitis from *Ruta chalepensis*. *Contact Dermatitis* **21**: 200–1.

Huxley A. & Taylor W. (1977) *Flowers of Greece and the Aegean*. Chatto & Windus, London.

Burseraceae

BOSWELLIA carterii

Boswellia *carterii* and *B. papyrifera* are native to India, Arabia and Somalia. Gum olibanum, used in incense, is derived by incision of the bark and leaves. Incense has been used in Christendom since the 5th century AD. Allergic contact dermatitis is reported in a 50-year-old housewife who applied a mixture of incense and brandy to her arthritic knee. Patch tests were positive using incense 'as is' and a 5% dilution in petrolatum (Basto & Azenha 1991). Previous reports of cutaneous reactions to incense refer to allergic dermatitis caused by musk ambrette in incense ('joss') sticks, e.g. Hayakawa *et al.* (1987).

Basto S.S. & Azenha A. (1991) Contact dermatitis due to incense. *Contact Dermatitis* **24**: 312–13.

Hayakawa R., Matsunaga K. & Arima Y. (1987) Airborne pigmented contact dermatitis due to musk ambrette in incense. *Contact Dermatitis* **16**: 96–8.

Vitaceae

VITIS vinifera (Fig. 7.5.17)

Common name: Grape vine
Distribution: Europe, widespread in cultivation in temperate zones

Although grape stems are irritant, allergy to grapes or the fermented product appears to be fortunately rare. Dermatitis due to grapes has been reported by Ramirez and Eller (1930) and Neshkov (1986). Ethanol and other related alcohols can cause allergic contact dermatitis (Van Ketel & Tan-Lim 1975). Grape-seed oil, used in aromatherapy, appears to be innocuous.

Neshkov N.S. (1986) (Dermatitis caused by grapes.) *Vestnik Dermatologii i venerologii* **2**: 66–7.

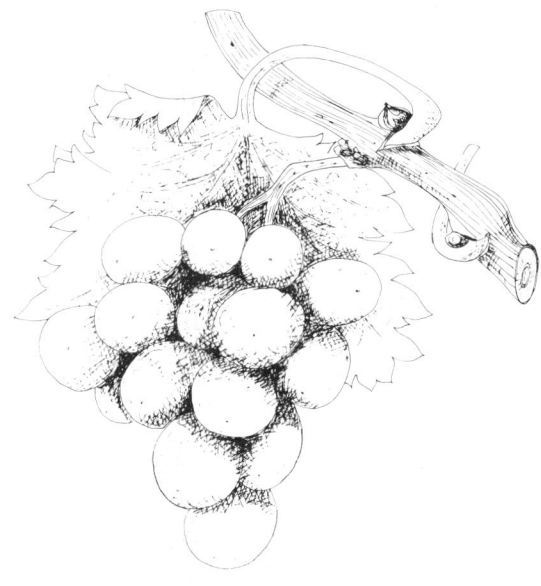

Fig. 7.5.17 *Vitis vinifera* (vine).

Ramirez M.A. & Eller J.T. (1930) The 'patch test' in 'contact dermatitis' (dermatitis venenata). *Journal of Allergy* **1**: 489–95.

Van Ketel W.G. & Tan-Lim K.N. (1975) Contact dermatitis from ethanol. *Contact Dermatitis* **1**: 7.

Hippocastanaceae

AESCULUS HIPPOCASTANUM

Common name: Horse chestnut
Distribution: Southeast Europe, widely planted

This handsome tree (Fig. 7.5.18) has a very large, domed crown. The bark is grey-brown. The brown leaf buds are sticky and open to form large, palm-like leaves, composed of 5–7 leaflets. 'Conkers' are the brown nuts, held in a spiny green capsule. Esculin (6-D-glucosyloxy-7-hydroxycoumarin sesquihydrate) is derived from the bark, leaves and seeds of horse chestnut. An anal preparation, Proctosedyl®, caused pruritus which proved on patch testing to be due to esculin (Comaish & Kersey 1980).

Comaish J.S. & Kersey P.J. (1980) Contact dermatitis to extract of horse chestnut (esculin). *Contact Dermatitis* **6**: 150–1.

Aceraceae

ACER negundo

Common name: Box elder (maple)
Distribution: North America. Maples and sycamores in general: Europe and Asia

Lovell *et al.* (1955) attribute air-borne contact dermatitis to this species (Fig. 7.5.19), a tall (up to 20 m) deciduous tree native to many parts of the USA. Aphids (greenfly) flourish on maples and may colonize the skin, causing a pseudo-phytodermatitis (Mitchell 1975).

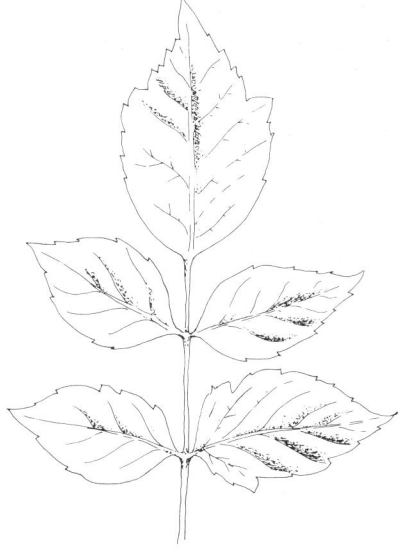

Fig. 7.5.19 *Acer negundo.*

Lovell R.G., Mathews K.P. & Sheldon J.M. (1955) Dermatitis venenata from tree pollen oils. *Journal of Allergy* **26**: 408–14.

Mitchell J.C. (1975) Pseudophytodermatitis from honeydew and aphides. *Dermatology International* **14**: 761.

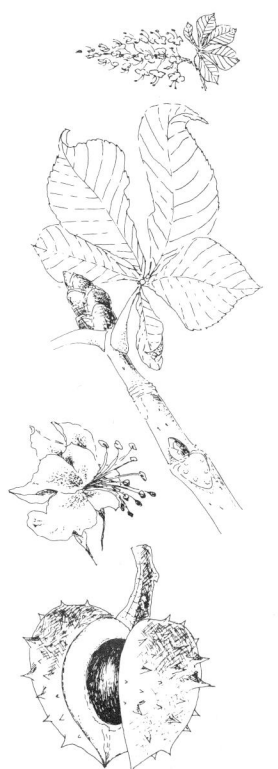

Fig. 7.5.18 *Aesculus hippocastanum* (horse chestnut).

Leguminosae (incl. Fabaceae, Papilionaceae, Mimosaceae)

Common name: Pea family

This large and important family (or group of families) includes several genera of economic importance and interest to the dermatologist. Vegetables, such as beans, and balsam of Peru, derived from *Myroxolon pereirae* (Fig. 7.5.20), cause contact urticaria. Cowhage (*Mucuna pruriens*) causes pruritus by mechanical and chemical irritation (p. 52). *Psoralea corylifolia*, the Bavachee, is phototoxic and has been used in the treatment of vitiligo for over three millenia (p. 67). Finally, allergic contact dermatitis may be caused by balsam of Peru. Several sensitizing hardwoods belong to this family, notably rosewoods, pao ferro and cocobolo (pp. 248–9).

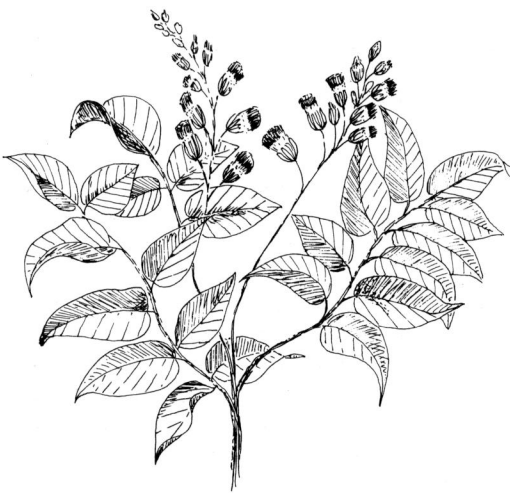

Fig. 7.5.20 *Myroxolon pereirae*.

ACACIA

Common name: Acacia; mimosa of florist
Distribution: Tropical and sub-tropical areas, especially in Australasia. Some spp. planted as ornamentals, and invading parts of South Africa

This large genus of trees and shrubs includes the Australian blackwood, a cause of allergic dermatitis (p. 248). Gum arabic is derived from *A. senegal*, although it may be contaminated with cashew gum. Gum arabic has been used in the printing trade and as a 'binding' agent in pharmacy. It is a respiratory allergen; hand dermatitis has been reported in patients who worked in the pottery industry. Patch tests were positive using a 1% aqueous solution of gum arabic (Ilchyshyn & Smith 1985).

Ilchyshyn A. & Smith A.G. (1985) Gum arabic sensitivity associated with epidemic hysteria dermatologica. *Contact Dermatitis* **13**: 202–3.

MYROXOLON PEREIRAE (*Toluifera pereirae*)/MYROXOLON TOLUIFERUM (*Toluifera Balsamum*)

Common names: Balsam of Peru (*M. pereirae*).
  Balsam of Tolu (*M. toluiferum*)
Distribution: Central America
Patch test: 25% pet.

Balsam of Peru is a sticky brownish gum obtained by lacerating the trunk. Its irritant aroma is derived from several constituents, including cinnamic acid and vanillin. It has several uses (Table 7.5.2), notably in perfumes and confectionery, and traditionally has been extensively used in pharmaceutical products. Allergy to balsam of Peru has been reviewed in detail by Hjorth (1961) and it is included in patch testing standard batteries. Because it shares several allergens with other plant

Table 7.5.2 Uses of balsam of Peru. (Hjorth 1961, Collins & Mitchell 1975.)

Medicaments
  Proprietary ointments
  Cough mixtures, throat lozenges
  Suppositories,
  Dental preparations
Cosmetics
  Perfumes,
  Hair tonics
  Toothpastes
Flavourings
  Caramel
  Cake flavouring
  'Cola' drinks
Liqueurs (e.g. Curacao)
  Fortified wines (e.g. Vermouths)

Table 7.5.3 Other possible sources of positive patch test reactions to balsam of Peru. (Hjorth 1961, Fisher 1974, Olholm-Larsen & Heydenreich 1976.)

Medicaments
 Balsam of tolu, benzyl benzoate, benzoic alcohol and acid

Flavourings
 Cinnamon, cloves, orange, vanilla

Perfume ingredients
 Cinnamyl acid, alcohol, cinnamates

Propolis (bee-keepers)

Colophony
 Conifers, violin rosin, wood tars

Laboratory chemicals

Baking (flavourings)

Plastics (cross-reaction with resorcinol monobenzoate in cellulose ester plastics, e.g. ball point pens, sunglasses)

---

extracts and cosmetic allergens, apparent cross-reactions are commonly seen on routine patch testing (Table 7.5.3), notably with perfume (Cronin 1980). It is a relatively important sensitizer in children (Fregert & Moller 1963). Contact urticaria has also been reported (Warin & Smith 1982).

Collins F.W. & Mitchell J.C. (1975) Aroma chemicals. Reference sources for perfumes and flavour ingredients with special reference to cinnamic aldehyde. *Contact Dermatitis* **1**: 43.
Cronin E. (1980) *Contact Dermatitis*. Churchill Livingstone, Edinburgh.
Fisher A.A. (1974) The chemical significance of positive patch test reactions to balsam of Peru. *Cutis* **13**: 909.
Fregert S. & Moller H. (1963) Contact allergy to balsam of Peru in children. *British Journal of Dermatology* **75**: 218–20.
Hjorth N. (1961) *Eczematous Allergy to Balsams*. Munksgaard, Copenhagen.
Olholm-Larsen O. & Heydenreich G. (1976) Allergy to balsam of Peru and wood tars: an increasing problem? *Contact Dermatitis* **2**: 293–4.
Warin R.P. & Smith R.J. (1982) Chronic urticaria: investigations with patch and challenge tests. *Contact Dermatitis* **8**: 117–21.

Saxifragaceae

TOLMIEA menziesii

Common name: Pick-a-back plant
Distribution: Northwest America, a common foliage house plant
Patch test: ? Leaf as is

This dwarf plant (Fig. 7.5.21) is hardy, but it is often grown as a house plant in Europe. It forms rosettes of jagged-edged leaves which are brown and green. New plants are formed on the edge of the stolons, like strawberry plants.

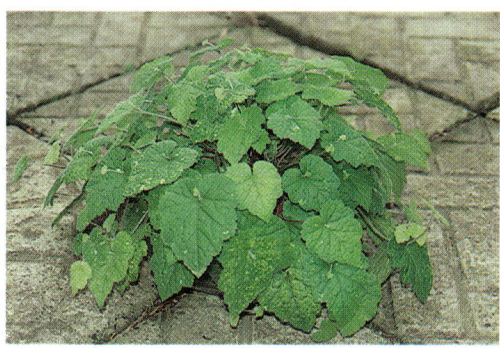

Fig. 7.5.21 *Tolmiea menziesii* (the pick-a-back plant); small plantlets develop on the leaf surfaces. (Grown by Ian & Mary Silcox.)

This endears it to amateur plant propagators and the plant appears frequently on produce stalls at fetes. It is probably a rare sensitizer, although Hjorth (1969) observed four positive patch tests in 93 cases of plant dermatitis. There is one well-documented case of allergic contact dermatitis on an elderly woman who developed a vascular eruption on the hands, followed by pruritus and erythema of eyelids and neck, only in the summer months. A patch test was positive but negative in controls (Calnan 1969). It may well be an under-reported sensitizer.

Calnan C.D. (1969) *Tolmiea menziesii*. *Contact Dermatitis Newsletter* **5**: 98.
Hjorth N. (1969) Plant dermatitis. *Contact Dermatitis Newsletter* **6**: 126.

Hydrangeaceae

HYDRANGEA MACROPHYLLA

Common name: Hydrangea (German: Hortensia)

Distribution: Far East and America, many species are very popular garden shrubs
Patch test: Hydrangea leaf as is (hydrangenol 0.1% pet.)

Although several species of *Hydrangea* are in cultivation in specialist collections, *H. macrophylla* (Fig. 7.5.22) is most widely grown. It appears to be a rare cause of allergic contact dermatitis, although it may be under-reported (Kuligowski *et al.* 1992). The flower

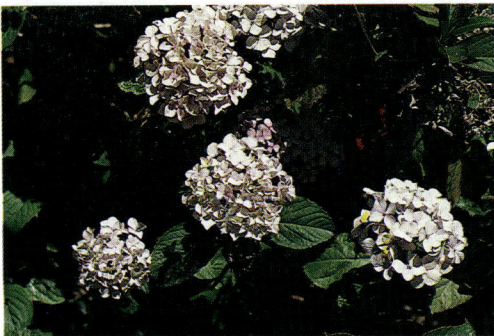

Fig. 7.5.22 *Hydrangea macrophylla.*

colour is deep pink, blue, white or an intermediate shade depending on soil pH and trace elements. An unconfirmed case of dermatitis was reported in 1926 (Broers 1926) and there have been sporadic cases subsequently confirmed by patch testing (Apted 1973, Burry *et al.* 1973, Hausen *et al.* 1982, Bruynzeel 1991). The hands are chiefly affected. The principal allergen appears to be hydrangenol (**7.VIII**), an isocoumarin (Schmalle *et al.* 1982, Hausen 1991). Affected individuals are usually professional gardeners, flower arrangers and nursery workers, and repeated exposure is probably necessary. A patient reported by Bruynzeel (1986) was also allergic to tulipalin A. A nursery gardener with hydrangea sensitivity was able to continue his work with the plants for 4 years by wearing rubber gloves (Meijer *et al.* 1990).

Apted J.H. (1973) Phytodermatitis from hydrangea. *Archives of Dermatology* **108**: 427.
Broers J.H. (1926) Beruflich erworbene Haut veran derungen. In Oppenheim M., Rille J.H. & Ullmann K. (eds) *Die Schadigungen der Haut durch Beruf und gewerbliche Arbeit*. Bdz Leipzig: Voss. Band **11**: 548.
Bruynzeel D.P. (1986) Allergic contact dermatitis to Hydrangea. *Contact Dermatitis* **14**: 128.
Bruynzeel D.P. (1991) Contact dermatitis from hydrangea (Letter). *Contact Dermatitis* **24**: 78.
Burry J.N., Kirk J., Reid J.G. & Turner T. (1973) Environmental dermatitis; patch tests in 1000 cases of allergic contact dermatitis. *Medical Journal of Australia* **11**: 681–5.
Hausen B.M. (1991) Hydrangenol, a strong contact sensitizer found in hydrangea (*Hydrangea* sp.; Hydrangeaceae). *Contact Dermatitis* **24**: 233–5.
Hausen B.M., Baurle L. & Schmalle H.W. (1982) Hortensienallergie. *Aktuelle Dermatologie* **8**: 141–5.
Kuligowski M.E., Chang A. & Leemreize J.H.M. (1992) Allergic contact hand dermatitis from Hydrangea: report of a 10th case. *Contact Dermatitis* **26**: 269–70.
Meijer P., Coenraads P.J. & Hausen B.M. (1990) Allergic contact dermatitis from hydrangea. *Contact Dermatitis* **23**: 59–60.
Schmalle H.W., Jarchow O.H., Hausen B.M. & Schulz K.H. (1982) 3,4-Dihydro-8-hydroxy-3-(4-hydroxyphenyl)isocoumarin, hydrangenol. *Acta Crystallographica, section B* **38**: 2938–41.

Hamamelidaceae

LIQUIDAMBAR orientalis

Common name: Storax (in part)
Distribution: Asia Minor
Patch test: Balsam of Peru. Perfume series

The gum storax (liquid storax) is obtained mostly from this deciduous tree, which has downy fragrant palm-like leaves and inconspicuous greenish-yellow flowers. The gum is used in perfumery and may cause allergic sensitization (Hjorth 1961). Storax of antiquity was derived from the unrelated genus, *Styrax officinalis* (q.v.).

Hjorth N. (1961) Eczematous allergy to balsams. *Acta Dermato-Venereologica* **41** (suppl. 46): 1–211.

Hydrangenol (5,4-dihydro-8 hydroxy-3-(4-hydroxyphenol)

7.VIII

Myrtaceae

MELALEUCA

Common names: Paper-bark. Cajuput. Tea-tree
Distribution: Australia
Patch test: Cajuput oil 2% pet. Niaouli oil 2% pet.

These shrubs or small trees mostly have a white bark which peels off in thin sheets. Several species are irritant. Cajuput oil is derived from twigs and fresh leaves of *M. leucadendron* (Fig. 7.5.23). It is used as a rubefacient, in aromatherapy and as a parasiticide in human and veterinary practice (Windholz *et al.* 1983). Tea-tree oil is gaining favour, particularly in Australia as a treatment for acne (Bassett *et al.* 1990).

This species is listed as a cause of dermatitis in Florida and Hawaii (Lampe 1986) and flowering specimens may even cause airborne contact dermatitis (Morton 1971). Oil of niaouli is derived from *M. viridiflora*.

Allergic dermatitis has been reported in a patient who applied a purified form of this oil (gomenol) (Sezary & Horowitz 1935). Both oils contain similar terpenes to those found in eucalyptus oil, and may cross-react. Again, most cutaneous reactions appear to be irritant (Greenberg & Lester 1954).

Bassett I.B., Pannowitz D.L. & Barretson R.St.C. (1990) A comparative study of tea-tree oil versus benzoyl peroxide in the treatment of acne. *Medical Journal of Australia* **153**: 455–8.
Greenberg L.A. & Lester D. (1954) *Handbook of Cosmetic Materials*. Interscience, New York.
Lampe K.F. (1986) Dermatitis-producing plants of south Florida and Hawaii. *Clinics in Dermatology* **4**: 83–93.
Morton J.F. (1971) *Plants Poisonous to People in Florida and Other Warm Areas.* (privately printed by) Hurricane House Publishers Inc., Miami, Florida.
Sézary A. & Horowitz A. (1935) Intolerance cutanée (eczema artificiel) au gomerol. *Bulletin de la Société Française de Dermatologie et Syphilologie* **42**: 425.
Windholz M., Budavari S., Blumetti R.F. & Otterbein E.S. (1983) *The Merck Index: An Encyclopedia of Chemicals, Drugs and Biologicals*. Merck & Co Inc., Rahway, NJ.

EUCALYPTUS

Common names: Eucalypt. Blue gum
Distribution: Chiefly Australia. A few species planted and naturalized in other temperate zones
Patch test: Eucalyptus oil 2% pet.

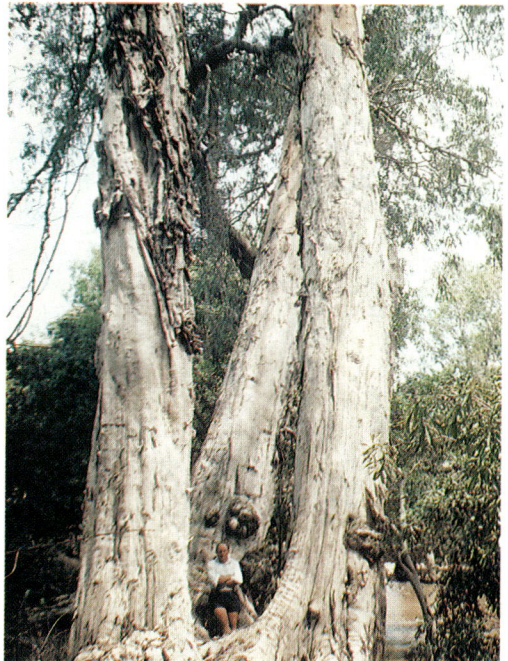

Fig. 7.5.23 *Melaleuca leucadendron*, McLeod's River, Australia. (Courtesy of T.R.N. Lothian.)

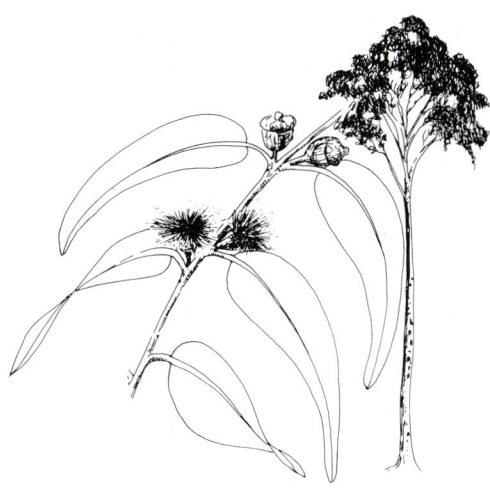

Fig. 7.5.24 *Eucalyptus* species.

Table 7.5.4 Uses of oil of cloves and types of eruption produced.

Baking	Hand dermatitis (Malten 1979)
Perfumes	May be irritant (Greenberg & Lester 1954)
Lipsticks	Cheilitis and stomatitis (Sulzberger & Goodman 1938)
Soaps	Dermatitis of hands and face (Sternberg 1937)
Clove cigarettes	A possible source of exposure (JAMA 1988)
Dentistry	Hand dermatitis (Koch et al. 1971 & 1973)

Gum trees (Fig. 7.5.24) are a familiar feature of the Australian bush, and they have been a source of inspiration to landscape painters such as Hans Heysen. Many species are distinguished by their bark, which may be deciduous, peeling off the trunk in strips, rough and fissured, rope-like (stringy) or scaly. The leaves are leathery, usually oval or lance-shaped and possess a resinous smell. *Eucalyptus globulus* in particular is the source of eucalyptus oil, which was distilled from the leaves. Most oil is now prepared synthetically. It is used medicinally as an inhalant, insect repellent or rubefacient. Although the oil is irritant, allergic sensitization has been reported following its application for soft tissue rheumatism (Löwenfeld 1932) and in food preparation (Peltonen et al. 1985). The wood of several species is durable and used for furniture, flooring, etc. It may cause contact dermatitis and an erythema multiforme-like eruption in carpenters and sawyers (Holst et al. 1976). The sensitizer is unknown.

7.IX Allergens in clove oil.

tree, cloves (Fig. 7.5.25), are used extensively in cooking and confectionery. Oil of cloves is derived by distillation of the buds and has numerous uses, several of which may lead to contact dermatitis (Table 7.5.4). The principal allergens are eugenol and isoeugenol (**7.IX**). Cross-reactions may occur with balsam of Peru (Hjorth 1961). Patch test reactions to cloves are commoner in individuals who react to fragrance mix (van den Akker et al. 1990).

Greenberg L.A. & Lester D. (1954) *Handbook of Cosmetic Materials*. Interscience, New York.
Hjorth N. (1961) Eczematous allergy to balsams. *Acta Dermato-Venereologica* (Suppl. 46): 1–216.
JAMA (1988) Council on scientific affairs. Evaluation of the health hazard of clove cigarettes. *JAMA* **260**: 3641–4.
Koch G., Magnusson B. & Nyquist G. (1971) Contact allergy to medicaments and material used in dentistry. *Odontological Review* **22**: 275.

Holst R., Kirby J. & Magnusson B. (1976) Sensitization to tropical woods giving erythema multiforme-like eruptions. *Contact Dermatitis* **2**: 295.
Löwenfeld W. (1932) Ekzematose Überempfindlichkeit gegen Eukalyptus Öl. *Dermatologische Wochenschrift* **95**: 1281.
Peltonen L., Wickström G. & Vaahtoranta M. (1985) Occupational dermatoses in the food industry. *Dermatosen* **33**: 166–9.

SYZYGIUM aromaticum (EUGENIA aromatica)

Common name: Clove
Distribution: Moluccan islands. Widely cultivated in tropical Africa and adjoining islands
Patch test: Clove oil 1% pet.

The aromatic dried flower buds of this small

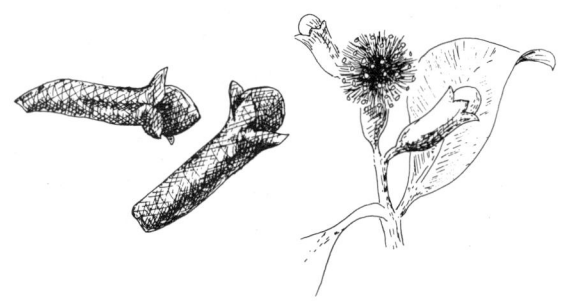

Fig. 7.5.25 Cloves.

Koch G., Magnusson B. & Nyquist G. (1973) Sensitivity to eugenol and colophony. *Odontological Review* **24**: 109.

Malten K.E. (1979) Four bakers showing positive patch tests to a number of fragrance materials which can be used as flavors. *Acta Dermato-Venereologica* **59** (suppl. 85): 117–21.

Sternberg L. (1937) Contact dermatitis cases caused by oil of cloves and by oil of camomile tea *Anthemis cotula*. *Journal of Allergy* **8**: 185–6.

Sulzberger M.B. & Goodman J. (1938) Acquired specific hypersensitivity to simple chemicals. *Archives of Dermatology and Syphilology* **37**: 597–615.

Van den Akker T.W., Roesyanto-Mahadi I.D., van Toorenenbergen A.W. & van Joost T.H. (1990) Contact allergy to spices. *Contact Dermatitis* **22**: 267–72.

Lecythidaceae

BERTHOLLETIA excelsa

Common name: Brazil nut
Distribution: Tropical South America, West Indies
Patch test: Paring of nut (as is)

The Brazil nut (Fig. 7.5.26) is a recognized cause of contact urticaria (p. 36). Delayed hypersensitivity has also been recorded in operators in a candy factory, who developed dermatitis after handling the nuts (Markson 1942).

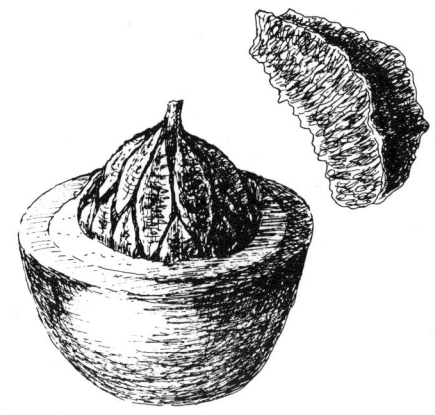

Fig. 7.5.26 Brazil nuts. Several nuts interlock in one fruit.

Markson L.S. (1942) Dermatitis from seed and oil of *Bertholletia excelsa* (Brazil nut). *Archives of Dermatology and Syphilology* **46**: 831–2.

Lythraceae

LAWSONIA inermis (*L. alba*)

Common name: Henna
Distribution: Tropical Africa, India. Naturalized, especially in India, North America and Sri Lanka
Patch test: Henna as is (lawsone 10% ethanol)

Henna, derived from the dried leaves, has been used as a red dye since ancient times. In tropical Asia, it is used to dye fingernails (Daniel & Osment 1982) but in the West is widely used as a hair dye. Considering this wide usage, cutaneous reactions are very rare and some cases of allergic contact dermatitis are more probably due to paraphenylenedramine, widely used in hair dyes (Greenberg & Lester 1954). Reactions suggestive of delayed hypersensitivity were reported by Pasricha *et al.* (1980), after henna leaves were applied as a compress to the skin. Similar cases were reported by Gupta *et al.* (1986) and Nigam and Saxena (1988). The allergen is a quinone, lawsone (2-hydroxy-1,4-naphthoquinone). Type I reactions may be severe (see p. 38).

Daniel C.R. & Osment L.S. (1982) Nail pigmentation abnormalities: their importance and proper examination. *Cutis* **2**: 348–60.

Greenberg L.A. & Lester D. (1954) *Handbook of Cosmetic Materials*. Interscience, New York.

Gupta B.N., Mathur A.K., Agarwal L. & Singh A. (1986) Contact sensitivity to henna. *Contact Dermatitis* **15**: 303–4.

Nigam P.K. & Saxena A.K. (1988) Allergic contact dermatitis to henna. *Contact Dermatitis* **18**: 55–6.

Pasricha J.S., Gupta R. & Panjwani S. (1980) Contact dermatitis to henna (*Lawsonia*). *Contact Dermatitis* **6**: 288–9.

Begoniaceae

BEGONIA

Several members of this attractive genus are irritant, notably the handsome foliage species, *Begonia rex*. However, one patch test to this species was considered to be a true allergic reaction (Agrup 1969).

Agrup G. (1969) Hand eczema and other dermatoses in South Sweden. *Acta Dermato-Venereologica* **49** (Suppl. 61): 1–91.

Table 7.5.5 Allergic reactions to members of the Umbelliferae.

Species	Common name	Comments & references
Anethum graveolens	Dill	Positive patch test in a sandwich maker (Hjorth & Weisman 1972)
Angelica spp.	Angelica	Used in Chinese medicine and perfumery. Contact sensitivity to root (Larsen 1975)
Apium graveolens	Celery	(Agrup 1969) Celery oil may sensitize (Gelfand 1936)
Carum carvi	Caraway	Major source of carvone (Hjorth 1967)
Centella asiatica (see text)		
Coriandrum sativum	Coriander	Seeds yield oil of coriander which may cause stomatitis (Loveman 1938)
Daucus carota v. sativa	Carrot (see text)	
Foeniculum vulgare	Fennel	Source of oil of anise (Loveman 1938)
Levisticum officinalis	Lovage root	Allergic dermatitis in a lab technician after making extracts and cleaning out vats of oil (Calnan 1969)
Opopanax spp.	Sweet myrrh (in part)	Gum opopanax used in perfumery. Six patients had positive patch tests, out of 11 sensitive to balsam of Peru (Hjorth 1961)
Pastinaca sativa	Parsnip	(Picardo et al. 1986)
Petroselinum crispum	Parsley	Dermatitis in sandwich maker (Hjorth & Weisman 1972, Stransky et al. 1980)
Pimpinella anisum	Aniseed	Major source of oil of anise (Hjorth 1967) which contains 90% anethole (**7.V**), a probable sensitizer (Loveman 1938). Oil of anise in lipstick may cause cheilitis (Zakon et al. 1947)

Umbelliferae

The allergic potential of many genera is overshadowed by their ability to cause florid phototoxic reactions (Chapter 6). The family includes many important vegetables and herbs, several of which are implicated in allergic contact dermatitis (see Table 7.5.5). The seeds of many species (notably caraway) contain D-carvone (**7.X**), an aromatic substance which has caused allergic dermatitis when used in toothpaste (Hjorth 1967). Allergic contact and photocontact dermatitis has been reported due to psoralens (Takashima et al. 1991).

Agrup G. (1969) Hand eczema and other hand dermatoses in south Sweden. *Acta Dermato-Venereologica* **49** (Suppl. 61): 1–91.
Calnan C.D. (1969) Lovage sensitivity. *Contact Dermatitis Newsletter* **5**: 99.
Gelfand H.H. (1936) Hypersensitiveness to celery. *Journal of Allergy* **7**: 590–3.
Hjorth N. (1961) *Eczematous Allergy to Balsams*. Munksgaard, Copenhagen.
Hjorth N. (1967) Toothpaste sensitivity. *Contact Dermatitis Newsletter* **1**: 14.
Hjorth N. & Weisman K. (1972) Occupational dermatitis in chefs and sandwich makers. *Contact Dermatitis Newsletter* **11**: 306.
Larsen W.G. (1975) Cosmetic dermatitis due to a perfume. *Contact Dermatitis* **1**: 142.
Loveman A.B. (1938) Stomatitis venenata. *Archives of Dermatology and Syphilology* **37**: 70.
Picardo M., Cristaudo A. & de Luca C. (1986) Contact

D-carvone

7.X

dermatitis to *Pastinaca sativa*. *Contact Dermatitis* **15**: 98–9.
Stransky L. & Tsankov N. (1980) Contact dermatitis from parsley (*Petroselinum*). *Contact Dermatitis* **6**: 233–4.
Takashima A., Yamamoto K., Kimura S., Takakuwa Y. & Mizuno N. (1991) Allergic contact and photocontact dermatitis due to psoralens in patients with psoriasis treated with topical PUVA. *British Journal of Dermatology* **124**: 37–42.
Zakon S.L., Goldbert A.L. & Kahn J.B. (1947) Lipstick cheilitis: common dermatitis. Report of 22 cases. *Archives of Dermatology and Syphilology* **56**: 499–505.

CENTELLA asiatica (HYDROCOTYLE asiatica)

Distribution: Asia

The fresh and dried leaves and stems of this species are extracted to produce Madecassol. This preparation has been used by dermatologists and plastic surgeons in Korea to promote wound healing and to prevent keloids. It is available in Europe (including Britain) as a 1% ointment or 2% powder to promote wound healing (Eun & Lee 1985). It is applied topically to broken areas of skin, including leg ulcers, graft sites and scars. There are several reports of sensitivity to this, and similar preparations (Huriez & Martin 1969, Santucci et al. 1985, Vena & Angelini 1986, Izu et al. 1992). The potential allergens include madecassic acid, asiatic acid and asiaticoside (Huriez & Martin 1969). Propylene glycol may contribute to the irritancy of Madecassol ointment (Eun & Lee 1985).

Eun H.C. & Lee A.Y. (1985) Contact dermatitis due to Madecassol. *Contact Dermatitis* **13**: 310–11.
Huriez C.L. & Martin P. (1969) L'allergie de contact a l'asiaticoside. *Giornale Ital Dermatol* **44**: 463–4.
Izu R., Aguirre A., Gil N. & Diaz-Perez J.L. (1992) Allergic contact dermatitis from a cream containing *Centella asiatica* extract. *Contact Dermatitis* **26**: 192–3.
Santucci B., Picardo M. & Cristaudo A. (1985) Contact dermatitis due to Centelase®. *Contact Dermatitis* **13**: 39.
Vena G.A. & Angelini G. (1986) Contact allergy to Centelase. *Contact Dermatitis* **15**: 108–9.

DAUCUS carota vars

Common name: Carrot

Distribution: Temperate areas. Several cultivated forms
Patch test: Carrot as is

Dermatitis from carrots particularly affects individuals working in canning factories. It is chiefly localized to the hands (Klauder & Kimmich 1956) although the face, neck and forearms may also be affected (Vickers 1941). Sinha *et al.* (1977) noted positive patch test reactions to carrot in food handlers with fingertip dermatitis. Allergic reactions to carrot have been reported in two housewives with hand dermatitis. Methanol and ethanol extracts were positive, as was an eluate from reverse-phase HPLC (high pressure liquid chromatography) (Foulds & Sadhra 1990). *Daucus carota* contains falcarinol, an allergen also present in ivy (*Hedera helix*) (Hansen *et al.* 1986).

Foulds I. & Sadhra S. (1990) Allergic contact dermatitis from carrots (meeting extract). *Contact Dermatitis* **23**: 261.
Hansen L., Hammershøy O. & Boll P.M. (1986) Allergic contact dermatitis from falcarinol isolated from *Schefflera arboricola*. *Contact Dermatitis* **14**: 91–3.
Klauder J.V. & Kimmich J.M. (1956) Sensitization dermatitis to carrots. *Archives of Dermatology* **74**: 149–58.
Sinha S.M., Pasricha J.S., Sharma R.C. & Kandhari K.C. (1977) Vegetables responsible for contact dermatitis of the hands. *Archives of Dermatology* **113**: 776–9.
Vickers H.R. (1941) The carrot as a cause of dermatitis. *British Journal of Dermatology* **53**: 52–7.

Araliaceae

HEDERA HELIX

Common names: *H. helix* ssp. *helix* — ivy, English ivy (USA). *H. helix* ssp. *canariensis* — Canary Island ivy, Algerian ivy (USA)
Distribution: Temperate Old World in woods and hedgerows. Commonly grown as a wall climber or ground cover
Patch test: Leaf as is (falcarinol ? 0.1% pet.)

Hedera is the only member of the family which is native to Britain. It is a woody evergreen plant which is very common, found scrambling over rocks and through hedges or climbing up trees and walls. The type species,

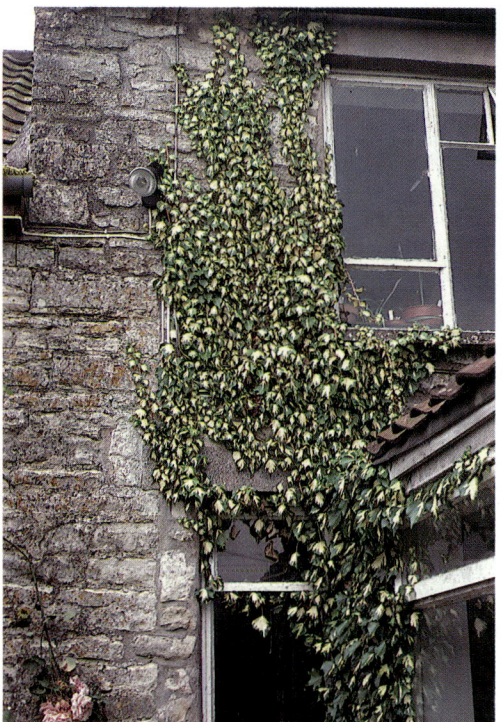

Fig. 7.5.27 *Hedera helix* 'Gold Heart'.

Table 7.5.6 Although popularly called 'ivy' the following species are unrelated.

Devil's ivy	*Scindapsus aureus*
German ivy	*Senecio mikanoides*
Grape ivy	*Rhoicissus rhomboidea*
Ground ivy	*Glechoma hederacea*
Poison ivy	*Toxicodendron* spp.

berries. Several unrelated plants are given the common name 'ivy' (Table 7.5.6). The berries and leaves are poisonous, although death has not been reported. Extracts of the plant have been used medicinally as tonics and expectorants and are applied to bruises. Culpeper states that 'the fresh leaves boiled in wine, and old filthy ulcers hard to be cured washed therewith, do wonderfully help to cleanse them'. 'Helancyl' cream contains ivy extract and is claimed to 'remove disadvantageous curves in females' (Gafner *et al.* 1988).

H. helix ssp. *helix*, has five-lobed glossy green leaves (Fig. 7.5.27) with slight veining. Variegated cultivars of *H. helix* ssp. *helix* (including 'gold heart') and *H. helix canariensis*, which has trilobed leaves (Fig. 7.5.28), are grown on house walls and as pot plants. All forms of the species are vigorous and need regular pruning. The flowers, seen chiefly in the wild in late autumn, are yellowish-green, held in groups of almost globular umbels, followed by black globular

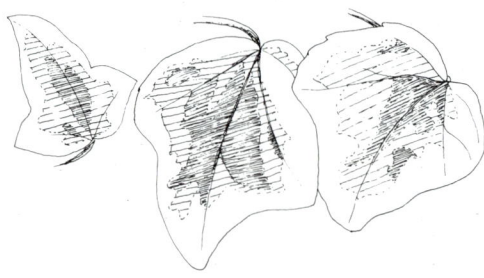

Fig. 7.5.28 Leaves of *Hedera helix* ssp. *canariensis*.

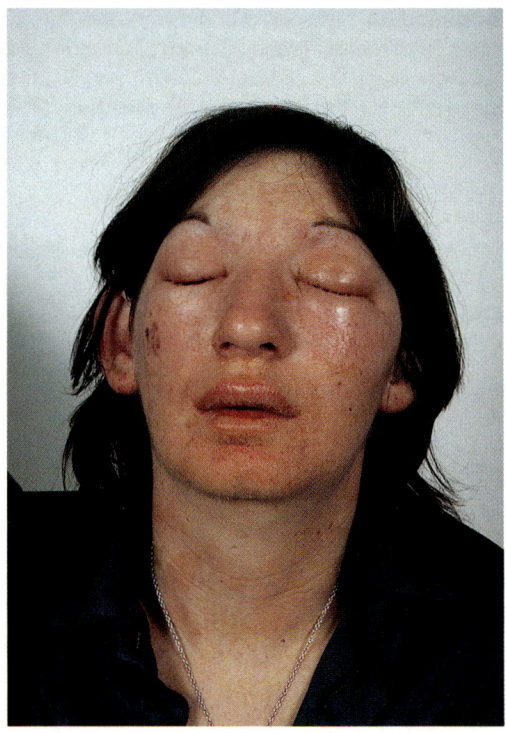

Fig. 7.5.29 Allergic contact dermatitis from ivy. (Courtesy of Dr J. Boyle.)

Dermatitis (Fig. 7.5.29), both irritant and allergic, has been reported from both *Hedera helix* ssp. *helix* and ssp. *canariensis* (Calnan 1981a, Boyle & Harman 1985, Hausen *et al.* 1987), usually after pruning the plants in spring, or in children who climb walls or trees covered with ivy (Massmanian *et al.* 1988). Patch tests with both sub-species are positive in the majority of patients. Cross-reaction has been reported with *Brassaia (Schefflera) actinophylla*, the 'Queensland umbrella tree' (Mitchell 1981). Detailed studies by Hausen *et al.* (1987) have revealed that two fractions derived from a short ether extract of ivy are both irritant and sensitizing. The major allergen is falcarinol (heptadeca-1,9-diene-4,6-diyne-3-ol) which sensitizes guinea pigs at a concentration of only 0.03% (**7.XI**). The second, didehydrofalcarinol, is a weaker sensitizer (1% required in guinea pig testing).

7.XI Allergens in ivy.

The concentrations of these two antigens vary during the season and are affected by other variables such as climate and soil. Falcarinone, a ketone oxidation product of falcarinol, is detected in *H. helix* among other members of the Araliaceae (Hansen & Boll 1986). Its role as a sensitizer in ivy dermatitis is unproven. Falcarinols are found in other members of the Araliaceae — including *Schefflera arboricola* (q.v.). Both falcarinol and falcarinone are found in members of the carrot and celery family (Umbelliferae). The concentration of falcarinol is increased in celery root when plants are grown in soil infected with *Fusarium*, an important fungal disease of root vegetables, suggesting that falcarinol may have an antifungal action.

SCHEFFLERA actinophylla

Common name: Umbrella tree
Distribution: Australasia, a common foliage house plant

This attractive shrub is a popular 'green' plant for houses and offices. The deep glossy leaves are divided into up to five narrow, oval pointed leaflets (Fig. 7.5.30). The stem eventually reaches a height of 2.5 m. Calnan (1981b) and Hammershøy (1981) report allergic contact dermatitis due to this plant. Cross-reaction occurs with *Hedera helix* (see above) (Mitchell 1981) and falcarinols have been isolated from *S. arboricola* (Hansen & Boll 1986a, b, Hansen *et al.* 1986).

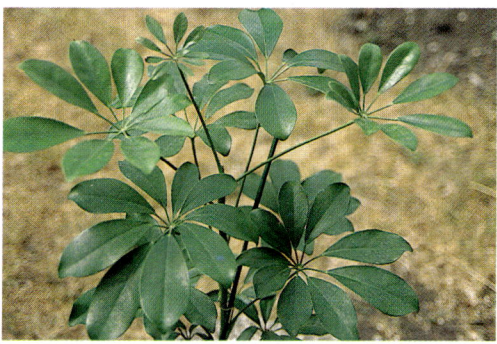

Fig. 7.5.30 *Schefflera actinophylla*, a popular foliage house plant.

Boyle J. & Harman R.R.M. (1985) Contact dermatitis to *Hedera helix* (common ivy). *Contact Dermatitis* **12**: 111–12.
Calnan C.D. (1981a) Dermatitis from ivy *Hedera canariensis variegata*. *Contact Dermatitis* **7**: 124.
Calnan C.D. (1981b) Dermatitis from *Schefflera*. *Contact Dermatitis* **7**: 341.
Gafner F., Epstein W., Reynolds G. & Rodriguez E. (1988) Human maximization test of falcarinol, the principal contact allergen of English ivy and Algerian ivy (*Hedera helix, H. canariensis*). *Contact Dermatitis* **19**: 125–8.
Hammershøy O. (1981) Allergic contact dermatitis from *Schefflera*. *Contact Dermatitis* **7**: 57–8.
Hansen L. & Boll P.M. (1986a) Polyacetylenes in Araliaceae: their chemistry, biosynthesis and biological significance. *Phytochemistry* **25**: 285–93.

Hansen L. & Boll P.M. (1986b) Polyacetylenic falcarinol as the major allergen in *Schefflera arboricola*. *Phytochemistry* **25**: 529–30.

Hansen L., Hammershøy O. & Boll P.M. (1986) Allergic contact dermatitis from falcarinol isolated from *Schefflera arboricola*. *Contact Dermatitis* **14**: 91–3.

Hausen B.M., Brohan J., Konig W.A., Faasch H., Hahn H. & Bruhn G. (1987) Allergic and irritant contact dermatitis from falcarinol and didehydrofalcarinol in common ivy (*Hedera helix* L.). *Contact Dermatitis* **17**: 1–9.

Massmanian A., Valcuende Cavero F., Ramirez Bosca A. & Castells Rodellas A. (1988) Contact dermatitis from variegated ivy (*Hedera helix* subsp. *canariensis* Willd). *Contact Dermatitis* **18**: 247–8.

Mitchell J.C. (1981) ACD from *Hedera helix* and *Brassaia actinophylla* (Araliaceae). *Contact Dermatitis* **7**: 158–9.

Rubiaceae

This family, of mostly tropical genera, includes several species of economic and medical importance. The root of *Cephaelis ipecacuanha* yields the familiar emetic. Its properties are due to the alkaloid, emetine. Pharmacists are at risk of an irritant papulopustular eruption after handling ipecacuanha powder (Mitchell & Rook 1979).

The bark of the Andean tree *Cinchona* sp. yields several alkaloids including quinine, a familiar cause of fixed drug eruption. Allergic reactions to quinine appear to be increasingly rare; a 2% aqueous solution is suitable for patch testing (Calnan & Caron 1961).

Several species of *Coffea*, notably *C. arabica* (Fig. 7.5.31), are cultivated as a source of coffee beans, chiefly in Africa but also in Central America. Operatives sorting, roasting and milling are at risk of dermatitis and respiratory symptoms, including an allergic alveolitis (Morgan & Seaton 1975). Recently finger and palm dermatitis has been described on a coffee bar worker, whose symptoms worsened when preparing espresso coffee; a patch test was positive to coffee powder and the drink, negative on 20 controls (Piraccini *et al.* 1990). Green coffee beans appear to be more allergenic than the final product; presumably some allergens are lost during roasting (Leher *et al.* 1978). Coffee dermatitis in the consumer is rare, although cheilitis (Lupton 1953) and mucosal contact dermatitis (Sonnex *et al.* 1981) have been recorded. In the latter case, a positive patch test was obtained with the coffee.

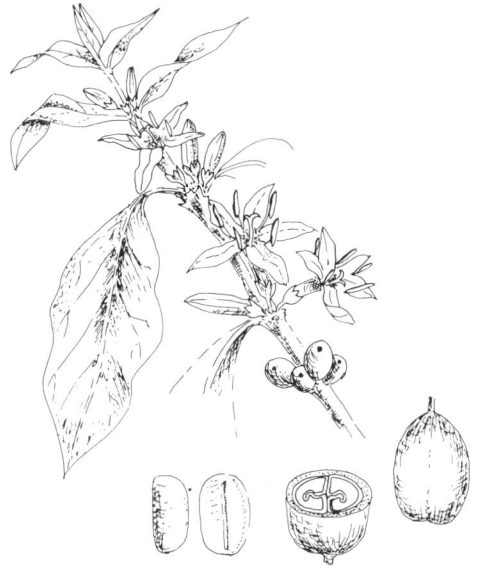

Fig. 7.5.31 *Coffea arabica* (the coffee plant).

Gardenia jasminoides (*G. florida*) is a beautiful greenhouse shrub, native to Japan, China and Taiwan. The leaves are dark green, glossy, long oval. The waxy white flowers, up to 8 cm diameter, are sweetly perfumed. A double-flowered form is sometimes grown. The petals are added to flavour tea — 'jasmine tea'. Powdered gardenia fruits are used as a folk remedy, applied to bruises. This caused allergic contact dermatitis in a male patient; patch tests were positive, using the fruit and pericarp (fruit wall) and an ethanol extract. The allergen is unknown, although the fruit contains iridoid-glucosides, carotenoids, flavonoids, mannitol and β-sitosterol (Kubo *et al.* 1990).

The root of *Rubia tinctoria*, madder (Fig. 7.5.32), yields alizarin, recorded as a sensitizer (Greenberg & Lester 1954). Madder was previously used as a red pigment, notably to dye French military uniforms. In two women who developed dermatitis after weeding madder, one patient was positive on patch testing with the root (Castelain & Ducombs 1988).

Calnan C.D. & Caron G.A. (1961) Quinine sensitivity. *British Medical Journal* **2**: 1750.

Castelain M. & Ducombs G. (1988) Contact dermatitis from madder. *Contact Dermatitis* **19**: 228–9.

Greenberg L.A. & Lester D. (1954) *Handbook of Cosmetic Materials*. Interscience, New York.

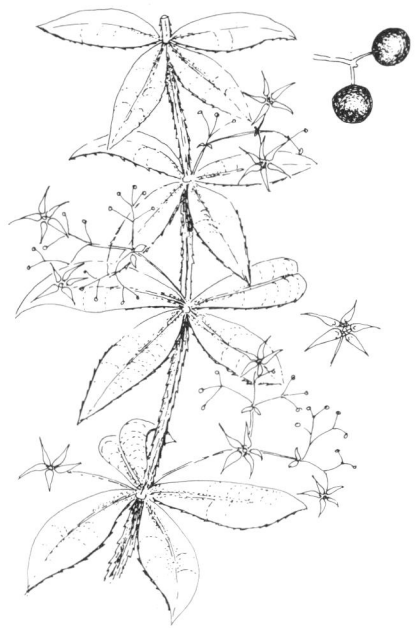

Fig. 7.5.32 *Rubia tinctoria* (madder).

Kubo Y., Nonaka S. & Yoshida M. (1990) Allergic contact dermatitis from gardenia fruit. *Contact Dermatitis* **22**: 65–7.

Leher S.B., Karr R.M. & Salvaggio J.E. (1978) Extraction and analysis of coffee bean allergens. *Clinical Allergy* **89**: 217–26.

Lupton E.S. (1953) Cheilitis due to coffee. *Archives of Dermatology and Syphilology* **68**: 333–4.

Mitchell T. & Rook A. (1979) *Botanical Dermatology*. Greengrass, Vancouver.

Morgan W.K.C. & Seaton A. (1975) *Occupational Lung Diseases*. Saunders, Philadelphia.

Piraccini B.M., Bardazzi F., Vincenzi C. & Tardio, M.P. (1990) Occupational contact dermatitis due to coffee. *Contact Dermatitis* **23**: 114.

Sonnex T.S., Dawber R.P.P. & Ryan T.J. (1981) Mucosal contact dermatitis due to instant coffee. *Contact Dermatitis* **7**: 298–300.

Compositae (Asteraceae)

The daisy family is one of the largest and most important in the plant kingdom. It includes many troublesome weeds (e.g. dandelion), ornamental annuals (e.g. sunflower) and herbaceous perennials, such as *Dahlia* and chrysanthemum; many species and cultivars are grown as pot plants or cut flowers. The family includes several vegetables, including lettuce, chicory and artichokes and herbs, including the chamomiles and tarragon. Many species are used in herbal medicine, notably feverfew (*Tanacetum parthenium*). The pot marigold (*Calendula*) is an ingredient of several herbal ointments used for eczema, and tincture of arnica is applied to bruises and wound swellings. In the past, many species were used industrially, e.g. *Carthamnus tinctorius*, the safflower, an inferior substitute for saffron. Pyrethrum (*Tanacetum cinerariifolium*) is still grown as a source of 'natural' insecticide.

Compositae are mostly herbaceous plants. The flower head (capitulum) is made up of numerous small flowers (florets), surrounded by bracts (the involucre). In some genera (e.g. *Taraxacum*, the dandelion), all the florets are similar. In many genera the flower head is divided into an inner 'disc' of short, tubular florets; the outer 'ray' florets are long and strap-like (e.g. the daisy, *Bellis perennis*).

Compositae are an important cause of dermatitis worldwide. Cultivation of the florist's chrysanthemum (X *Dendranthema* cultivars) is a major cause of allergic sensitization. Additionally, locally growing weeds can induce or elicit allergic reactions. The principal allergenic weeds in different regions of the world are summarized in Table 1.1.3. Contact with weeds may occur during many activities, including lawn-mowing and golfing. Many Compositae are aggressive invaders in the USA and Mexico, rapidly colonizing prairie and pastureland. *Parthenium hysterophorus*, an uncommon allergen in Texas, where it is native, was introduced accidentally to India where it has become a common weed, causing dermatitis of epidemic proportions.

Irritant dermatitis

Many members of the family can induce irritant reactions. These may be mechanical: several species, particularly thistles, possess sharp spines and others, notably the bur marigold (*Bidens tripartita*), have prickly or barbed fruits. A mechanical irritant dermatitis may be compounded by chemical irritancy and also allergenic reactions in susceptible individuals, e.g. Bindii (jo-jo) dermatitis in Australia, due to *Soliva pterosperma* (Commens *et al.* 1984). Some species, including dandelion, lettuce and chicory, possess a milky latex (sap). Thus, the mass production of chicory may cause irritant contact dermatitis due to sap exuding from the broken end of the chicon (Fig. 2.1.3) and Fig. 7.5.45 (Rycroft et al. 1987).

Contact urticaria
Several members of the family can cause hayfever via an IgE-mediated response due to water-soluble proteins in the pollen. Cutaneous Type I hypersensitivity is rarely reported, although it may be caused by salad plants such as lettuce in food handlers (Fregert & Sjoborg 1982, Krook 1977). Ingestion of food products containing Compositae pollen, e.g. honey, can cause angio-oedema (Bousquet et al. 1984). Cross-sensitivity does not occur between Type I and Type IV allergens (Wrangsjö et al. 1990).

Allergic contact dermatitis
This affects chiefly exposed areas such as the face, 'V' of the neck, forearms and hands. Although classically regarded as more prevalent in men, recent studies suggest an equal sex distribution (reviewed by Paulsen 1992). Airborne contact dermatitis is due to plant hairs or dust from dried plant material (Arlette & Mitchell 1981) or, in the case of *P. hysterophorus*, to pollen (Mitchell 1981). The allergens may be spread manually to other parts of the body by contaminated finger tips (Howell 1978). The clinical pattern differs from photosensitive eczema in that photoprotected areas, such as the eyelids, nasolabial folds and 'Wilkinson's triangle' (behind the ears), are involved in Compositae dermatitis (Figs 7.5.34, 7.5.46, 7.5.51, 7.5.60, 7.5.68). Early in the disease process acute exudative flares occur during the growing season but, with repeated exposure, they merge to produce a chronic lichenified dermatitis. Lichenification of flexures can mimic atopic eczema. Severely affected individuals may become erythrodermic and *P. hysterophorus* has been reported to cause death in India, due to intercurrent infection and respiratory complications (Lonkar et al. 1974). Other routes of sensitization or elicitation, of allergic contact dermatitis include ingestion (e.g. in herbal teas) or the use of plant extracts in ointments or in aromatherapy. Indirect contact via formites, such as a hat band (Shelmire 1946) may elicit dermatitis.

Photosensitivity and Compositae dermatitis
Chronic actinic dermatitis occurs typically in the middle-aged to elderly male. The clinical spectrum ranges from mild photosensitive eczema to 'actinic reticuloid', where lymphoma-like infiltration of the skin occurs in a light-exposed distribution. Several authors report an association with Compositae allergy (e.g. Hjorth et al. 1976). Frain-Bell et al. (1979) found nine out of 69 patients with this syndrome to be allergically sensitive to an oleo-resin extract of florist's chrysanthemum and 47 out of 55 to oleoresin extracts of several Compositae (Frain-Bell & Johnson 1979). Similarly, White et al. (1990), using the 0.1% sesquiterpene lactone mix (Ducombs et al. 1990), demonstrated an association between positive patch tests and abnormal monochromator readings, particularly in males.

Although airborne Compositae dermatitis may be associated with photosensitivity, compositae rarely cause photoallergic reactions and photosensitivity may be a non-specific consequence of bombardment with airborne allergens. One case of photosensitivity, to *P. hysterophorus*, has been reported by Bhutani and Rao (1978). However, the majority of individuals with airborne dermatitis to *P. hysterophorus* improve when removed from the allergen, even if they are still exposed to sunlight (Lonkar et al. 1974). The major allergens in Compositae, sesquiterpene lactones, are not photoactive, although several Compositae (notably *Tagetes*) contain polyacetylenes and their thiophene derivatives (Bohlmann et al. 1973, Towers et al. 1979). These could theoretically cause phototoxic reactions in humans.

The allergens
Sesquiterpene lactones, the predominant allergens in Compositae, are found especially in fragile hairs (trichomes). They are 15-carbon atom molecules in which a methylene group is attached to a lactone ring. Skeletons of important allergenic groups are shown (see **7.XII**. In general, the antigenic portion of the molecule is the α-methylene which is bonded

7.XII Typical sesquitepene lactones.

exocyclically to the γ-lactone ring (Mitchell 1970), although this is lacking in several allergenic sesquiterpene lactones (Hausen et al. 1985). Over 600 sesquiterpene lactones have been synthesized or extracted (Epstein et al. 1980). At least 50 are allergenic. As well as their widespread occurrence in Compositae, sesquiterpene lactones are found in other genera, notably *Frullania* (a liverwort), the tulip tree (*Liriodendron*, Magnoliaceae) and sweet bay (*Laurus nobilis*). Not surprisingly, cross-reaction can occur both within different Compositae and with these genera. Cross-sensitivity depends in part on the *cis*- or *trans*-configuration of the α-methylene ring junction (Schaeffer et al. 1990). The chemistry of allergenic sesquiterpene lactones has been studied in detail by Hausen and Benezra and colleagues (see Hausen et al. 1976 & 1985, Benezra et al. 1986, Schaeffer et al. 1990) and the allergenic molecules are illustrated by Evans and Schmidt (1980). The detailed function of these molecules is unclear, although alantolactone has an inhibitory effect on seed germination (Dalvi et al. 1971).

Patch testing
There is no ideal substance for patch testing for Compositae dermatitis. Where possible, it is desirable to include pollen, stems and leaves of the suspected plants, but beware of irritancy. Because many species share allergenic sesquiterpene lactones, a piece of chrysanthemum or feverfew (*Tanacetum parthenium*) leaf is often used as a simple screen. However, false negative results are likely. Formerly, a large series of ethanolic extracts chiefly of North American Compositae was supplied by Hollister–Stier International (Spokane, Washington, USA). Open testing often yielded false negative reactions and Hjorth et al. (1976) recommended their use in petrolatum as closed tests. Hausen (1977) describes a technique for extraction of sesquiterpene lactones using purified diethyl ether. The extract is then dried, evaporated and diluted 1% in petrolatum for patch testing (see also section 7.3). Alantolactone, the major sesquiterpene lactone in the elecampane (*Inula helenium*), is available commercially in 0.25%, although it can fail to detect allergy to several Compositae (Hjorth et al. 1976). In addition, it can actively sensitize and should not be used as a screening test (Aberer & Hausen 1990). Recently, a sesquiterpene lactone mix, a mixture of alantolactone, dehydrocostus lactone and costunolide (0.1% pet.) has been reported to be valuable in screening patients with suspected compositae dermatitis (Ducombs et al. 1990). Although it may fail to detect dermatitis due to some Compositae, such as dandelion (*Taraxacum officinale*) (Lovell & Rowan 1991), this mixture should be of considerable value. It will be available commercially by mid 1992. However if patch tests with the mixture are negative, the patient should be patch tested with suspected plant parts or extracts thereof. A careful history is essential in order to interpret the results.

Treatment of Compositae dermatitis
Avoidance of weeds is rarely practicable. Commercial or keen amateur chrysanthemum growers should be patch tested sequentially with a range of cultivars: many varieties are less likely to elicit allergic contact dermatitis. Topical or systemic corticosteroids are often of limited value (Lonkar et al. 1974). Sunscreens are helpful if there is associated photosensitivity. Roed-Petersen and Thomsen (1980) report good results following the use of azathioprine (100–150 mg a day) in two patients with photosensitivity associated with compositae allergy. These authors have used photochemotherapy (PUVA) in the summer months.

As in poison ivy dermatitis, oral hyposensitization has been attempted in patients with weed dermatitis (Shelmire 1940, Storrs et al. 1976). The oleoresin(s) must be taken daily in gradually increasing doses. Side-effects are common and include pruritus ani and a widespread eczematous or urticarial eruption. The treatment is thought to deplete memory T-cells (Srinivas et al. 1988). If the course of treatment is discontinued, sensitivity may rapidly recur. At present, this hazardous mode of therapy is of limited value and oleoresins should certainly not be used prophylactically.

Aberer W. & Hausen B.M. (1990) Active sensitisation to elecampane by patch testing with a crude plant extract. *Contact Dermatitis* **22**: 53–5.

Arlette J. & Mitchell J.C. (1981) Compositae dermatitis. *Contact Dermatitis* **7**: 129–36.

Benezra C. (1986) Molecular recognition patterns of sesquiterpene lactones in costus-sensitive patients. *Contact Dermatitis* **15**: 223–30.

Bhutani J.K. & Rao D.S. (1978) Photocontact dermatitis caused by *Parthenium hysterophorus*. *Dermatologica* **157**: 206–9.

Bohlmann F., Burkhardt T. & Zdero C. (1973) *Naturally Occurring Acetylenes*. Academic Press, London.

Bousquet J., Campos J. & Michel F.B. (1984) Food intolerance to honey. *Allergy* **39**: 73–5.

Commens C., McGeogh A.H. & Bartlett B. (1984) Bindii (jo-jo) dermatitis (*Soliva pterosperma* (Compositae)). *Journal of the American Academy of Dermatology* **10**: 768–73.

Dalvi R.R., Singh B. & Salunkie D.K. (1971) A study on phototoxicity of alantolactone. *Chemico-Biological Interactions* **3**: 13.

Ducombs G., Benezra C., Talaga P. et al. (1990) Patch testing with the 'sesquiterpene lactone mix'. *Contact Dermatitis* **22**: 249–52.

Epstein W.L., Reynolds G.W. & Rodriguez E. (1980) Sesquiterpene lactone dermatitis. Cross-sensitivity in costus-sensitised patients. *Archives of Dermatology* **116**: 59–60.

Evans F.J. & Schmidt R.J. (1980) Plants and plant products that induce contact dermatitis. *Planta Medica: Journal of Medicinal Plant Research* **38**: 289–316.

Frain-Bell W. & Johnson B.E. (1979). Contact allergic sensitivity to plants and the photosensitivity dermatitis and actinic reticuloid syndrome. *British Journal of Dermatology* **101**: 503–12.

Frain-Bell W., Hetherington A. & Johnson B.E. (1979) Contact allergic sensitivity to chrysanthemum and the photosensitivity dermatitis and actinic reticuloid syndrome. *British Journal of Dermatology* **101**: 491–501.

Fregert S. & Sjoborg S. (1982) Unsuspected lettuce: immediate allergy in a case of delayed metal allergy. *Contact Dermatitis* **8**: 265.

Hausen B.M. (1977) A simple method of extracting crude sesquiterpene lactones from Compositae plants for skin tests, chemical investigations and sensitizing experiments in guinea pigs. *Contact Dermatitis* **3**: 58–60.

Hausen B.M. (1985) Structure-activity aspects of 4 allergenic sesquiterpene lactones lacking the exocyclic alpha-methylene at the lactone ring. *Contact Dermatitis* **13**: 329–32.

Hausen B.M. & Schulz K.H. (1976) Chrysanthemum allergy III. Identification of the allergens. *Archives of Dermatological Research* **255**: 111–21.

Hjorth N., Roed-Petersen J. & Thomsen K. (1976) Airborne contact dermatitis from Compositae oleoresins simulating photodermatitis. *British Journal of Dermatology* **95**: 613–20.

Howell J.B. (1978) Contact dermatitis from weeds: facts and fallacies (letter). *Contact Dermatitis* **4**: 365–9.

Krook G. (1977) Occupational dermatitis from *Lactuca sativa* (lettuce) and *Cichorium* (endive); simultaneous occurrence of immediate and delayed allergy as a cause of CD. *Contact Dermatitis* **3**: 27–36.

Lonkar A., Mitchell J.C. & Calnan C.D. (1974) Contact dermatitis from *Parthenium hysterophorus*. *Transactions of the St John's Hospital Dermatological Society* **60**: 43–53.

Lovell C.R. & Rowan M. (1991) Dandelion dermatitis. *Contact Dermatitis* **25**: 185–8.

Mitchell J.C. (1970) Allergic contact dermatitis from *Frullania* and Compositae. The role of sesquiterpene lactones. *Journal of Investigative Dermatology* **54**: 233–9.

Mitchell J.C. (1981) *Parthenium* pollen — *Parthenium* dermatitis. *Contact Dermatitis* **7**: 212–17.

Paulsen E. (1992) Compositae dermatitis: a survey. *Contact Dermatitis* **26**: 76–86.

Roed-Petersen J. & Thomsen K. (1980) Azathioprin in treatment of airborne dermatitis from Compositae oleoresins and sensitivity to UVA. *Acta Dermato-Venereologica* **60**: 275–7.

Rycroft R.J.G., Lovell C.R., Harries P.G., Winter P. & Mallet A.I. (1987) Occupational irritant contact dermatitis from chicory. *Bollettino di Dermatologia Allergologica e Professionale* **2**: 77–82.

Schaeffer M., Talaga P., Stampf J.-L. & Benezra C. (1990) Cross-reaction in allergic contact dermatitis from α-methylene γ-butyrolactones; importance of the *cis* or *trans* ring junction. *Contact Dermatitis* **22**: 32–6.

Schmidt R.J. (1986) Compositae. In *Clinics in Dermatology*, 4, No. 2. J.B. Lippencott, Philadelphia, pp. 46–61.

Shelmire B. (1940) Contact dermatitis from vegetation. *Southern Medical Journal* **33**: 337–46.

Srinivas C.R., Krupashankar D.S., Singh K.K., Balachandran C. & Shenoi S.D. (1988) Oral hyposensitization in *Parthenium* dermatitis. *Contact Dermatitis* **18**: 242–3.

Storrs F.J., Mitchell J.C. & Rasmussen J.E. (1976) Contact hypersensitivity to liverwort and the compositae family of plants. *Cutis* **18**: 681–6.

Towers G.H.N., Arnason T., Wat C.-K. et al. (1979) Phototoxic polyacetylenes and their thiophene derivatives. *Contact Dermatitis* **5**: 140–4.

White I.R., Norris P.G. & Hawk J.L.M. (1990) Sesquiterpene lactone sensitivity and chronic actinic dermatitis. *Contact Dermatitis* **23**: 260. (Abstract.)

Wrangsjö K., Ros A.M. & Wahlberg J.E. (1990) Contact allergy to Compositae plants in patients with summer-

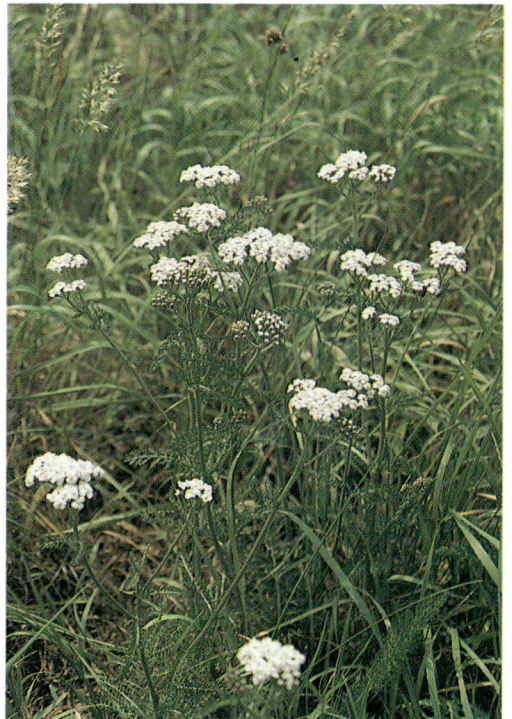

Fig. 7.5.33 *Achillea millefolium* (yarrow).

exacerbated dermatitis. *Contact Dermatitis* **22**: 148–54.

ACHILLEA millefolium

Common names: Yarrow. Milfoil
Distribution: Europe (very common, especially in Britain). Introduced to other temperate areas

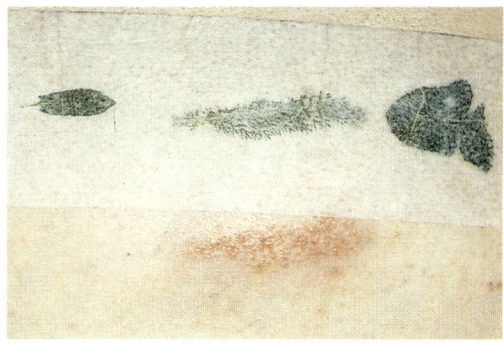

Fig. 7.5.35 Open patch test with yarrow (Courtesy of Dr M.G. Davies.)

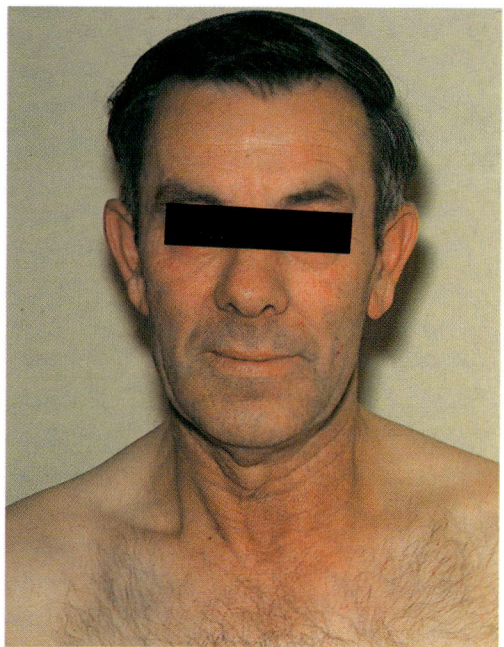

Fig. 7.5.34 Allergic contact dermatitis caused by yarrow. (Courtesy of Dr M.G. Davies.)

This low-growing perennial (Fig. 7.5.33) has dark-green finely divided leaves and congested heads of small white (rarely pale pink or purple) flowers. It is common on roadsides, hedge banks, or waste grounds and is a common lawn weed. Achilles reputedly used it to treat wounds caused by iron weapons and Culpeper recommends it for 'green wounds' and also for 'ulcers and fistulas, especially such as abound with moisture'. Allergic contact dermatitis (Figs 7.5.34, 7.5.35) in an airborne distribution may occur through grass cutting (Davies & Kersey 1986) or through ingestion, e.g. yarrow tea (Gans 1929). Desacetylmatricarin has been isolated from a related species, *A. lanulosa* (Yoshioka *et al.* 1973) Recently several sensitizing sesquiterpene lactones, notably α-peroxyachifolide (**7.XIII**), have been isolated from *A. millefolium*. The concentration increases as the plant withers (Hausen *et al.* 1991).

Davies M.G. & Kersey P.J.W. (1986) Contact allergy to yarrow and dandelion. *Contact Dermatitis* **14**: 256–7.
Gans O. (1929) Uber die Dermatitis durch *Achillea*

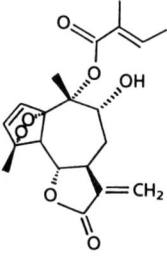

α-peroxyachifolide

7.XIII

millefolium. *Deutsche Medische Wochenschrift* **55**: 1213.

Hausen B.M., Brewer J., Weglewski J. & Rucker G. (1991) α-Peroxyachifolid and other new sensitizing sesquiterpene lactones from yarrow (*Achillea millefolium* L., Compositae). *Contact Dermatitis* **24**: 274–80.

Yoshioka H., Mabry T.J. & Timmermann B.M. (1973) *Sesquiterpene Lactones. Chemistry, NMR and Plant Distribution*. University of Tokyo Press, Tokyo.

AMBROSIA spp.

Common name: Ragweeds

Distribution: North America. Naturalized in Australia and India. Occasional in Europe

Several members of this genus are weeds in North America and Mexico. Of the 40 or so species, the major ones causing allergic contact dermatitis in North America are listed in Table 7.5.7 (Brunsting & Williams 1936, Shelmire 1940, Mitchell *et al.* 1971). These weeds are able rapidly to colonize recently cleared land and followed the pioneers as they cut down the forest in North America.

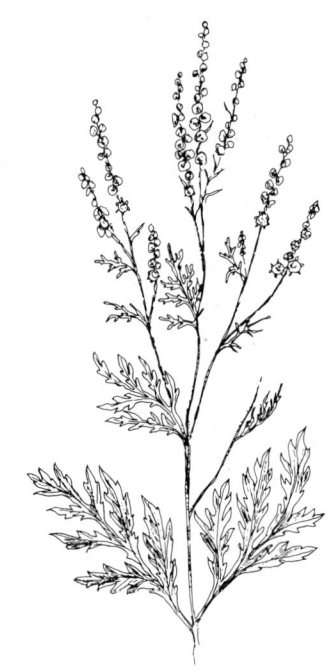

Fig. 7.5.36 *Ambrosia artemisiaefolia*.

Table 7.5.7 Sensitizing ragweeds (*Ambrosia* spp.).

Common name	Botanical name(s)	Notes
Short/low/common ragweed Roman wormwood	*Ambrosia artemisiaefolia* (*A. elatior*)	Annual. Especially common in eastern USA, but found over most of the country. A troublesome weed in gardens and yards. Ornamental light green, cut leaves like *Artemisia*. Numerous greenish flowers in slender spikes
Western ragweed	*Ambrosia psilostachya* (*A. coronopifolia*)	Perennial. Thick leaves. Variable. Chiefly in western states. Naturalized in Australia. Cross-sensitivity with turpentine
Great/tall/high ragweed	*Ambrosia trifida* (*A. aptera*)	Very tall (up to 18 ft recorded!). Stout stem, three-lobed sharp pointed leaves. Flowers insignificant. Common in moist soil, especially in southern and eastern states
Lance-leaved ragweed	*Ambrosia bidentata*	Annual. Hairy stems. Lance-shaped leaves. Small greenish flowers
False ragweed Hooker's gaertneria	*Ambrosia acanthicarpa* (*Franseria acanthicarpa*)	Annual. Grows in sandy soil in northern USA. Spiny fruiting heads

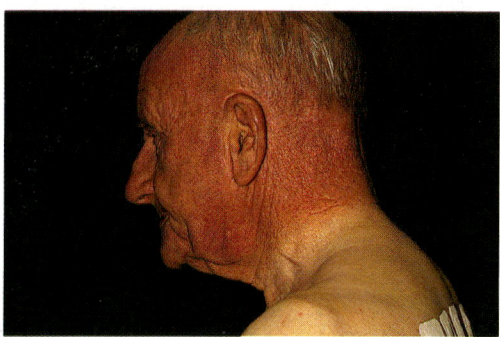

Fig. 7.5.37 Ragweed sensitivity. (Courtesy of Dr J.N. Burry.)

A. artemisiaefolia (Fig. 7.5.36) is the most ubiquitous species and is a high sensitizer. The oleoresin in *Ambrosia* spp. is borne by specialized canals to the leaf surface. Although the pollen of several species is an important cause of Type I hypersensitivity, it does not appear to be involved in causing contact dermatitis (Shelmire 1940). Allergic reactions can occur at any time during the plant's growing season (spring to frost) and have a typically 'airborne' distribution, affecting the face, neck and arms (Fig. 7.5.37). Several sesquiterpene lactones are found in different species. Δ-3-carene has been found in *A. psilostachya* and cross-sensitivity with turpentine has been reported by Fisher (1952).

Brunsting L.A. & Williams D.H. (1936) Ragweed (contact) dermatitis. Observations in 48 cases and report of unsuccessful attempts at desensitisation by injection of specific oils. *Journal of the American Medical Association* **106**: 1533–5.
Fisher A.A. (1952) Some immunologic phenomena in treatment of and patch testing for ragweed oil dermatitis. *Journal of Investigative Dermatology* **19**: 271–9.
Mitchell J.C., Roy A.K., Dupuis G. & Towers G.H.N. (1971) Allergic contact dermatitis from ragweeds (*Ambrosia* species); the role of sesquiterpene lactones. *Archives of Dermatology* **104**: 73–6.
Shelmire B. (1940) Contact dermatitis from vegetation. *Southern Medical Journal* **33**: 337–46.

ANTHEMIS arvensis

Common names: Corn chamomile. Field chamomile
Distribution: Europe. Naturalized in other temperate areas

This annual weed of fields or wastelands is similar in appearance to *A. cotula* but only slightly, and pleasantly, scented. Allergic contact dermatitis has been attributed to this plant. Patch tests were positive to all plant parts; weaker patch test results were obtained in the same individuals to *Matricaria recutita* (Moslein 1963).

Moslein P. (1963) Pflanzen als Kontakt-Allergene. *Berufsdermatosen* **11**: 24–8.

ANTHEMIS cotula

Common names: Stinking mayweed. Stinking chamomile. Dog fennel (USA)
Distribution: Europe; introduced to other temperate areas where it commonly escapes

This annual, fetid plant is one of the many species loosely referred to as 'chamomile' (see Table 7.5.8, p. 171). The white flowers, with a yellow central disc, are held on 40–50 cm stems on basic soil in southern England and western Europe. It has become a major weed in the USA. Several cases of bullous irritant contact dermatitis have been reported in farm workers and harvesters who were hand-weeding (e.g. Adams & O'Malley 1990). Because of its irritant properties, open rather than closed patch tests are preferable with this species and should be interpreted with caution. In a large North American series of patients with weed dermatitis, *A. cotula* gave the most frequent positive results (Menz & Winkelmann 1987). It contains anthecotulide (**7.XIV**), a sesquiterpene lactone with irritant as well as sensitizing properties (Hausen *et al.* 1984).

Anthecotulide

7.XIV

Adams R.M. & O'Malley M. (1990) Severe bullous dermatitis from *Anthemis cotula* (stinking mayweed) in a crew of agricultural field workers. *Contact Dermatitis* **23**: 259.

Hausen B.M., Busker E. & Carle R. (1984) Uber das Sensibilisierungsvermogen von Compositearten VII. Experimentelle Untersuchungen mit Auszugen und Inhaltsstoffen von *Chamomilla recutita* (L.) Rauschert und *Anthemis cotula* L. *Planta Medica* **50**: 229–34.

Menz J. & Winkelmann R.K. (1987) Sensitivity to wild vegetation. *Contact Dermatitis* **16**: 169–73.

ARCTOTHECA calendula (syn. CRYPTOSTEMMA)

Common name: Capweed
Distribution: Cape Province, South Africa. Naturalized in Australia

This showy annual (Fig. 7.5.38) is common on roadsides and waste places in South Africa and forms extensive colonies in pastures in

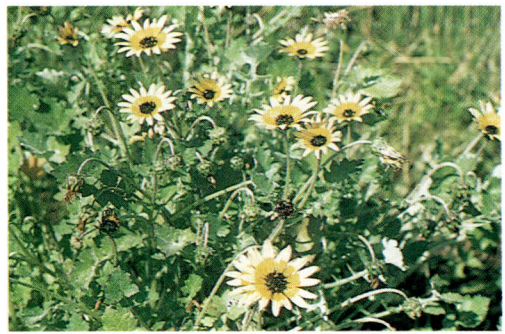

Fig. 7.5.38 *Arctotheca calendulacea*. (Courtesy of Dr J.N. Burry.)

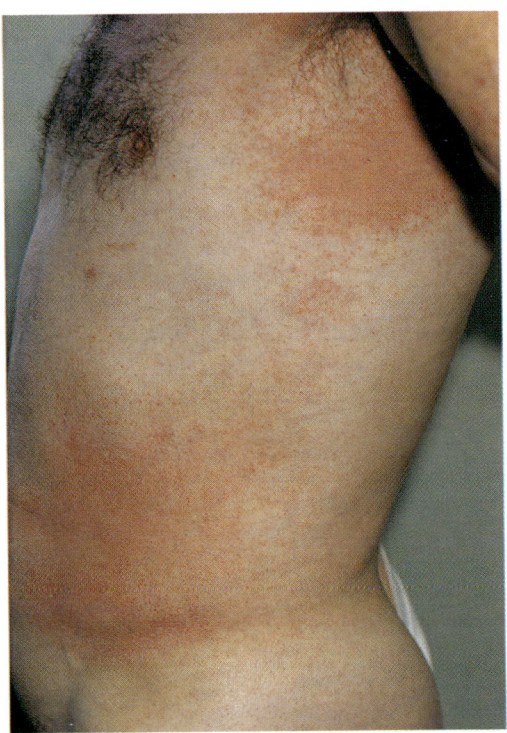

Fig. 7.5.39 Dermatitis in a sheep shearer handling fleeces contaminated with *Arctotheca*. (Courtesy of Dr J.N. Burry.)

southern Australia. The light green leaves are long, soft and jagged. The juicy, ribbed stems, up to 20 cm, bear bright yellow 8–10 cm flowers with a dark centre. It is reported as a cause of bush dermatitis in Australia (Burry 1973). A sheep-shearer developed contact dermatitis of the trunk after handling fleeces contaminated with *Arctotheca* (Fig. 7.5.39) (Kloot & Burry 1982/3).

Burry J.N., Kuchel R., Reid J.G. & Kirk J. (1973) Australian bush dermatitis; compositae dermatitis in South Australia. *Medical Journal of Australia* **1**: 110–16.

Kloot P.M. & Burry J.N. (1982/3) Some botanical aspects of compositae dermatitis in South Australia. *Australian–Weeds* **2**: 61–70.

ARNICA

Common names: Arnica. Mountain tobacco. Wolf's bane
Distribution: Northern hemisphere – temperate zone
Patch test: Tincture of arnica 10% MEK.

This genus of yellow-flowered aromatic herbaceous perennials occurs throughout the northern temperate regions in meadows, prairies and light woodland, often at high altitude. *Arnica montana* (Fig. 7.5.40) is the major source of tincture of arnica, which is

Helenalin   Carabron

7.XV Allergens in *Arnica* spp.

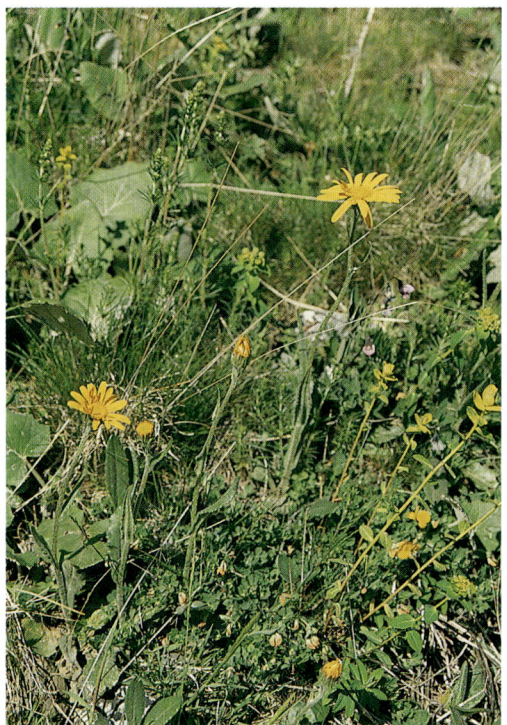

Fig. 7.5.40 *Arnica montana*, photographed in the Spanish Pyrenees.

helenalin and its esters (Hausen *et al.* 1978, Hausen 1980) (**7.XV**). Passreiter *et al.* (1988) have isolated other allergens, 8, 9-epoxythymoldiesters, from *A. sachalinensis* (**7.XVI**). These allergens are chemically unrelated to sesquiterpene lactones and do not cross-react. Cross-reaction between *Arnica* spp. and florists' chrysanthemum may occur, and also with *Tagetes* (Pirker *et al.* 1992).

Hausen B.M. (1980) Arnikaallergie. *Der Hautarzt* **31**: 10–17.
Hausen B.M., Herrman H.D. & Willuhn G. (1978) The sensitizing capacity of Compositae plants. I. Occupational contact dermatitis from *Arnica longifolia* Eaton. *Contact Dermatitis* **4**: 3–10.
Passreiter C.M., Florack M., Willuhn G. & Goerz G. (1988) Allergische Kontakt dermatitis auf Asteraceae. Identifizierung eines 8,9-Epoxythymoldiesters als Kontaktallergie von *Arnica sachalinensis*. *Dermatosen in Beruf und Umwelt* **27**: 141–2.
Pirker C., Moslinger T., Koller D.Y., Gotz M. & Jarisch R. (1992) Cross-reactivity with *Tagetes* in *Arnica* contact eczema. *Contact Dermatitis* **26**: 217–19.
Wrangsjö K., Ros A.M. & Wahlberg J.E. (1990) Contact allergy to Compositae plants in patients with summer-exacerbated dermatitis. *Contact Dermatitis* **22**: 148–54.

still frequently applied to bruises. Contact dermatitis due to the tincture has been recognized since the mid 19th century (Hausen 1980). Other species, including *A. longifolia*, *chamissonis* and *sachalinensis*, have also been used as sources for the tincture. Tincture of arnica diluted 10% in MEK (methylethyl ketone) can be used for patch testing. Wrangsjö *et al.* (1990) used a 0.5% ether extract of the plant in petrolatum. The major allergens appear to be sesquiterpene lactones, notably

10-acetoxy-8,9-epoxy-thymolisobutyrate

7.XVI

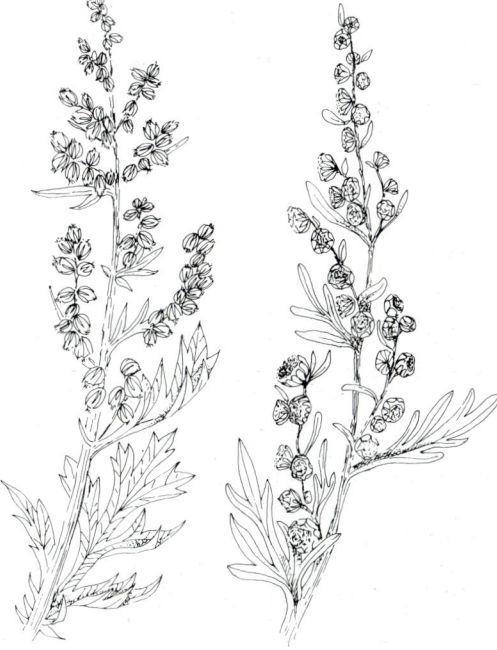

Fig. 7.5.41 *Artemisia absinthum*.

ARTEMISIA spp.

Common names: Mugwort. Wormwood. Motherwort. Prairie sage
Distribution: Northern temperate regions. Central and South America. Naturalized in Australia

This large genus (over 400 species) includes *A. absinthum* (wormwood), a highly aromatic herb with silvery green much-divided leaves (Fig. 7.5.41). It was used in the past to banish fleas from the house and as a vermifuge. It is used to flavour absinthe and some vermouths. It has caused allergic contact dermatitis in the USA (due to a proprietary ointment used for pre-existing dermatitis; Underwood & Gaul 1948) and in Australia (quoted in Burry *et al.* 1973). Like *Ambrosia*, it is wind-pollinated and oleoresins may be disseminated on pollen, causing airborne dermatitis.

Artemisia vulgaris (mugwort) (Fig. 7.5.42) is a perennial weed found in hedgerows and roadsides in western Europe (including southern Britain). It has become widely naturalized in the USA. It has aromatic leaves, coarser than *A. absinthum*, white on the upper surface and dark green below. The inconspicuous greenish-yellow flowers are held erect on a leafy spike. It has many herbal uses and Culpeper recommends that 'being made up with hog's grease into an ointment, it takes away wens and hard knots and kernels that grow about the neck and throat'. Kurz and Rapaport (1979) reported allergic contact dermatitis in a Japanese male who applied tea made from this species to his arm affected with poison oak dermatitis.

Artemisia ludoviciana, the prairie sage, and its var. *mexicana*, have caused allergic dermatitis in a gardener (Mitchell & Rook 1979) and contain ludovicins A, B and C, which are sesquiterpene lactones (Mitchell *et al.* 1971).

Burry J.N., Kuchel R., Reid J.G. & Kirk J. (1973) Australian bush dermatitis: Compositae dermatitis in South Australia. *Medical Journal of Australia* **1**: 110–16.
Kurz G. & Rapaport M.J. (1979) External/internal allergy to plants (*Artemisia*). *Contact Dermatitis* **5**: 407–8.
Mitchell J. & Rook A. (1979) *Botanical Dermatology*. Greengrass, Vancouver.
Mitchell J.C., Geissman T.A., Dupuis G. & Towers G.H.N. (1971) Allergic contact dermatitis caused by *Artemisia* and *Chrysanthemum* species. *Journal of Investigative Dermatology* **56**: 98–101.
Underwood G.B. & Gaul L.E. (1948) Overtreatment dermatitis in dermatitis venenata due to plants. *JAMA* **138**: 570–82.

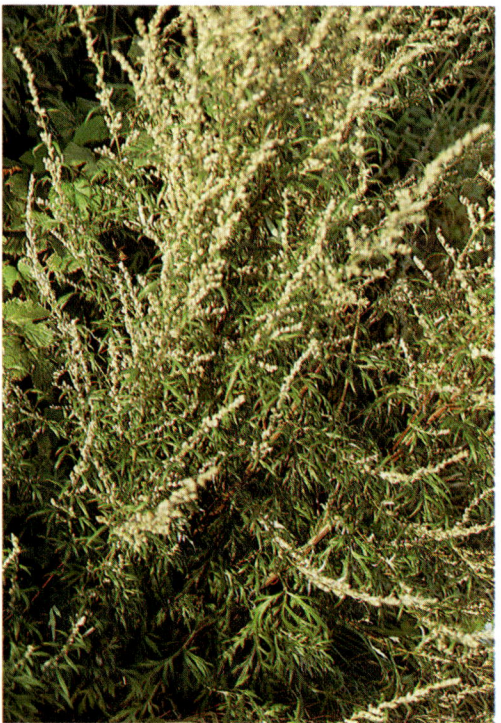

Fig. 7.5.42 *Artemisia vulgaris* (mugwort), a common roadside weed.

CALENDULA officinalis

Common names: Pot marigold. English marigold
Distribution: Mediterranean; a commonly grown garden annual

Several cultivars of this popular orange-flowered annual are in cultivation. It is widely used in herbal medicines for the treatment of eczema and warts and is a component of many 'skin ointments'. Allergic contact dermatitis appears to be rare and chiefly attributed to use of the ointment (Underwood & Gaul 1948).

Underwood G.B. & Gaul L.E. (1948) Overtreatment dermatitis in dermatitis venenata due to plants. *JAMA* **138**: 570–82.

CARTHAMNUS tinctorius

Common name: Safflower
Distribution: Africa; Asia (Middle East to India). Grown as an ornamental annual and as a source of red/yellow dyes

This tall (60–80 cm) annual has showy fluffy blooms, each about 3–4 cm in diameter. The dried flower yields the red dye carthamin, used to adulterate saffron. The meal has been used as a protein supplement for livestock and oil derived from the plant is used in 'low fat' margarines. A female inspector in a flower auction developed allergic dermatitis with positive patch tests to the flower but not to the leaf or other Compositae. The allergen has not been determined, but it may not be a sesquiterpene lactone (van der Willigen *et al.* 1987).

Van der Willigen A.H., Van Joost T., Stolz E. & Van der Hoek J.C.S. (1987) Contact dermatitis to safflower. *Contact Dermatitis* **17**: 184–6.

CHAMAEMELUM nobile
(syn. *Anthemis nobilis*)

Common name: Sweet (Roman) chamomile
Distribution: Europe. Grown as a lawn plant

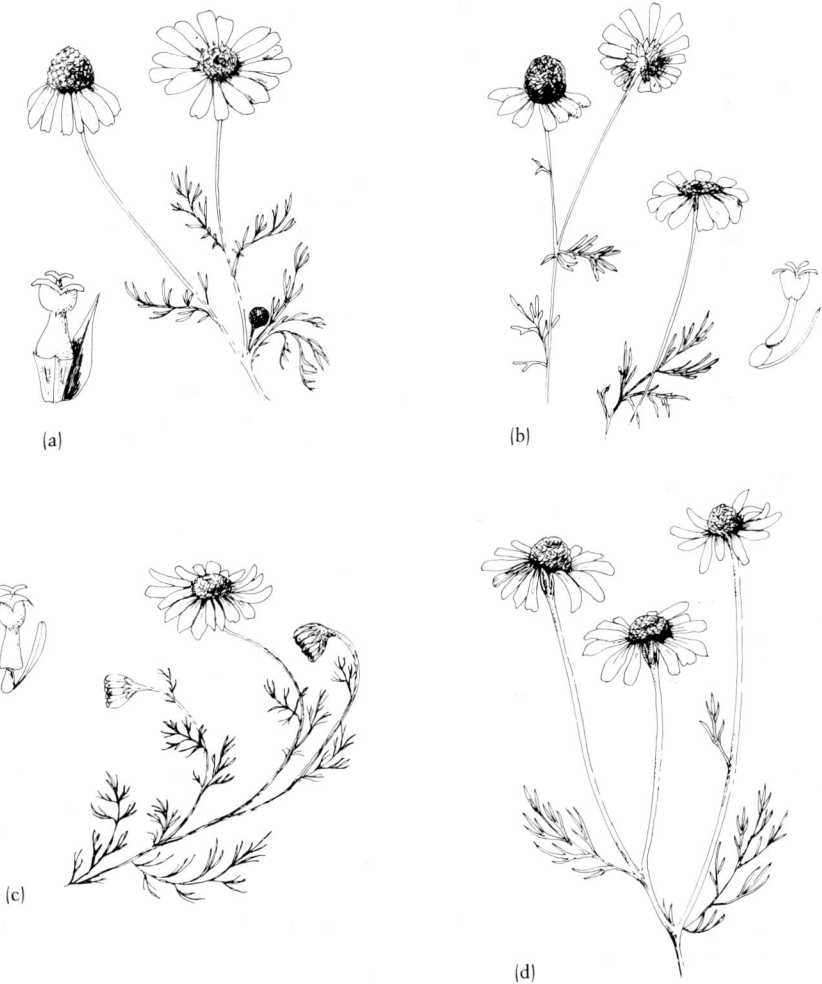

Fig. 7.5.43 Chamomiles; (a) *Anthemis arvensis*, (b) *A. cotula*, (c) *Chamaemelum nobile* and (d) *Matricaria recutita*.

This sweetly scented plant (Fig. 7.5.43) has been used to make lawns since the 17th century. (Sir Francis Drake was reputed to have played bowls on a chamomile lawn on the eve of the Armada.) The double-flowered form is particularly useful, requiring less trimming than the single form. The dried flowers are used to make chamomile tea, which has caused anaphylaxis (Benner & Lee 1963), and exacerbation of contact dermatitis (Babini 1949). Culpeper states that the oil applied topically 'helps stitches and pains in the sides', among many other uses. A proprietary ointment, Kamillosan®, is made from *C. nobile* and has caused allergic dermatitis (van Ketel 1982). This preparation is promoted for the prevention and treatment of nappy rash and as a nipple cream. McGeorge and Steele (1991) report two patients who developed allergic contact dermatitis of the nipples after using this preparation. To add confusion, the same proprietary preparation, marketed in Germany, can be made from German chamomile (*Matricaria chamomilla*)! (McGeorge & Steele 1991). Possible allergens include nobilin, a sesquiterpene lactone (Yoshioka *et al.* 1973).

Babini G. (1949) A not uncommon form of allergy to chamomile. *Minerva Medicine* **2**: 917.
Benner M.H. & Lee H.W. (1973) Anaphylactic reaction to chamomile tea. *Journal of Allergy and Clinical Immunology* **52**: 307–8.
McGeorge B.C.C. & Steele M.C. (1991) Allergic contact dermatitis of the nipple from Roman chamomile ointment. *Contact Dermatitis* **24**: 139–40.
Van Ketel W.G. (1982) Allergy to *Matricaria chamomilla*. *Contact Dermatitis* **8**: 143.
Yoshioka H., Mabry T.J. & Timmermann B.N. (1973) *Sesquiterpene Lactones: Chemistry, NMR and Plant Distribution*. University of Tokyo Press, Tokyo.

CHRYSANTHEMUM

This genus has been mostly disbanded. The florist's chrysanthemum is, strictly speaking, X *Dendranthema* (q.v.), although often incorrectly referred to as *Chrysanthemum* X *morifolium*. The ox-eye daisy (*C. leucanthemum*) is now *Leucanthemum vulgare* (q.v.). The true *Chrysanthemum* spp. include *C. coronarium* and *C. segetum*, attractive, and apparently harmless, weeds of European cornfields.

CICHORIUM intybus

Common names: Chicory, witloof, escarole
Distribution: Native to west and central Europe. Naturalized in South Africa, Australia, USA and South America
Patch test: Leaf, as is, or ether extracts

Cichorium intybus is a herbaceous plant (Fig. 7.5.44) with tough, grooved stems up to a metre in height. The clear blue flowers,

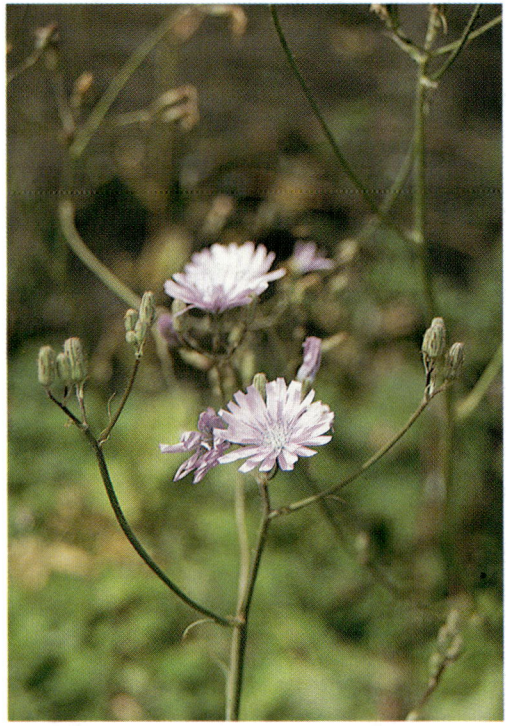

Fig. 7.5.44 *Cichorium intybus* (chicory).

resembling dandelions, are borne in clusters in the leaf axils. It grows by roadsides, and in fields, often in dry calcareous soil. Although native to southern Britain and the Euro-Mediterranean region, it has been introduced to Scotland, Ireland and all other temperate regions.

The blanched shoots are grown popularly as a winter salad in continental Europe. Chicory shoots (chicons) have become increasingly popular in the UK and a major producer uses a

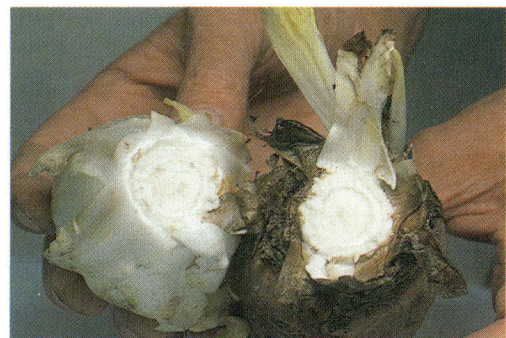

Fig. 7.5.45 Broken chicon, exuding sap.

hydroponic (soil-less) process for blanching. Operatives, who snap off or stack the chicons in trays, develop irritant contact dermatitis, conjunctivitis and bronchospasm from the milky sap which exudes from the broken ends (Fig. 7.5.45) (Rycroft et al. 1987). Greengrocers and market gardeners are also exposed to the plant occupationally.

The roots were used in the Second World War as a coffee substitute and Bonnevie (1948) recorded eczema following exposure to the vapour and juice of roasted chicory. Friis (1973) reported the first fully proven case of allergic contact dermatitis in a 55-year-old shopkeeper with hand eczema. Patch tests were positive using the leaf and ether extracts. Vail and Mitchell (1973) reported a similar case in a patient who reacted also to endive, Romaine lettuce and 1% alantolactone (Friis et al. 1975). Although this may represent true cross-reaction with alantolactone (the major sesquiterpene lactone in *Inula helenium*) Rycroft et al. (1987) found that even 0.1% alantolactone produced irritant reactions in some individuals.

Positive patch tests are elicited using the leaf or portion of chicon. The mature stem and flower appear not to be allergenic (Vail & Mitchell 1973).

The major allergens in chicory are the sesquiterpene lactones, lactucin and lactopicrin, also found in lettuce (Yoshioka et al. 1973). No helenin (alantolactone) or isohelenin could be isolated from chicory (Rycroft et al. 1987). Cross-reaction may occur with chrysanthemum (Hausen 1979) and several American Compositae oleoresins

(Krook 1977). The allergens penetrate gloves (Malten 1983). Rycroft et al. (1987) found that rubber gloves with plastic armlets were insufficient to prevent the irritant effects of the sap; however, symptoms improved after the operatives wore polyester cotton overalls with absorbent oversleeves and extractor fans were installed above the sites of aerosol release.

CICHORIUM endivia

Common name: Endive
Distribution: ? Mediterranean area

Cichorium endivia is an annual or biennial plant; the narrow leaves form a rosette and the flower spike is similar to *C. intybus*. Endive leaves are used in salads, chiefly in continental Europe. Allergic contact dermatitis to the leaves affects salad makers and cross-reactions are observed with chicory (Vail & Mitchell 1973, Krook 1977). The allergens are unknown.

Krook (1977) reported immediate hypersensitivity in two patients who also had delayed hypersensitivity to endive and lettuce. This association of immediate and delayed hypersensitivity to the same allergen is very rare.

Bonnevie P. (1948) Some experiences of war-time industrial dermatoses. *Acta Dermato-Venereology* **28**: 231–7.
Friis B. (1973) Occupational dermatitis from chicory salad (*Cichorium intybus var foliosum*). *Contact Dermatitis Newsletter* **13**: 349.
Friis B., Hjorth N., Vail J.T., Jr. & Mitchell J.C. (1975) Occupational contact dermatitis from *Cichorium* (chicory, endive) and *Lactuca* (lettuce). *Contact Dermatitis* **1**: 311–13.
Hausen B.M. (1979) The sensitizing capacity of Compositae plants. III Test results and cross-reactions in Compositae-sensitive patients. *Dermatologica* **159**: 1–11.
Krook G. (1977) Occupational dermatitis from *Lactuca sativa* (lettuce) and *Cichorium* (endive). *Contact Dermatitis* **3**: 27–36.
Malten K.E. (1983) Chicory dermatitis from September to April. *Contact Dermatitis* **9**: 232.
Rycroft R.J.G., Lovell C.R., Harries P.G., Winter P. & Mallet A.I. (1987) Occupational irritant contact dermatitis from chicory. *Bollettino di Dermatologia Allergologica e Professionale* **2**: 77–82.
Vail J.T., Jr. & Mitchell J.C. (1973) Occupational dermatitis from *Cichorium intybus*, *Cichorium endivia* and *Lactuca sativa* var *longifolia*. *Contact Dermatitis Newsletter* **14**: 413–14.

Yoshioka H., Mabry T.J. & Timmerman B.N. (1973) *Sesquiterpene Lactones: Chemistry, NMR and Plant Distributions.* University of Tokyo Press, Tokyo.

CNICUS benedictus

Common name: Blessed thistle
Distribution: Southern Europe

This somewhat spiny annual, with yellow flowers, was extensively used in herbal medicine in the past. Although there are no definite reports of allergic contact dermatitis, the species contains an allergenic sesquiterpene lactone, cnicin (Zeller *et al.* 1985).

Zeller W., De Gols M. & Hausen B.M. (1985) The sensitizing capacity of Compositae plants. *Archives of Dermatological Research* **277**: 28–35.

CONYZA bonariensis
(syn. ERIGERON bonariensis)

Common names: Fleabane. Horseweed
Distribution: North and South America. Naturalized weed in Australia

Conyza bonariensis and the closely related *C. canadensis* are tall annuals, with very small white and green flower heads; the small rays are connected together like a colander. The leaves are stalkless and velvety. There is only circumstantial evidence that *C. canadensis* may sensitize (Lovell *et al.* 1955). However, *C. bonariensis* is well recognized as a cause of allergic dermatitis in South Australia (Fig. 7.5.46), where it is a widespread naturalized weed along roadsides and waste places (Burry 1979), and in southern Europe (Sertoli *et al.* 1978).

Burry J.N. (1979) Dermatitis from fleabane: compositae dermatitis in South Australia. *Contact Dermatitis* **5**: 51–64.
Lovell R.G., Mathews K.P. & Sheldon J.M. (1955) Dermatitis venenata from tree pollen oils. *Journal of Allergy* **26**: 408–14.
Sertoli A. (1978) Allergic contact dermatitis to *Salvia officinalis*, *Inula viscosa* and *Conyza bonariensis*. *Contact Dermatitis* **4**: 314–15.

CYNARA scolymus

Common name: Globe artichoke

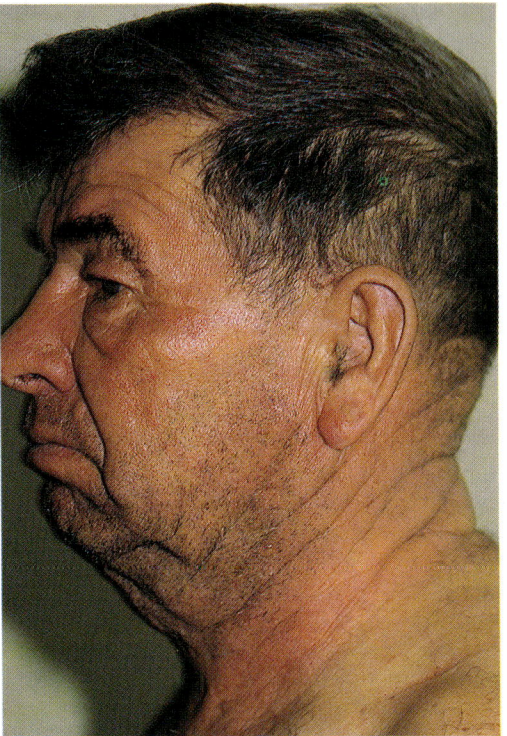

Fig. 7.5.46 Facial airborne contact dermatitis. *Conyza bonariensis* is a major cause in Australia. (Courtesy of Dr J.N. Burry.)

Distribution: Unknown in the wild. Widely cultivated in Mediterranean regions and other temperate areas

The globe artichoke is an imposing herbaceous plant with enormous flower heads (15 cm diameter); the purple flowers are surrounded by fleshy bracts (Fig. 7.5.47). The buds are consumed as a vegetable. (The 'Jerusalem' artichoke is a different species, *Helianthus tuberosus*.) *Cynara scolymus* may be an old cultivar of the cardoon, *C. cardunculus*, which has spiky bracts. Burry *et al.* (1973) reported a widespread bullous contact dermatitis in a woman who picked artichokes while scantily clad. Artichoke dermatitis may affect pickers, market gardeners and flower arrangers (Sidi *et al.* 1950, Turner 1980, Meding 1983). Positive patch test reactions are obtained to freshly cut stems or roots but not to the bracts (Sidi *et al.* 1950). Cross-reactions occur with

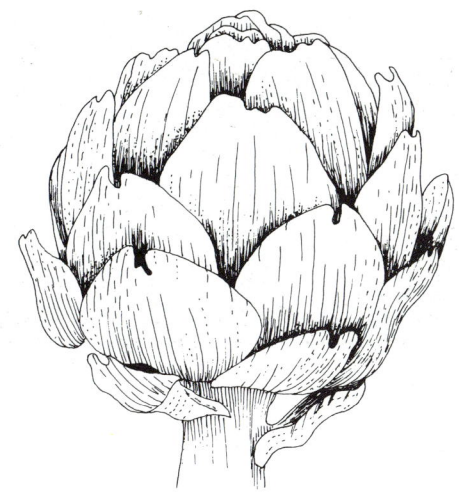

Fig. 7.5.47 Artichoke head.

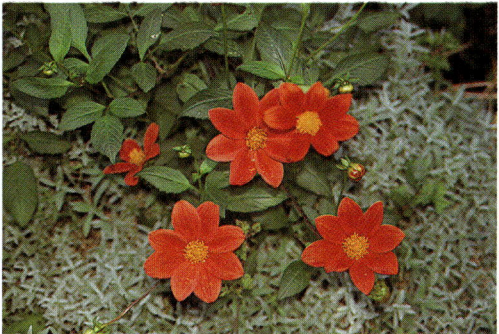

Fig. 7.5.48 *Dahlia coccinea*, one of the attractive species from which the modern dahlia hybrids are derived.

other Compositae (Burry *et al.* 1973) and the allergen is probably cynaropicrin, a sesquiterpene lactone (Schneider & Thiele 1974).

Burry J.N., Kuchel R., Reid J.G. & Kirk J. (1973) Australia bush dermatitis. Compositae dermatitis in South Australia. *Medical Journal of Australia* **1**: 110–16.
Meding B. (1983) Allergic contact dermatitis from artichoke, *Cynara scolymus*. *Contact Dermatitis* **9**: 314.
Schneider von G. & Thiele K. (1974) Eigenschaften und bestimmung des artischoken — bitterstoffen, cynaropicrin. *Planta Medica* **25**: 149.
Sidi E., Morrill-Dobkevitch S. & Godechot R. (1950) Les dermites provoquees par les artichauts. *Presse Medicale* **58**: 382.
Turner T. (1980) Compositae dermatitis in South Australia: contact dermatitis from *Ixodia archillaeoides* and *Cynara cardunculus* or the tribulations of a dry flower arranger. *Contact Dermatitis* **6**: 444.

DAHLIA cvs

Common name: Dahlia
Distribution: Mexico. Widely cultivated

This popular genus of half-hardy tuberous perennials (Fig. 7.5.48) has been in cultivation for nearly 300 years. The genus ranges from dwarf species to tree-like species such as *D. arborea*. The species are rarely cultivated, although attractive. Most of the modern hybrids are derived from *D. variabilis*. Bedding dahlias are cultivars of *D. pinnata*. Calnan (1978) reported dermatitis of the face, particularly around the mouth, extensor forearms and hands, in professional market gardeners. Patch tests were positive to the leaf. Vryman (1933) described dermatitis of the hands, and later the face, in a gardener's boy. Patch tests were negative to the leaf, but positive to the tuber. Sharma and Kaur (1989) obtained positive patch tests using a 1:10 ether dilution of *D. pinnata* (whole plant) in 18% of Indian patients with airborne contact dermatitis and in a later study (Sharma & Kaur 1990) obtained positive patch tests to *D. pinnata* alone in 20 out of 32 patients with suspected dahlia dermatitis. Cross-reaction occurs with florist's chrysanthemum (Calnan 1978) and the allergen is presumably a sesquiterpene lactone.

Calnan C.D. (1978) Sensitivity to dahlia flowers. *Contact Dermatitis* **4**: 168.
Sharma S.C. & Kaur S. (1989) Airborne contact dermatitis from Compositae plants in northern India. *Contact Dermatitis* **21**: 1–5.
Sharma S.C. & Kaur S. (1990) Contact dermatitis from *Dahlia pinnata*. *Contact Dermatitis* **23**: 204–5.
Vryman L.H. (1933) Dahlienwurzelrinden-Dermatitis. *Archivs fur Dermatologie und Syphilologie* **168**: 233–4.

X DENDRANTHEMA cvs

Common name: Chrysanthemum
Distribution: Asia. Widely cultivated

The 'chrysanthemum' (Fig. 7.5.49) is a hybrid genus which has been in cultivation for over

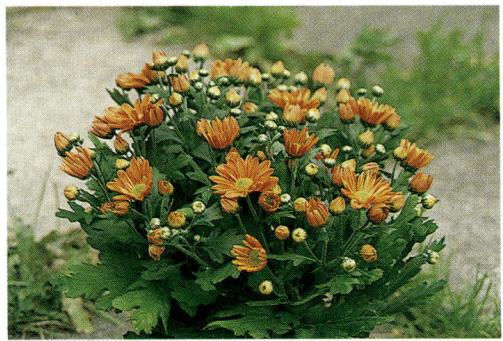

Fig. 7.5.49 X *Dendranthema* cultivar, 'chrysanthemum'.

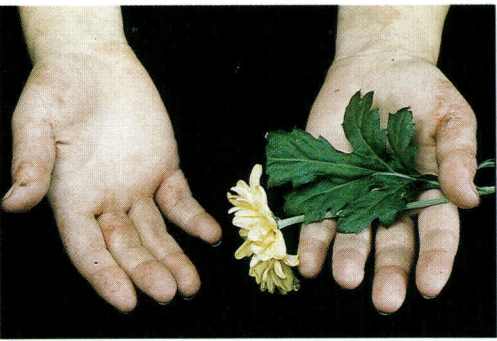

Fig. 7.5.50 Allergic contact dermatitis of the hands caused by chrysanthemum.

two millenia. Its origins are unclear and specific names such as *Chrysanthemum 'indicum'* and *C. 'morifolium'* are spurious (Schmidt et al. 1985). Cultivars are grown as pot plants, herbaceous border subjects and for cut flowers. Allergic contact dermatitis occurs in the enthusiastic amateur, who may spend several hours 'disbudding' the plants to encourage larger blooms, and also in the professional grower (Hausen & Schulz 1976) and florist (Illuminati et al. 1988). Chrysanthemums represent the commonest cause of occupational dermatitis due to compositae (Hausen & Oestmann 1988). Chrysanthemums are commonly grown and exhibited in India, where Sharma et al. (1989) have reported 32 cases of allergic contact dermatitis. Contact urticaria to chrysanthemum has been reported (Tanaka et al. 1987) but delayed hypersensitivity is of much greater importance.

The clinical presentation of allergic contact dermatitis is variable (Figs 7.5.50 & 7.5.51). Initially, the fingertips only may be involved. Later, the process may spread to involve the whole palm, forearms and face in a 'pseudo-photosensitive' distribution (however, finger webs and eyelid margins are affected). Airborne contact dermatitis is common (Sharma et al. 1989), perhaps due to fine dust from the plant rather than pollen. Alternatively, the allergens themselves may be volatile (Schmidt 1986).

Although photocontact allergy to chrysanthemum does not occur, patch test positivity to chrysanthemum oleoresin (Fig. 7.5.52) was found in nine of 69 patients with chronic actinic dermatitis (Frain-Bell et al.

1979). These authors found no evidence of phototoxic substances in chrysanthemum, using a *Candida albicans* system.

Patch tests should be carried out using the patient's own cultivars: some are much more likely to cause allergic dermatitis than others (Schmidt 1986). Cross-reaction may occur with colophony, tars and turpentine (Frain-Bell et al. 1979), also with other Compositae. Schmidt et al. (1985) obtained positive reactions using feverfew (*Tanacetum parthenium*) extract in all patients with chrysanthemum dermatitis. All parts of the suspected plant should be tested: Sharma et al. (1989), for example, obtained positive results in all 32 patients using ethanolic extracts of the flowers but only in six using extracts of the stems.

The allergens are sesquiterpene lactones, which are borne on the surface of the flowers and leaves, usually in trichomes (plant hairs). Although positive patch tests can be obtained using alantolactone and parthenolide in

Arteglasin-A

7.XVII

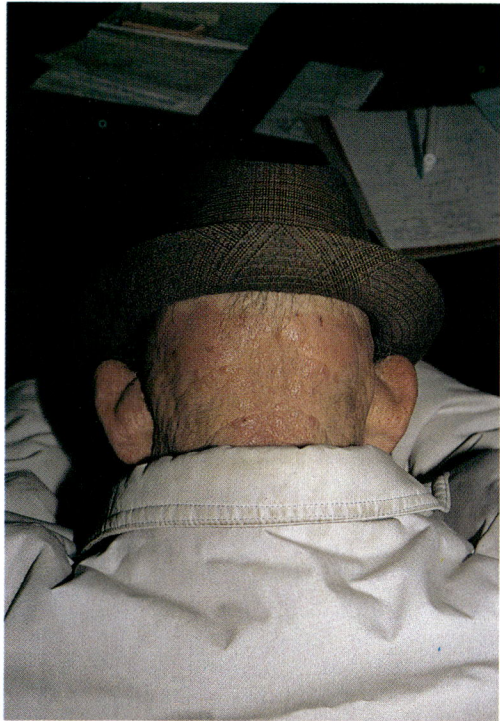
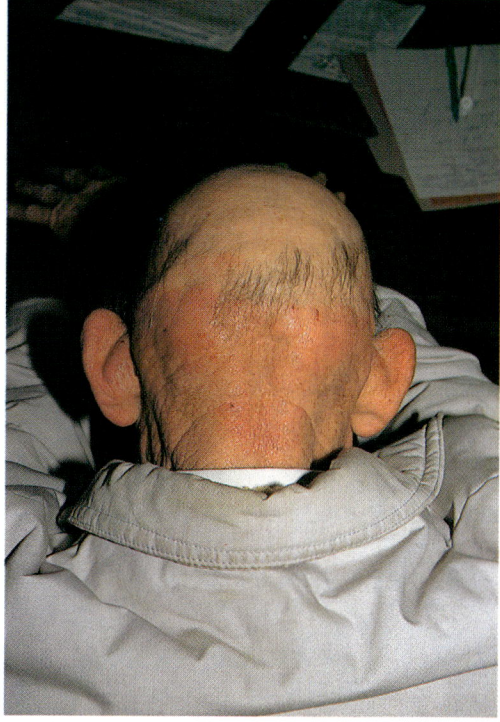

Fig. 7.5.51 Airborne contact dermatitis mimicking photosensitivity. This elderly chrysanthemum grower always wore his hat when gardening. A patch test was positive with chrysanthemum leaf and his eruption improved considerably when he changed to African violets.

patients with chrysanthemum dermatitis, neither of these sesquiterpene lactones was found in the cultivars tested by Schultz et al. (1975). The major allergen appears to be arteglasin A (**7.XVII**), a guaianolide (Hausen et al. 1976), also present in *Artemisia* spp. In addition, Osawa et al. (1973) have isolated an unusual chlorinated sesquiterpene lactone chlorochrymorin in a cultivar named 'Otomezakura'. It is not known if this is allergenic.

When available, the sesquiterpene lactone mix (Ducombs et al. 1990) would appear to serve as a useful screen for chrysanthemum sensitivity. Patch testing with a random chrysanthemum is unreliable and all the patient's cultivars should ideally be tested. There may be cultivars which can be safely cultivated. An ethanolic (Bluemink et al. 1973) or benzene/chloroform/ethanol extract (Hausen & Schultz 1976) of flowers would be time-consuming but more reliable. The use of feverfew extract (Schmidt et al. 1985) merits further study. (An extensive bibliography on X *Dendranthema* is given by Mitchell & Rook 1979.)

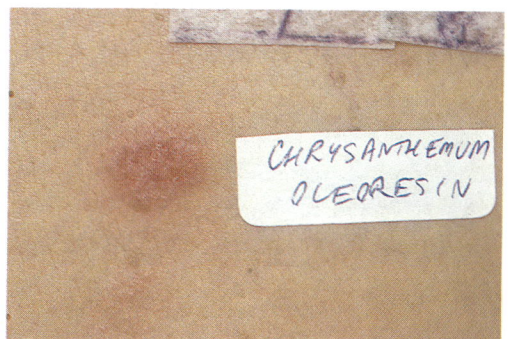

Fig. 7.5.52 Positive patch test with chrysanthemum oleoresin.

Bluemink E., Mitchell J.C. & Nater J.P. (1973) Contact dermatitis due to chrysanthemums. *Archives of Dermatology* **108**: 220–2.

Ducombs G., Benezra C., Talaga P. *et al.* (1990) Patch testing with the 'sesquiterpene lactone mix'. *Contact Dermatitis* **27**: 249–52.

Frain-Bell W., Hetherington A. & Johnson B.E. (1979) Contact allergic sensitivity to chrysanthemum and the photosensitivity dermatitis and actinic reticuloid syndrome. *British Journal of Dermatology* **101**: 491–501.

Hausen B.M. & Oestmann G. (1988) Untersuchungen uber die Haufigkeit berufsbedingter allergischer Hauterkrankungen auf einen Blumengrossmarkt. *Dermatosen in Beruf und Umwelt* **36**: 117–24.

Hausen B.M. & Schulz K.H. (1976) Chrysanthemum allergy III. Identification of the allergens. *Archives of Dermatological Research* **255**: 111–21.

Illuminata R., Russo R., Guerra L. & Melino M. (1988) Occupational airborne contact dermatitis in a florist. *Contact Dermatitis* **18**: 246.

Mitchell J. & Rook A. (1979) *Botanical Dermatology*. Greengrass, Vancouver.

Osawa T., Suzuki A., Tamura S., Ohashi Y. & Sasada Y. (1973) Structure of chlorochrymorin, a novel sesquiterpene lactone from *Chrysanthemum morifolium*. *Tetrahedron Letters* **51**: 5135–8

Schmidt R.J. & Kingston T. (1985) Chrysanthemum dermatitis in south Wales: diagnosis by patch testing with feverfew (*Tanacetum parthenium*) extract. *Contact Dermatitis* **13**: 120–1.

Schmidt R.J. (1986) Compositae. *Clinics in Dermatology* **4**(2): 46–61.

Schulz K.H., Hausen B.M., Wallhofer L. & Schmidt-Loffler P. (1975) Chrysanthemen — Allergie II. Experimentalle Untersuchungen zur Identifizierung der Allergene. *Archiv fuer Dermatologische Forschung* **251**: 235–44.

Sharma S.C., Tanwar R.L. & Kaur S. (1989) Contact dermatitis from chrysanthemums in India. *Contact Dermatitis* **21**: 69–71.

Tanaka T., Moriwaki S.-I. & Horio T. (1987) Occupational dermatitis with simultaneous immediate and delayed allergy to chrysanthemum. *Contact Dermatitis* **16**: 152–4.

DITTRICHIA viscosa (graveolens) (syn. *Inula viscosa*)

Common names: Sticky elecampane. Stinkwort
Distribution: A weed of Mediterranean regions. Naturalized in Australia
Patch test: Dried leaf. 0.5% ether extract in petrolatum

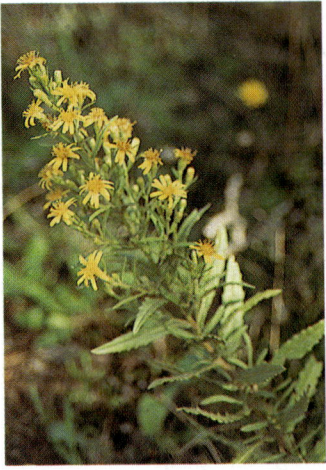

Fig. 7.5.53 *Dittrichia viscosa* photographed in Euboea; a common roadside weed in the Mediterranean region, particularly on acid soils.

This woody-based plant has leafy stems and long (up to 1 m) sprays of small yellow flowers in the autumn (Fig. 7.5.53). The whole plant is sticky and rank-smelling. The stems and leaves are coarse, causing mechanical irritation. In the Mediterranean area it is a common and troublesome weed. It has been used in folk medicine and is believed to keep away fleas (and wild beasts!). Allergic contact dermatitis has been reported in both Europe (Gonçalo & Gonçalo 1991) and Australia (Burry *et al.* 1975). Gonçalo and Gonçalo (1991) report nine cases, mostly exhibiting an airborne pattern of contact sensitivity, although one female patient developed lesions resembling erythema multiforme on the trunk and arms. Although most cases occur in farm workers or gardeners, one patient was sensitized after using the stem as a toothpick! (Gonçalo & Gonçalo 1991). All their patients were positive to the fresh leaf and to ether extracts dilute to 0.5% or 1% in petrolatum. The dried leaf appears not to give false positive irritant reactions (Burry *et al.* 1975). The allergens are sesquiterpene lactones, inuviscolide and 2-deacetoxyxanthinin (**7.XVIII**) (Pinedo *et al.* 1987) and cross-reactions occur with other Compositae, *Frullania* and *Laurus nobilis*.

Inuviscolide   Deacetoxyxanthinin

7.XVIII Allergens in *Dittrichia*.

Burry J.N., Reid J.G. & Kirk J. (1975) Australian bush dermatitis. *Contact Dermatitis* **1**: 263–4.
Gonçalo M. & Gonçalo S. (1991) Allergic contact dermatitis from *Dittrichia viscosa* (L.) Greuter. *Contact Dermatitis* **24**: 40–4.
Pinedo J.M., Decanales F.G., Hinojosa J.L., Llama P. & Hausen B.M. (1987) Contact dermatitis to sesquiterpene lactones in *Inula viscosa* Aiton. *Contact Dermatitis* **17**: 322–3.

FRANSERIA acanthicarpa (AMBROSIA acanthicarpa)

Common names: False ragweed. Franserioid ragweed. Hooker's gaertneria
Distribution: USA

This ragweed is common in sandy soils in North America and derives its specific name from the long spikes on the fruiting heads. Like the true ragweeds (*Ambrosia*) it is a cause of weed dermatitis (Mackoff & Dahl 1951). Cross-reaction occurs with other North American weeds (Mitchell 1972).

Mackoff S. & Dahl A.O. (1951) A botanical consideration of the weed oleoresin problem. *Minnesota Medicine* **34**: 1169.
Mitchell J.C. (1972) Plant dermatitis — note on inadequacy of some plant extracts. *Contact Dermatitis Newsletter* **11**: 271.

GAILLARDIA

Common names: Blanket flower. Kokardenblume (German)
Distribution: USA. A popular herbaceous plant in temperate areas

Two species of *Gaillardia* are commonly grown in borders for their ornamental flowers. *Gaillardia pulchella* (Fig. 7.5.54) is an annual with large red and yellow flowers on stems up to a metre in height. *Gaillardia aristata*, a perennial species, has yellow flowers on 0.5 m stems. Dermatitis due to *G. pulchella* was first reported by Rostenberg and Good (1935) and more recently by Hausen (1985). Dermatitis due to *G. aristata* has been reported in South Australia by Burry (1980). The major allergen is spathulin (**7.XIX**) (Hausen 1985).

Spathulin

7.XIX

Burry J.N. (1980) Dermatitis from *Gaillardia aristata*: Compositae dermatitis in South Australia. *Contact Dermatitis* **6**: 157.
Hausen B.M. (1985) Kokardenblumen — Allergie. *Dermatosen in Beruf und Umwelt* **33**: 62–5.
Rostenberg A., Jr. & Good C.K. (1935) *Gaillardia* dermatitis. *JAMA* **104**: 1496–7.

GERAEA viscida

A research worker handling leaf trichomes of this plant became sensitized to the exudate, as well as achieving a publication (Rodriguez et al. 1979).

Rodriguez E., Sanchez B., Grieco P.A. *et al.* (1979) Gerin, a eudesmane methyl ester in trichome exudates of *Geraea viscida*. *Phytochemistry* **18**: 1741–2.

HELENIUM autumnale, microcephalum, amarum (syn. tenuifolium)

Common names: Sneezeweed. Small-head sneezeweed. Bitterweed
Distribution: USA. Occasionally grown as border plants

This genus of ornamental herbaceous plants is native to the USA. *Helenium autumnale* is a vigorous perennial reaching a height of 80 cm. The stems are much-branched and leafy, bearing in late autumn numerous yellow flowers, each 2–3 cm in diameter. The disk is

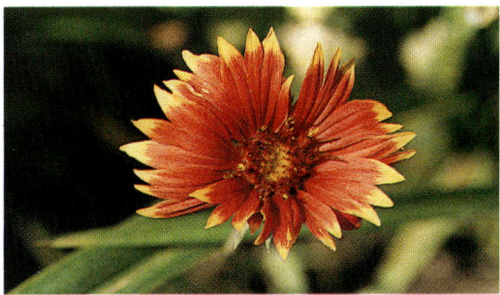

Fig. 7.5.54 *Gaillardia* cultivar.

orange-yellow and the rays are often somewhat drooping. It is a widespread species, favouring most habitats. It is especially prevalent in the swamps of Louisiana. As its common name suggests, the whole plant is pungent, inducing sneezing. Allergic contact dermatitis was first reported by Balyeat *et al.* (1932). Subsequent cases have been described by Mitchell (1972) and Calnan (1978). Cross-reaction occurs with other Compositae (Mackoff & Dahl 1951), suggesting that the allergens are sesquiterpene lactones. Shelmire (1940) reports that the related species, *H. microcephalum* and *H. amarum* are strong sensitizers. *Helenium amarum* is sometimes grown as an ornamental annual.

Balyeat R.M., Rinkel H.J. & Stemen T.R. (1932) Contact dermatitis (venenata). Distribution and importance of the heleniums as a cause of contact dermatitis in the United States. *American Journal of Medical Science* **184**: 547.
Calnan C.D. (1978) Dermatitis from *Helenium*. *Contact Dermatitis* **4**: 115–16.
Mackoff S. & Dahl A.O. (1951) A botanical consideration of the weed oleoresin problem. *Minnesota Medicine* **34**: 1169–73, 1188.
Mitchell J.C. (1972) Plant dermatitis — note on inadequacy of some plant extracts. *Contact Dermatitis Newsletter* **11**: 271.
Shelmire B. (1940) Contact dermatitis from vegetation. *Southern Medical Journal* **33**: 337–46.

HELIANTHUS annuus

Common name: Sunflower
Distribution: Southern USA and Central America. Commonly grown in gardens and as a food crop, especially in Eastern Europe

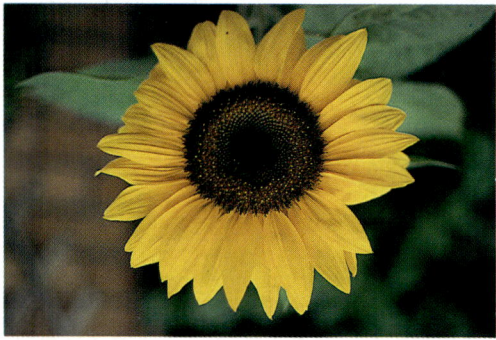

Fig. 7.5.55 *Helianthus annuus* (the sunflower).

This familiar annual has tall (up to 3–4 m) stems, bearing one or more massive yellow flower with a dark disk (Fig. 7.5.55). It is popularly grown as an ornamental plant (competitively by schoolchildren!). In addition, it is an important commercial crop. Sunflower seed oil is widely used in cooking and margarines derived from it are increasingly popular because of their high content of polyunsaturated fats. There are reports of several cases of allergic contact dermatitis, chiefly occupationally acquired; these are reviewed in detail by Hausen and Spring (1989). Numerous antigenic sesquiterpene lactones (**7.XX**) are secreted by fine capitate glandular hairs (trichomes) on the leaf surface.

1-0-methyl 1-4,
5-dihydroniveusin A
(hemiketal form)

7.XX The major allergen in *Helianthus* annus.

Frequent brushing against the leaves (e.g. during harvesting) is sufficient to cause allergic contact dermatitis. The allergens remain stable after drying and wind-blown trichomes from dry plant material may cause airborne dermatitis. 90% of the sesquiterpene lactones can be isolated by a brief (90 sec) ether extract of the plant material (Hausen & Spring 1989).

Hausen B.M. & Spring O. (1989) Sunflower allergy. *Contact Dermatitis* **20**: 326–34.

HELICHRYSUM diosmifolium

Common names: Ball everlasting. Straw flower
Distribution: Australia, in open forest. Ornamental annual. Dried flowers used in arrangements

The genus *Helichrysum* occurs worldwide, and includes the Mediterranean 'curry plant'. Several species, notably those from Australia, are popularly grown as 'everlasting' flowers

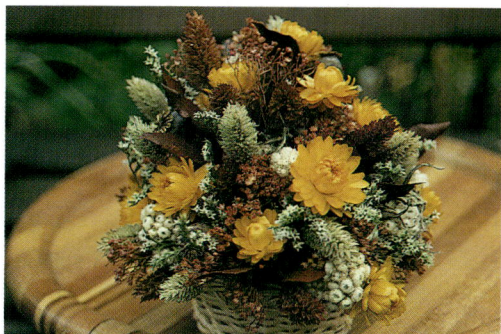

Fig. 7.5.56 *Helichrysum* species in a dried flower arrangement.

(Fig. 7.5.56), maintaining their colour and texture when dried. The plants are handled frequently by florists and flower arrangers. *Helichrysum diosmifolium* is an erect, somewhat branched plant, with sticky leaves and flat or domed clusters of globular white to pale pink flowers. Mitchell and Rook (1979) describe an anecdotal report of eczema from contact with the plant. More recently, allergic contact dermatitis has been reported by McMahon and Freeman (1986).

McMahon R. & Freeman S. (1986) Allergic contact dermatitis to *Helichrysum diosmifolium*. *Australian Journal of Dermatology* **27**: 138–40.
Mitchell J. & Rook A. (1979) *Botanical Dermatology*. Greengrass, Vancouver.

HUMEA elegans
(syn. CALOMERIA amaranthoides)

Common names: Amaranth feathers. Crimson shower. Plume bush. Incense bush
Distribution: Australia (Victoria and New South Wales) in forests. Cultivated occasionally as an ornamental biennial

This impressive plant has soft aromatic leaves which are dark green and lance-shaped. The 2–3 m stem bears a greatly branched feathery head of tiny bell-shaped amber or red flowers on thread-like stalks. Superficially, the individual flower spikes resemble love-lies-bleeding (*Amaranthus*). Humea is occasionally grown as an ornamental pot plant. Allergic contact dermatitis was first reported by Hearnden (1902) in a woman who rubbed the leaves on her veil for their scent. Airborne dermatitis occurs in its native habitat (Maiden 1914). Two more recent reports (Cronin 1968, Rook 1970) describe allergic contact dermatitis in gardeners.

Cronin E. (1968) Sensitivity to *Humea elegans*. *Contact Dermatitis Newsletter* **3**: 39.
Hearnden L.V.C. (1902) A case of contact dermatitis caused by *Humea elegans*. *Lancet* **ii**: 216.
Maiden J.H. (1914) On some plants which cause inflammation or irritation of the skin. *Agricultural Gazette New South Wales* **25**: 611.
Rook A. (1970) Contact dermatitis from *Humea elegans*. *Contact Dermatitis Newsletter* **7**: 164.

INULA helenium, brittanica (see also DITTRICHIA)

Common names: Elecampane. Meadow elecampane
Distribution: Continental Europe, Asia, in damp areas. *Inula helenium* naturalized in parts of Britain. Occasionally grown in herb gardens and borders
Patch test: Alantolactone 0.1% pet.

The genus *Inula* contains several species of herbaceous perennials with bright yellow flowers (Fig. 7.5.57). *Inula helenium*, the elecampane, has branched heads of flowers, each 5–7 cm in diameter. It was grown by the Romans, who used its scented root medicinally. Culpeper is enthusiastic in praise of the roots which help 'all sorts of filthy old putrid sores or cankers whatsoever'. It is still used in herbal medicine, particularly in

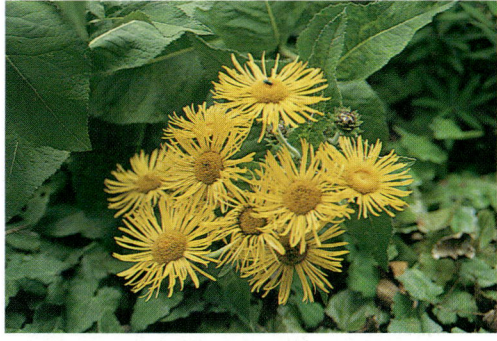

Fig. 7.5.57 *Inula ensifolia*. This border perennial is typical of the genus.

ointments (Pinyankova & Nugmanova 1975) and as a vermifuge (Hjorth 1970). Although the plant itself has not been reported to cause allergic contact dermatitis, it contains the allergenic sesquiterpene lactone alantolactone-I (7.XXI). Crude extracts of the plant may

Alantolactone-1

7.XXI

sensitize (Hjorth 1970, Aberer & Hausen 1990) and should not be used as a screening agent in patch testing, even though alantolactone cross-reacts with other sesquiterpene lactones. Even low concentrations of alantolactone itself (0.1%) may cause false positive patch test reactions (Rycroft et al. 1987).

Inula brittanica does not occur in Britain, despite its specific name. Allergic contact dermatitis was reported in a stable-lad who handled hay contaminated with it. The allergen is unknown, but there was no cross-reaction with other Inula spp. (Hegyi 1967).

Aberer W. & Hausen B.M. (1990) Active sensitisation to elecampane by patch testing with a crude plant extract. Contact Dermatitis 22: 53–5.
Hegyi E.A. (1967) Plant dermatitis: Inula brittanica. Contact Dermatitis Newsletter 2: 4.
Hjorth N. (1970) Active sensitisation with alantolactone. Contact Dermatitis Newsletter 8: 175–6.
Pinyankova Z.P. & Nugmanova M.L. (1975) Dermatitis due to elecampane. Vesta. Derm. Vener. 51: 52.
Rycroft R.J.G., Lovell C.R., Harries P.G., Winter P. & Mallet A.I. (1987) Occupational irritant contact dermatitis from chicory. Bollettino di Dermatologia Allergologica e Professionale 2: 77–82.

IVA xanthifolia

Common name: Marshelder
Distribution: USA, particularly Gulf States. Central America

This relatively uncommon plant is reported as a cause of allergic contact dermatitis (Williams et al. 1960). Positive patch test reactions using oleoresins from *Iva* species often occur in patients with a diagnosis of 'weed dermatitis' (Shelmire 1940); however, this may represent cross-reaction with other genera.

Shelmire B. (1940) Contact dermatitis from vegetation. Southern Medical Journal 33: 337–46.
Williams O., Spears R. & Beggs H.W. (1960) Hypersensitivity to marshelder. Difficulties encountered in patch testing. Journal of the Louisiana State Medical Society 112: 216.

IXODIA achillaeoides

Common name: Ixodia
Distribution: Southeast Australia and Tasmania. An 'everlasting' used in dry flower arrangements

Ixodia is closely related to Helichrysum (q.v.). It is an erect, sticky shrub with long-stalked small white flowers in clusters. Allergic contact dermatitis has been recorded in a patient who handled the dried flowers (Turner 1980).

Turner T. (1980) Compositae dermatitis in South Australia: contact dermatitis from Ixodia achillaeoides and Cynara cardunculus or the tribulations of a dry flower arranger. Contact Dermatitis 6: 444.

LACTUCA sativa

Common name: Lettuce
Distribution: Unknown in wild state. Widely cultivated
Patch test: Leaf as is

This annual salad vegetable may be derived from *L. serriola* (*scariola*), an Asiatic species found wild, or possibly naturalized, in eastern England. The common and Latin name derive from the milky sap (latex) found in all parts of the plant (lac, lactis = milk). Numerous cultivars are grown, including vars. *asparagina* (asparagus lettuce), *capitata* (cabbage lettuce), *crispa* (curled lettuce), *longifolia* or *romana* (cos or Romaine lettuce). The latex has a milky sedative effect and lettuce has been grown as a herb, although Culpeper warns that 'it is chiefly forbidden to those that are short-winded, or have any imperfection in the lungs, or spit blood'.

Lettuce is an occasional cause of allergic contact dermatitis in food handlers such as salad makers, greengrocers and market gardeners. Cross-reaction occurs with chicory and endive (q.v.). The hands and forearms are affected typically (Krook 1973, Friis et al. 1975, Helander 1984). In a recent report by Mitchell et al. (1989), a 16-year-old atopic male developed hand dermatitis after starting work as a chef. Patch tests were positive to lettuce, chicory, and, curiously, to cabbage (which is botanically unrelated). The eczema cleared after he discontinued work as a chef.

Both lactucin (**7.XXIIa**) and lactucopicrin

Lactucin

7.XXIIa

(**7.XXIIb**) have been isolated from lettuce (Hausen & Hjorth 1984); these are also present in chicory, doubtless explaining the typical 'cross-reaction' between the two plants. In guinea pigs, lactucopicrin is the chief sensitizer (Hausen et al. 1986), although in the case of Mitchell et al. (1989) positive patch tests were obtained with lactucin, but not lactucopicrin.

Lactupicrin
(lactucopicrin)

7.XXIIb

There are also several reports of immediate hypersensitivity to lettuce, typically occurring in association with delayed hypersensitivity (e.g. Rinkel & Balyeat 1932, Krook 1977, Fregert & Sjoborg 1982). In one patient reported by Krook (1973) a patient with contact urticaria induced by lettuce developed alarming throat swelling after eating endive.

Both prick and patch testing can be performed using the mature leaf and are negative in controls (Krook 1977); immature leaves are innocuous (Krook 1973).

Fregert S. & Sjoborg S. (1982) Unsuspected lettuce: immediate allergy in a case of delayed metal allergy. *Contact Dermatitis* **8**: 265.
Friis B., Hjorth N., Vail J.T., Jr. & Mitchell J.C. (1975) Occupational contact dermatitis from *Cichorium* (chicory, endive) and *Lactuca* (lettuce). *Contact Dermatitis* **1**: 311–13.
Hausen B.M. & Hjorth N. (1984) Skin reactions to topical food exposure. *Dermatologic Clinics* **2**: 567–8.
Hausen B.M., Anderson K.E., Helander I. & Gensch K.H. (1986) Lettuce allergy: sensitising potency of allergens. *Contact Dermatitis* **15**: 246–9.
Helander I. (1984) Contact dermatitis to lettuce. *Contact Dermatitis* **11**: 249.
Krook G. (1973) Contact dermatitis due to lettuce (*Lactuca sativa*). *Contact Dermatitis Newsletter* **13**: 346.
Krook G. (1977) Occupational dermatitis from *Lactuca sativa* (lettuce) and *Cichorium* (endive). *Contact Dermatitis* **3**: 27–36.
Mitchell D., Beck M.H. & Hausen B.M. (1989) Contact sensitivity to lettuce in a chef. *Contact Dermatitis* **20**: 398–9.
Rinkel H.J. & Balyeat R.M. (1932) Occupational dermatitis due to lettuce. *JAMA* **98**: 137.

LEUCANTHEMUM vulgare (syn. CHRYSANTHEMUM leucanthemum)

Common names: Ox-eye daisy. Marguerite
Distribution: Europe, Asia. Naturalized in USA. Occasionally cultivated
Patch test: Leaf, stalk and petal

This perennial plant is common on basic soil in pastures and meadows. The leaves are typically linear and undivided. The 50 cm stems each bear a solitary daisy-like flower with white rays and a central disk (Fig. 7.5.58). Contact dermatitis may occur in gardeners or florists (Scarzella 1958). Usually, the stems and leaves are allergenic, although Ducombs and Geniaux (1982) report a case of a young woman in whom only the petals elicited a positive patch test reaction.

Ducombs G. & Geniaux M. (1982) Personal communication referred to in Benezra C., Ducombs G., Sell Y. & Foussereau J. (1985) *Plant Contact Dermatitis*. B.C. Decker, Toronto, p. 112.
Scarzella M. (1958) A case of contact dermatitis due to *Leucanthemum vulgare*. *Minerva Pediatrica* **10**: 34.

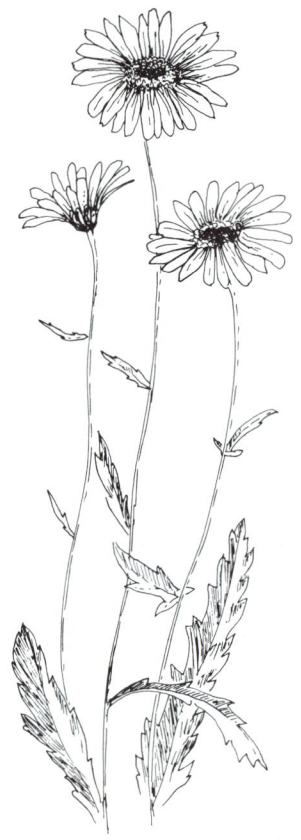

Fig. 7.5.58 *Leucanthemum vulgare* (ox-eye daisy).

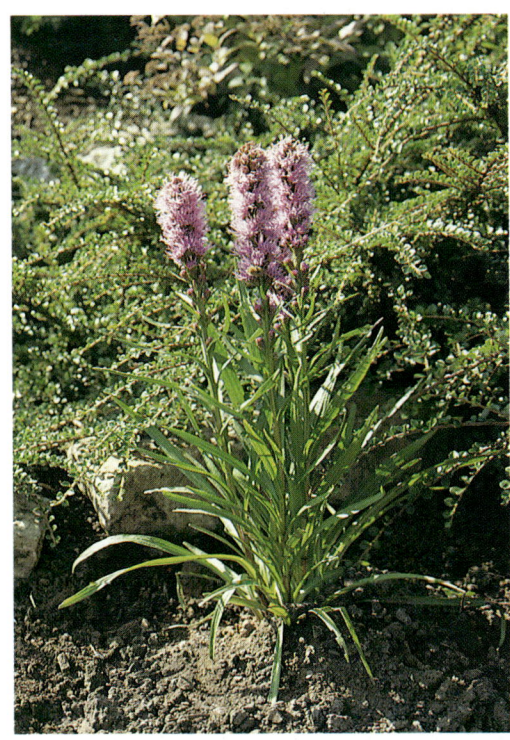

Fig. 7.5.59 *Liatris spicata.*

LIATRIS spicata

Common name: Blazing star
Distribution: USA. Cultivated as a border perennial

This popular ornamental plant (Fig. 7.5.59) has erect, leafy stems, up to 1.5 m, with a plume-like spike of purple flowers in mid-summer. The buds open in reverse order, i.e. from the top downwards. Allergic contact dermatitis appears to be rare, although Goerz *et al.* report positive patch tests in a patient with allergic contact dermatitis due to other Compositae.

Goerz G., Wirth G., Maas B. & Willuhn G. (1985) Allergische Kontaktdermatitis auf Asteraceae (Kompositen) Kreuzreaktion mit *Liatris spicata*. *Dermatosen in Beruf und Umwelt* **33**: 95–8.

MATRICARIA chamomilla (CHAMOMILLA recutita)

Common names: Wild chamomile. German chamomile
Distribution: Europe
Patch test: Leaf and petal

This annual weed is one of many plants known as 'chamomile' (see Table 7.5.8 & Fig. 7.5.43). It is a fragrant herb, common on waste ground and cultivated areas. The leaves are finely divided and there are numerous 2 cm flowers, each with white rays and a conical yellow disk. The rays soon reflex after opening. In a detailed review of the literature of chamomile dermatitis by Hausen *et al.* (1984) only five cases could be attributed definitely to *M. chamomilla*. Van Ketel (1987) reported allergy to this species in a part-time florist. Patch tests were positive in this patient to petals and stems, although Moslein (1963) obtained positive reactions only to the petals.

Table 7.5.8 The chamomiles (see Fig. 7.5.43).

Common name	Botanical name	Notes
Sweet chamomile	Chamaemelum nobile (Anthemis nobilis)	European native. Perennial. Pleasantly scented. Usually double-flowered form grown in chamomile lawns. Source of chamomile tea. Allergenic
Wild (German) chamomile	Matricaria recutita (chamomilla)	Annual weed of cultivated areas and waste grounds. Allergenic
Scentless mayweed (chamomile)	Matricaria inodora	Tall annual weed commonly found on roadsides and by the sea. Allergenic
Stinking mayweed (dog fennel)	Anthemis cotula	Europe: naturalized in USA, South Africa and Australia. Annual weed of waste and arable land. Has a strong, sickly smell; strongly irritant causing bullous reactions. ? Also allergenic
Corn chamomile (field mayweed)	Anthemis arvensis	Annual. Sweetly scented (like C. nobile). Found in chalky soils; relatively uncommon. Allergenic
Yellow chamomile	Anthemis tinctoria	European biennial, naturalized as a garden escape in parts of Britain. Source of a yellow dye. Apparently not allergenic

Cross-reaction occurs with other Compositae, including florist's chrysanthemum (van Ketel 1987). A positive allergen is the sesquiterpene lactone, desacetylmatricarin (Moslein 1963).

Hausen B.M., Dusker E. & Carle R. (1984) Uber das Sensibilisierungsvermogen von Compositearten VII. Experimentelle Untersuchungen mit Auszugen und Inhaltsstoffen von *Chamomilla recutita* (L.) Raischert und *Anthemis cotula* L. *Planta Medica* **50**: 229–34.
Moslein P. (1963) Pflanzen als Kontakt-Allergene. *Berufsdermatosen* **11**: 24–8.
Van Ketel W.G. (1987) Allergy to *Matricaria chamomilla*. *Contact Dermatitis* **16**: 50–1.

OLEARIA axillaris

Common name: Coast daisy bush
Distribution: Australasia

This large genus of shrubs or small trees is indigenous to Australasia. *Olearia axillaris* is a large, bushy, grey shrub with strongly aromatic narrow leaves, white on the undersurface. The tiny cream flowers often lack ray florets and are clustered around branches. It grows particularly in coastal areas of New South Wales and Victoria. Burry *et al.* (1975) report four positive patch tests using this plant in 13 individuals with Compositae dermatitis in South Australia.

Burry J.N., Reid J.G. & Kirk J. (1975) Australian bush dermatitis. *Contact Dermatitis* **1**: 263–4.

OXYTAENIA acerosa

Common name: Copperweed
Distribution: Southwest USA

Schwartz and Warren (1940) report allergic contact dermatitis in a plant chemist who was working with this plant. Patch tests were positive to the plant itself and to an alcohol extract; however, an ether extract gave negative results.

Schwartz L. & Warren L.H. (1940) Dermatitis caused by contact with copperweed (*Oxytaenia acerosa*). *Journal of Allergy* **12**: 63–8.

PARTHENIUM argentatum

Common names: Mexican rubber plant. Guayule

Allergic contact dermatitis was first reported by Smith and Hughes (1938). *Parthenium argentatum* contains the potent allergens, guayulins A and B, which elicit allergic contact dermatitis in experimental animals (Rodriguez 1981).

Rodriguez E. (1981) Potent contact allergen in the rubber plant guayule (*Parthenium argentatum*). *Science* **211** (4489): 1444–5.
Smith C.M. & Hughes R.P. (1938) Dermatitis caused by Mexican Rubber Plant. *Archives of Dermatology and Syphilology* **38**: 780.

PARTHENIUM hysterophorus

Common names: Congress grass. Carrot weed. Feverfew (NB. this name is also used for *Tanacetum parthenium*)
Distribution: Central and south America. Southwest USA (may be naturalized) on waste ground. A major weed in India
Patch test: Leaf as is. Parthenin ?0.1%

This annual, or short-lived perennial, herb has 40–80 cm stems covered in fine hairs. The thin greyish leaves are fern-like, often with toothed margins. The numerous flowers are each about 0.5 cm in diameter, with a few narrow white rays. Large amounts of sticky pollen are produced (Mitchell 1981).

It is recorded as an important cause of allergic contact dermatitis and respiratory symptoms in the southern states of the USA (Shelmire 1940, Ogden 1957). In 1956 it was accidentally introduced to the Maharastea State on the west coast of India, in a consignment of wheat from the USA. Conditions in India have proved to be favourable to its growth and the plant has spread rapidly along canal banks (often assisted by floods), roads and railways, sometimes obliterating the tracks. It has become a major field weed. Several thousands of cases of allergic contact dermatitis have occurred in India, some of them fatal (Lonkar et al. 1974). One outbreak of epidemic proportion followed a dam burst (Mitchell & Calnan 1978).

There are several possible reasons for the extent of allergic contact dermatitis in India, as compared with America. The plant grows much more vigorously in India and contains large amounts of the sesquiterpene lactone, parthenin, which is absent from plants in South America (Lonkar et al. 1976, Towers et al. 1977). Much agriculture in the USA is mechanized, whereas in India the operatives and inhabitants of rural communities come in closer contact with the plants.

Typically, *Parthenium* dermatitis affects adult males in both USA and India (Towers & Mitchell 1983). This cannot be explained in terms of degree of exposure, since Indian women and children also work in the fields. Other Compositae, including chrysanthemum, also tend to cause dermatitis more commonly

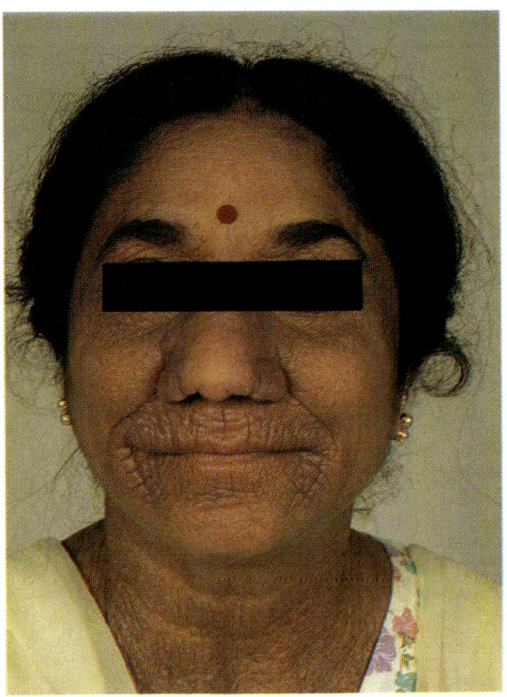

Fig. 7.5.60 Leonine facies attributed to *Parthenium hysterophorus*. (Courtesy of Dr R.R.M. Harman.)

in males. Initially, the face, neck and flexures are affected. Often the distribution shows a typical 'airborne' pattern, involving the eyelids and nasolabial folds in contradistinction to photosensitive eczema (Lonkar et al. 1974, Sharma & Kaur 1989). Later, the affected skin becomes lichenified; the individual may develop a 'leonine' facies (Fig. 7.5.60) and a persistent generalized eruption may develop, resembling severe atopic dermatitis (Behl & Captain 1979). Singh et al. (1987) noted sparing of vitiliginous skin, perhaps due to vacuolization of Langerhans cells in the vitiliginous areas. Skin or respiratory infection may be fatal (Lonkar et al. 1974).

In India, the major allergenic sesquiterpene lactone is parthenin (**7.XXIII**) (Lonkar et al. 1976). The allergen is borne in glandular trichomes on the plant surface (Rodriguez et al. 1976). This allergen is absent in South American material. Other sesquiterpene lactones isolated from *Parthenium hysterophorus* include the diasteriomer of parthenin, hymenin, which does not cross-

Parthenin **Hymenin**

7.XXIII Allergens in *P. hysterophorus*.

react with parthenin (Subba Rao *et al.* 1977).

Jeanmougin *et al.* (1988) report 'photo-aggravation' of *Parthenium* contact dermatitis. This may be a non-specific reaction; persistent light reactivity can follow airborne contact dermatitis to a variety of different allergens. Most of the patients reported by Lonkar *et al.* (1974) improve if they avoid further exposure to the plant, even if they move to a sunny coastal area.

To date, there is only one well-documented case of photocontact dermatitis caused by this species (Bhutani & Rao 1978). The patient, a 70-year-old retired agricultural labourer, exhibited a typical photosensitive eruption, sparing the eyelids. Closed patch testing to the plant was negative, but subsequent irradiation with UVA yielded a positive reaction. Histology of the eruption revealed elastotic degeneration with a histiocytic infiltrate, resembling actinic reticuloid.

Various materials have been used for patch testing, including the leaf itself, acetone and benzene extracts, and 1% parthenin in petrolatum (Lonkar *et al.* 1976). Subba Rao *et al.* (1977) elicited positive patch test reactions in 56% of a group of adult males exposed to the plant, only 4% of whom developed clinical features of dermatitis. This is difficult to interpret; a similar phenomenon can be observed when screening for other occupational allergens (e.g. epoxy resin) in a workforce. Active sensitization is also a real problem; Benezra *et al.* (1985) recommend a 0.1% concentration of parthenin for patch testing. Alantolactone is an unsatisfactory screening material (Lonkar *et al.* 1974).

Treatment is notoriously difficult: even potent topical corticosteroids and prednisolone are relatively ineffective. Ogden (1957) reported some response to ACTH. Azathioprine may be effective. Attempts have been made to achieve oral hyposensitization. Srinivas *et al.* (1988) report a 50-year-old female school teacher with erythoderma requiring systemic steroids, who was successfully desensitized by daily ingestion of *Parthenium* leaf diluted in maize starch and dispersed in corn starch. A daily starting dose of 0.1 mg was increased gradually to 1 mg after 2 weeks. She remained symptom-free until discontinuing the capsules. Continued therapy appears to be necessary (Srinivas *et al.* 1988).

Behl P.N. & Captain R.M. (1979) *Skin-Irritant and Sensitising Plants Found in India*. S. Chand, Ram Naga, New Delhi.
Benezra C., Ducombes G., Sell Y. & Foussereau J. (1985) *Plant Contact Dermatitis*. B.C. Decker, Toronto.
Bhutani J.K. & Rao D.S. (1978) Photocontact dermatitis caused by *Parthenium hysterophorus*. *Dermatologica* **157**: 206–9.
Jeanmougin M., Taieb M., Mancieb J.R., Moulin J.P. & Ciratte J. (1988) Photo-aggravation d'un eczema de contact à *Parthenium hysterophorus*. *Annales de Dermatologie et Venerelogie* **115**: 1238–40.
Lonkar A., Mitchell J.C. & Calnan C.D. (1974) Contact dermatitis from *Parthenium hysterophorus*. *Transactions of the St John's Hospital Dermatological Society* **60**: 43–53.
Lonkar A., Nagasampagi B.A., Narayanan C.R., Landge A.B. & Sawaikar D.D. (1976) An antigen from *Parthenium hysterophorus* Linn. *Contact Dermatitis* **2**: 151–4.
Mitchell J.C. (1981) *Parthenium* pollen – *Parthenium* dermatitis. *Contact Dermatitis* **7**: 212–17.
Mitchell J.C. & Calnan C.D. (1978) Scourge of India: *Parthenium* dermatitis. *International Journal of Dermatology* **17**: 303–4.
Ogden H.D. (1957) Diagnosis and treatment of *Parthenium* dermatitis. *Journal of the Louisiana Medical Society* **109**: 378.
Rodriguez E., Dillon M.O., Mabry T.J., Mitchell J.C. & Towers G.H.N. (1976) Dermatologically active sesquiterpene lactones in trichomes of *Parthenium hysterophorus* L. (Compositae). *Experientia* **32**: 236.
Sharma S.C. & Kaur S. (1989) Airborne contact dermatitis from Compositae plants in northern India. *Contact Dermatitis* **21**: 1–5.
Shelmire B. (1940) Contact dermatitis from vegetation. *Southern Medical Journal* **33**: 337–46.
Singh K.K., Srinivas C., Balachandran C. & Menon S. (1987) *Parthenium* dermatitis sparing vitiliginous skin. *Contact Dermatitis* **16**: 174.
Srinivas C.R., Krupashankar D.S., Singh K.K., Balachandran C. & Shenoi S.D. (1988) Oral hyposensitization in *Parthenium* dermatitis. *Contact Dermatitis* **18**: 242–3.
Subba Rao P.V., Mangala A., Subba Rao B.S. & Prakash K.M. (1977) Clinical and immunological studies on persons exposed to *Parthenium hysterophorus* L. *Experientia* **33**: 1387–8.

Towers G.H.N. & Mitchell J.C. (1983) The current status of the weed *Parthenium hysterophorus* L. as a cause of allergic contact dermatitis. *Contact Dermatitis* **9**: 465–9.

Towers G.H.N., Mitchell J.C., Rodriguez E. *et al.* (1977) Biology and chemistry of *Parthenium hysterophorus* L.; a problem weed in India. *Journal of Scientific and Industrial Research* **36**: 672–84.

PYRETHRUM

See *Tanacetum cinerariifolium*.

RUDBECKIA hirta

Common names: Black-eyed Susan.
   Coneflower
Distribution: North American prairies

This attractive plant (Fig. 7.5.61) has 0.5–1 m stems with yellow to orange flowers with a conspicuous, often cone-shaped, dull brown disk. Lovell *et al.* (1955) and Mackoff and Dahl (1951) report cases of allergic contact dermatitis to this species and positive patch tests were obtained using the oleoresin in the survey of photosensitive eczema by Frain-Bell and Johnson (1979).

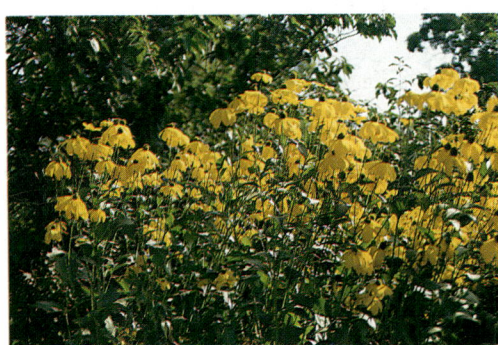

Fig. 7.5.61 *Rudbeckia hirta*.

Frain-Bell W. & Johnson B.E. (1979) Contact allergic sensitivity to plants and the photosensitivity dermatitis and actinic reticuloid syndrome. *British Journal of Dermatology* **101**: 503–12.

Lovell R.G., Mathews K.P. & Sheldon J.M. (1955) Dermatitis venenata from tree pollen oils. *Journal of Allergy* **26**: 408–14.

Mackoff S. & Dahl A.O. (1951) A botanical consideration of the weed oleoresin problem. *Minnesota Medicine* **34**: 1169–73, 1188.

SAUSSUREA lappa (S. costus)

Common name: Costus root
Distribution: India

This plant is native to the Himalayas, although other members of the genus, such as *S. alpina*, the alpine saw-wort, are native to Britain and northern Europe. Superficially the purple flower heads resemble those of artichokes (*Cynara* spp.). *Saussurea lappa* root is the source of costus root oil, which was used extensively in perfumes, particularly in India (Mitchell & Epstein 1974). It contains many sesquiterpene lactones, including costunolide (a germacranolide), which is a potent sensitizer. Costus root oil cross-reacts with many other sesquiterpene lactones and, therefore, with other Compositae such as florist's chrysanthemum, lettuce, chicory, etc. (Epstein *et al.* 1980). Two of its constituent sesquiterpene lactones, costunolide and dehydrocostus lactone (a guaianolide), were used in the 'sesquiterpene lactone mix', a possible screen for Compositae sensitivity (Ducombs *et al.* 1990) (**7.XXIV**). Although it was unclear how important Compositae extracts were in perfume dermatitis (Rodriguez & Mitchell 1977), attempts have been made to remove the sesquiterpene lactones by hydrogenation or binding to aminated polystyrenes (Cheminat *et al.* 1981). It has now been removed from perfumes.

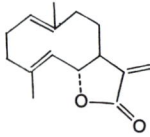 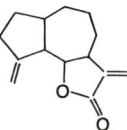

Costunolide   Dehydrocostus lactone

7.XXIV

Cheminat A., Stampt J.-L., Benezra C., Farrall M.J. & Frechet J.M.J. (1981) Allergic contact dermatitis to costus: removal of haptens with polymers IV. *Acta Dermato-Venereologica* **61**: 525–9.

Ducombs G., Benezra C., Talaga P. *et al.* (1990) Patch testing with the 'sesquiterpene lactone mix': a marker for contact allergy to compositae and other sesquiterpene lactone-containing plants. *Contact Dermatitis* **22**: 249–52.

Epstein W.L., Reynolds G.W. & Rodriguez E. (1980) Sesquiterpene lactone dermatitis: cross-sensitivity in costus-sensitised patients. *Archives of Dermatology*

116: 59–60.

Mitchell J.C. & Epstein W.L. (1974) Contact sensitivity to a perfume material, costus absolute. *Archives of Dermatology* **110**: 871–3.

Rodriguez E. & Mitchell J.C. (1977) Absence of contact hypersensitivity to some perfume materials derived from compositae species. *Contact Dermatitis* **3**: 168.

SOLIDAGO spp.

Common name: Golden rod
Distribution: *Solidago virgaurea* Europe (including Britain). Many other spp. in USA. Cultivated as ornamental perennials

The golden rods are mostly North American natives, although *S. virgaurea* (Fig. 7.5.62) is found on dry banks, cliffs and heathland in southern and western Britain. The stems (usually 1–1.5 m tall) bear a large terminal head of numerous yellow daisy-like flowers. *Solidago canadensis* and *gigantea* are commoner garden plants, with pyramidal heads of numerous tiny yellow tubular flowers; they are commonly naturalized as a garden escape, on river and stream banks, and on waste ground. Shelmire (1939) demonstrates positive patch test reactions to an extract of *S. gigantea*. Schwartz *et al.* (1957) reported maculopapular dermatitis in farm workers who were handling hay presumed to be contaminated with S. *virgaurea*. Underwood and Gaul (1948) described three cases of allergic contact dermatitis to *Solidago* spp. with positive patch tests. The allergens are probably sesquiterpene lactones. A 10% oleoresin gave positive patch test reactions in eight of 55 patients with photosensitivity dermatitis (Frain-Bell & Johnson 1979); however, this may represent cross-reaction with other Compositae.

Frain-Bell W. & Johnson B.E. (1979) Contact allergic sensitivity to plants and the photosensitivity dermatitis and actinic reticuloid syndrome. *British Journal of Dermatology* **101**: 503–12.

Schwartz L., Tulipan L. & Birmingham D.J. (1957) *Occupational Diseases of the Skin*, 3rd edn. Lea & Febiger, Philadelphia.

Shelmire B. (1939) Contact dermatitis from weeds: patch testing with their oleoresins. *JAMA* **113**: 1085–90.

Underwood G.B. & Gaul L.E. (1948) Over treatment dermatitis in dermatitis venenata due to plants. *JAMA* **138**: 570–82.

SOLIVA pterosperma

Common names: Bindii, jo-jo. Stalkless *Soliva*
Distribution: Australia — especially coastal regions in turf

This annual weed has finely divided grey leaves which form a downy mat. Minute pink daisy-like flowers are borne at the leaf bases. The fruits are needle-sharp and can penetrate the skin, even through thick clothing. Children, in particular, develop a maculopapular, sometimes pustular, eruption during the late spring and summer. It affects chiefly the areas that come into contact with the ground, such as palms, soles, knees and elbows. Although there is a clear mechanical irritant component to the eruption, Commens *et al.* (1984) found that lesions could be induced only in susceptible individuals, suggesting an additional component of allergic dermatitis (Commens *et al.* 1982, 1984).

Commens C., Bartlett B.H., McGeoch A.H. *et al.* (1982) Bindii (jo-jo) dermatitis: the clinical and histopathological spectrum. *Australasian Journal of Dermatology* **23**: 110–15.

Commens C., McGeoch A.H., Bartlett B. *et al.* (1984) Bindii (jo-jo) dermatitis (*Soliva pterosperma*

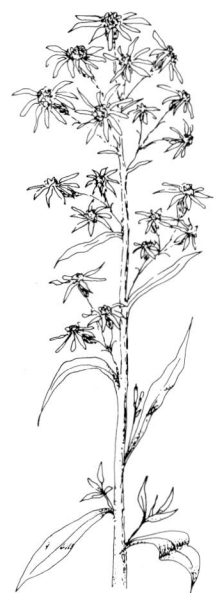

Fig. 7.5.62 *Solidago virgaurea* (golden rod).

[Compositae]). *Journal of the American Academy of Dermatology* **10**: 768–73.

TAGETES spp.

Common name: Marigold
Distribution: Central and South America. Many species cultivated as ornamental annuals. *Tagetes minuta* is an important weed in southeast Africa (see Table 7.5.9)

The garden marigolds (Fig. 7.5.63) are derived from several species of *Tagetes*. Pot marigold, often used in homoeopathic preparations, is a separate genus, *Calendula*. Several species of *Tagetes* are strongly, even offensively, aromatic and are potently irritant. Gerard warns that the African marigold (*T. erecta*) 'is of a most ranke and unwholesome smell' and that it 'is of a venomous and poysonsome facultie'. The roots of *Tagetes* species yield α-terthienyl and bithienyl (Bohlmann *et al.* 1973), both of which are phototoxic in experimental models; however, there are no reported cases of phytophotodermatitis due to the genus. *Tagetes indica* has been implicated in airborne contact dermatitis in India (Sharma & Kaur 1989).

Tagetes minuta has become a major weed

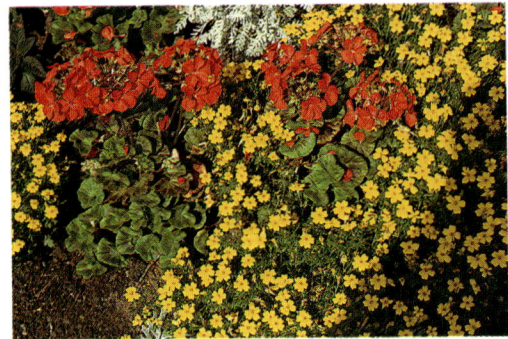

Fig. 7.5.63 A *Tagetes* cultivar planted with a *Pelargonium* cultivar.

in parts of Africa; the sap causes chemical irritation, even blistering, and the seeds and rough stems are mechanical irritants (Watt & Breyer-Brandwijk 1962). In addition, Verhagen and Nyaga (1974) report allergic patch test reactions to acetone extracts of leaf and flower head in three farmers who presented with chronic lichenified dermatitis. There was no augmentation of the patch test reactions by UV irradiation (Verhagen & Nyaga 1974).

Tagetes patula oil has been used in perfumery and a 1% dilution in grape seed oil has caused bilateral hand eczema in an

Table 7.5.9 *Tagetes* species and cultivars.

Species	Common name	Description	Notes
T. erecta	African marigold	Large, fully double flowers on 50 cm stems	Cultivars include Guinea Gold, Toreador, Inca hybrids, Tom Thumb (dwarf)
T. lucida	Mexican marigold	Orange/yellow sweet-scented flowers on 25–30 cm stems	Occasionally cultivated
T. minuta (syn. *glandulifera*)	Stinking Roger Khaki weed	Erect herb up to 2 m. Very pungent. Divided toothed leaves. Congested terminal heads of narrowly cylindrical yellowish green flowers with a few white rays	A common naturalized weed in southeastern Africa, especially Kenyan highlands and Transvaal. Also found in Mediterranean regions and Australasia
T. patula	French marigold	Compact bushy plant with single or double flowers, ranging from yellow to chestnut, on 30 cm stems	Cultivars include Fire cross, Golden Ball, Spanish Brocade
T. signata v. *pumila*	'Tagetes' of nursery gardeners	Mound-like dwarf plants with numerous small, usually single, flowers, on branching stems (about 20 cm)	Cultivars include Golden Gem, Paprika, and Starfire

aromatherapist (Bilsland & Strong 1990). The allergen is unknown, no sesquiterpene lactones have so far been isolated (Pirker *et al.* 1992).

Bilsland D. & Strong A. (1990) Allergic contact dermatitis from the essential oil of French marigold (*Tagetes patula*) in an aromatherapist. *Contact Dermatitis* **23**: 55–6.
Bohlmann F., Burkhardt T. & Zdero C. (1973) *Naturally Occurring Acetylenes*. Academic Press, London.
Pirker C., Möslinger T., Koller D.Y., Götz M. & Jarisch R. (1992) Cross-reactivity with *Tagebes* in Arnica contact eczema. *Contact Dermatitis* **26**: 217–19.
Sharma S.C. & Kaur S. (1989) Airborne contact dermatitis from Compositae plants in northern India. *Contact Dermatitis* **21**: 1–5.
Verhagen A.R. & Nyaga J.M. (1974) Contact dermatitis from *Tagetes minuta*. *Archives of Dermatology* **110**: 441–4.
Watt J.M. & Breyer-Brandwijk M.G. (1962) *The Medicinal and Poisonous Plants of Southern Africa*, 2nd edn. E. & S. Livingstone, Edinburgh.

TANACETUM cinerariifolium (syn. CHRYSANTHEMUM or PYRETHRUM cinerariifolium)

Common name: Pyrethrum

Tanacetum cinerariifolium is the major source of the natural insecticide pyrethrum. It is a tufted perennial with silvery-grey silky leaves and a solitary 3–4 cm white flower. It grows on rocky ground on the western (Adriatic) coast of Jugoslavia. *Tanacetum roseum* and *T. coccineum* (native to the Caucasus) are other sources of pyrethrum. The powder is derived by grinding the flower heads.

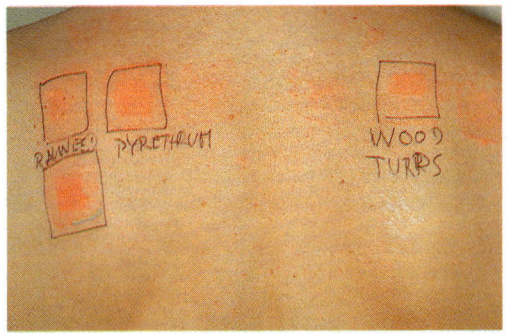

Fig. 7.5.64 Positive patch test with pyrethrum in a ragweed-sensitive patient. (Courtesy of J.N. Burry.)

Pyrethrum is cultivated commercially in Japan, parts of South America and east Africa. Historically, it was a major cause of allergic contact dermatitis (Fig. 7.5.64), particularly among workers harvesting the flower heads (Mitchell *et al.* 1972). The major allergen appears to be pyrethrosin (**7.XXV**), a sesquiterpene lactone, although many other sesquiterpene lactones have been isolated in alcoholic extracts of the flowers (Doskotch *et al.* 1971). Martin and Hester (1941) report accidental sensitization in a dermatologist who was preparing an extract of *T. cinerariifolium*.

7.XXV Allergens in *Pyrethrum*.

The pyrethins themselves, which have the insecticide activity, are chemically unrelated and are very rare sensitizers (Mitchell *et al.* 1972). Most pyrethroids, notably permethrin, are now prepared synthetically, although some natural pyrethrum insecticide is still available to satisfy the demand of 'organic' gardeners. Although synthetic pyrethroids themselves are not sensitizers, paraesthesia can follow contact. This can be counteracted by the application of vitamin E acetate (Flannigan & Tucker 1985). Recently permethrin has been released for the treatment of scabies.

Doskotch R.W., El-Feracy F.S. & Hufford C.D. (1971) Sesquiterpene lactones from *Pyrethrum* flowers. *Canadian Journal of Chemistry* **49**: 2103–10.
Flannigan S.A. & Tucker S.B. (1985) Variation in cutaneous sensation between synthetic pyrethroid insecticides. *Contact Dermatitis* **13**: 140–7.
Martin J.T. & Hester K.C. (1941) Dermatitis caused by insecticidal *Pyrethrum* flowers. *British Journal of Dermatology* **53**: 127–42.
Mitchell J.C., Dupuis G. & Towers G.H.N. (1972) Allergic contact dermatitis from *Pyrethrum* (*Chrysanthemum* spp.): the roles of pyrethrosin a sesquiterpene lactone, and of pyrethrin II. *British Journal of Dermatology* **86**: 568–73.

TANACETUM parthenium
(CHRYSANTHEMUM parthenium not PARTHENIUM hysterophorus)

Common names: Feverfew. Bachelor's buttons. Mutterkraut (German)
Distribution: Europe, including Britain, in cultivated areas and waste ground.

Commonly grown in herb collections
Patch test: 1% ether or brief water extract

This perennial has divided bright green (or golden yellow) leaves and many flower heads on 30–40 cm stems. The individual flowers are 1–2 cm in diameter, daisy-like, with bright yellow disk and white rays (Fig. 7.5.65). The whole plant is strong-smelling. Feverfew has been cultivated as a herb for many years and Culpeper attributes many virtues to it, particularly in obstetric practice ('it is chiefly used for the disease of the mother, whether it be the strangling or rising of the mother, or hardness, of inflammation of the same, applied outwardly thereunto'). Gerard recommends it for 'such as be melancholike, sad, pensive, and without speech'. Feverfew is popularly promoted as a 'natural cure' and prophylaxis against migraines and arthritis. The efficacy may correlate with its sesquiterpene lactone content (Johnson *et al.* 1985). Feverfew chewers develop allergic contact dermatitis as well as swelling of the lips and tongue, together with mouth ulcers (Johnson 1986). Airborne contact dermatitis from feverfew in a typical distribution may superficially mimic photosensitivity; several cases have been reported in Australia (Burry 1980) and Europe (Hausen 1981, Mensing *et al.* 1985).

Cross-reaction occurs with many other compositae, and feverfew extract can be used as a screening test for suspected dermatitis to florist's chrysanthemum (Schmidt & Kingston 1985). The major allergenic sesquiterpene lactone is parthenolide, a germacranolide (Hausen & Osmundsen 1983), although several other sesquiterpene lactones have been extracted from the plant growing in North America (Hausen 1981). Parthenolide (**7.XXVI**)

Parthenolide

7.XXVI

occurs in other Compositae as well as in botanically unrelated genera such as *Michelia compressa* and *Magnolia grandiflora*, both members of the Magnoliaceae (Wiedhopf *et al.* 1973, Ogura *et al.* 1978). Parthenolide is surprisingly water-soluble (Hausen 1991) and appears to be a major sensitizer in Compositae contact dermatitis.

Burry J.N. (1980) Compositae dermatitis in South Australia: contact dermatitis from *Chrysanthemum parthenium*. *Contact Dermatitis* **6**: 445.
Hausen B.M. (1981) Berufsbedingte Kontaktallergie auf Mutterkraut (*Tanacetum parthenium* (L.) Schultz-Bip; Asteraceae). *Dermatosen in Beruf und Umwelt* **29**: 18–21.
Hausen B.M. (1991) A simple method of isolating parthenolide from *Tanacetum* and other sensitising plants. *Contact Dermatitis* **24**: 153–5.
Hausen B.M. & Osmundsen P.E. (1983) Contact allergy to parthenolide in *Tanacetum parthenium* Schultz-Bip (feverfew, Asteracea) and cross-reactions to related sesquiterpene lactone containing compositae species. *Acta Dermato-Venerologica* **63**: 308–14.
Johnson E.S., Kadam N.P., Hylands D.M. & Heylands P.J. (1985) Efficacy of feverfew as prophylactic treatment of migraine. *British Medical Journal* **291**: 569–73.
Johnson S. (1986) *Feverfew*. Sheldon Press, London.
Mensing H., Kimmig W. & Hausen B.M. (1985) Airborne contact dermatitis. *Der Hautarzt* **36**: 398–402.
Ogura M., Cordell G.A. & Farnsworth N.C. (1978) Anticancer sesquiterpene lactones from *Michelia compressa* (Magnoliaceae). *Phytochemistry* **17**: 957–61.
Schmidt R.J. & Kingston T. (1985) Chrysanthemum

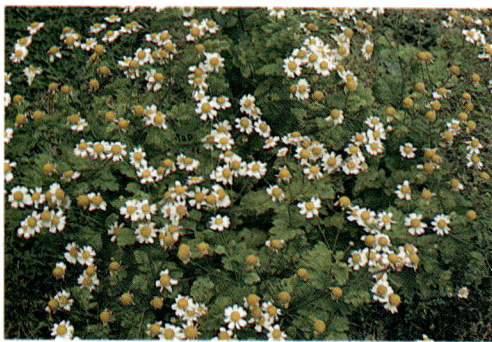

Fig. 7.5.65 *Tanacetum parthenium* (feverfew). (Courtesy of Miss M. Hansen.)

dermatitis in South Wales: diagnosis by patch testing with feverfew (*Tanacetum parthenium*) extract. *Contact Dermatitis* **13**: 120–1.

Wiedhopf R.M., Young M., Bianchi E. & Cole J.R. (1973) Tumour inhibitory agents from *Magnolia grandiflora*. *Journal of Pharmaceutical Sciences* **62**: 345.

TANACETUM vulgare

Common names: Tansy. Wurmkraut (German)

Distribution: Europe, including Britain, especially on hedge banks, railway tracks and waste ground. Sometimes cultivated. Naturalized in North America

This strongly aromatic perennial herb (Fig. 7.5.66) has a stem 0.5–1 m tall, with many linear, toothed leaves and heads of small golden-yellow flowers with no rays (Fig. 7.5.66). Like feverfew, it has a long history of use in herbal medicine. As the German name 'Wurmkraut' suggests, it was hung from ceilings as an insecticide. Culpeper attributes many properties to it, chiefly of a gynaecological nature. Thus 'Let those women that desire children love this herb, it is their best companion, their husbands excepted'. Its use as an abortifacient may lead to convulsions through over-dosage (Lampe & Fagerström 1968).

Cases of allergic contact dermatitis due to tansy have been reported by Huber and Harsh (1932), Greenhouse and Sulzberger (1933) and Rook (1960). Cross-reactions occur with other compositae, notably *T. parthenium* (Mackoff & Dahl 1951). Mitchell (quoted in Mitchell & Rook 1979) described a chrysanthemum grower whose dermatitis persisted after he discarded his chrysanthemum plants: a housecall revealed that he was weeding *T. vulgare* from his garden. Wrangsjo *et al.* (1990) obtained positive patch tests to *T. vulgare* oleoresin (1% pet.) in five of 15 patients with summer-exacerbated dermatitis. *Tanacetum vulgare* is reported to contain the sesquiterpene lactones arbusculin-A and tanacetin (Mitchell & Rook 1979). Like *T. parthenium*, *T. vulgare* also contains parthenolide (Nano *et al.* 1980); this may be the principal allergen.

Greenhouse C.A. & Sulzberger M.B. (1933) The common weed tansy (*Tanacetum vulgare*) as a cause of eczematous dermatitis. *Journal of Allergy* **4**: 523–6.

Huber H.L. & Harsh G.F. (1932) A summer dermatitis caused by a common weed. *Journal of Allergy* **3**: 578–82.

Lampe K.F. & Fagerström R. (1968) *Plant Toxicity and Dermatitis. A Manual for Physicians*. Williams and Wilkins, Baltimore.

Mackoff S. & Dahl A.O. (1951) A botanical consideration of the weed oleoresin problem. *Minnesota Medicine* **34**: 1169; 1173; 1188.

Mitchell J. & Rook A. (1979) *Botanical Dermatology*. Greengrass, Vancouver.

Nano G.M., Appendino G., Bicchi C. & Frattini C. (1980) On a chemotype of *Tanacetum vulgare* L. containing sesquiterpene lactones, with germacrane skeleton. *Fitoterapia* **L1**: 135–40.

Rook A. (1960) Plant dermatitis. *British Medical Journal* **2**: 1771–4.

Wrangsjo K., Ros A.M. & Wahlberg J.E. (1990) Contact allergy to compositae plants in patients with summer-exacerbated dermatitis. *Contact Dermatitis* **22**: 148–54.

TARAXACUM officinale

Common names: Dandelion. Piss-a-bed. Pissenlit (French)

Distribution: Europe, including Britain. A very common weed of fields and gardens. Naturalized in all temperate regions, including South Africa, USA and Australia

Patch test: Leaf as is. Oleoresin 0.1% pet.

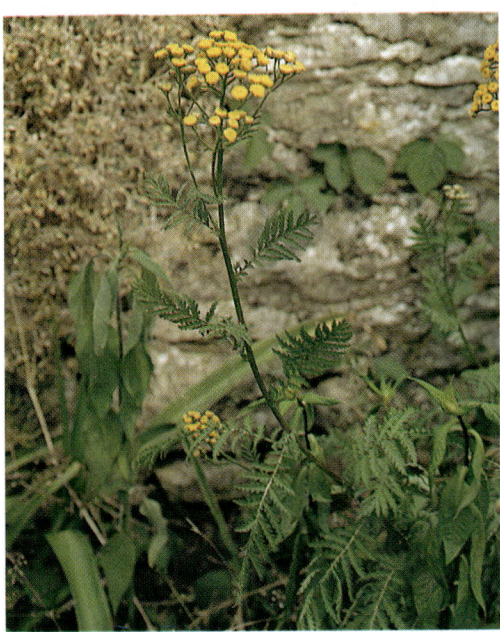

Fig. 7.5.66 *Tanacetum vulgare* (tansy).

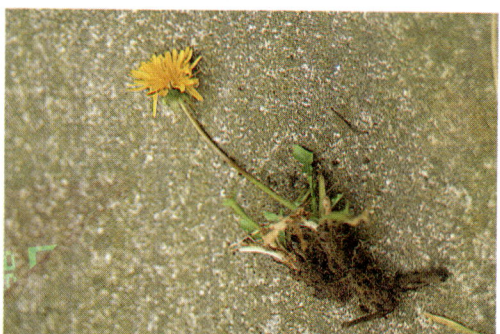

Fig. 7.5.67 *Taraxacum officinale* (dandelion) showing tap root.

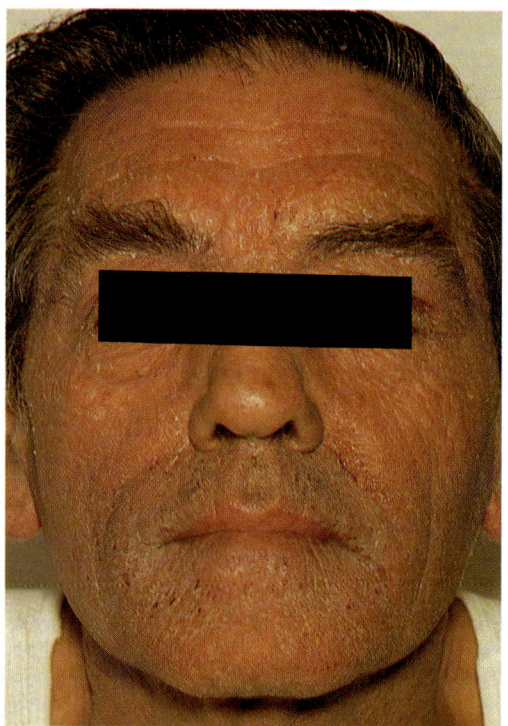

The vernacular name 'dandelion' may derive from 'dent de lion'; the immature seed resembles a lion's tooth. It is a perennial plant with a tuft of basal toothed leaves and large showy heads, about 4 cm diameter, of bright yellow flowers. It has a deep thick tap root (Fig. 7.5.67) which regenerates rapidly if not completely dug up. The leaves have a bitter taste and have been used in salads or given to the pet tortoise or rabbit. The tap root has been used, like chicory, as a coffee substitute. The diuretic effect of dandelion has given rise to the alternative name 'piss-a-bed' and was noted by Culpeper.

There are sporadic case reports of allergic contact dermatitis due to dandelion in Europe (Janke 1950, Hausen & Schultz 1978, Larregue *et al.* 1978, Davies & Kersey 1986) and Australia (Burry *et al.* 1973). During the exceptionally hot dry British summer of 1990 several patients presented with allergic contact dermatitis after mowing lawns contaminated with dandelions (Fig. 7.5.68) (Lovell & Rowan 1991). The hot weather selectively inhibited the growth of lawn grasses, whereas broad-leaved rosetting weeds, such as dandelion, flourished. Sensitization may also occur from picking the leaves as pet food (Davies & Kersey 1986), golf, or wine-making (Lovell & Rowan 1991). Dandelion dermatitis may be under-reported.

The allergen is taraxinic acid 1-0-β-glucopyranoside (**7.XXVII**), a sesquiterpene lactone linked to β-glucose via an ester linkage (Hansel *et al.* 1980, Hausen 1982). The sesquiterpene lactone mix (Ducombs *et al.*

Fig. 7.5.68 Airborne pattern of allergic contact dermatitis in a gardener whose eruption flared in the summer when he mowed the grass. A patch test was positive using a dandelion extract but negative with the sesquiterpene lactone mix.

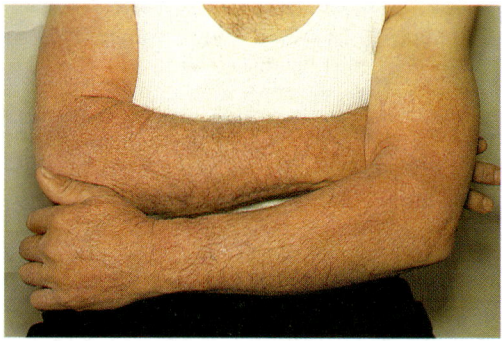

Taraxinic acid
1'-0-β-glucopyranoside

7.XXVII

1990) failed to detect all the patients with dandelion sensitivity reported by Lovell and Rowan (1991); this may be due to the β-glucose residue attached to the sesquiterpene lactone in the dandelion antigen.

Burry J.N., Kuchel R., Reid J.G. & Kirk J. (1973) Australian bush dermatitis: compositae dermatitis in S. Australia. *Medical Journal of Australia* **1**: 110–16.
Davies M.G. & Kersey P.J.W. (1986) Contact allergy to yarrow and dandelion. *Contact Dermatitis* **14**: 256–7.
Ducombs G., Benezra C., Talaga P. *et al.* (1990) Patch testing with the 'sesquiterpene lactone mix': a marker for contact allergy to compositae and other sesquiterpene lactone-containing plants. *Contact Dermatitis* **22**: 249–52.
Hansel R., Kartarahardja M., Huang J.-T. & Bohlmann F. (1980) Sesquiterpenlacton-β-D-glucopyranoside sowie ein neues Eudesmanolid aus *Taraxacum officinale*. *Phytochemistry* **19**: 857–61.
Hausen B.M. (1982) Taraxinsaure-1-0-β-glucopyranosid, das Kontaktallergen des Lowenzahns (*Taraxacum officinale* Wiggers). *Dermatosen in Beruf und Umwelt* **30**: 51–3.
Hausen B.M. & Schultz K.H. (1978) Allergische Kontaktdermatitis durch Lowenzahn (*Taraxacum officinale* Wiggers). *Dermatosen in Beruf und Umwelt* **26**: 198.
Janke D. (1950) Durch Lowenzahn (*Taraxacum officinale*) verursachtes Ekzem. *Hautarzt* **1**: 177.
Larregue M., Rat J.P., Gallet P., Bressieux J.M. & Pousset J.L. (1978) Eczema de contact au pissenlit, a l'huile de laurier noble et au frullania par allergie croisse. *Annales de Dermatologie et de Venereologie* **105**: 547–8.
Lovell C.R. & Rowan M. (1991) Dandelion dermatitis. *Contact Dermatitis* **25**: 185–8.

WEDELIA trilobata

Distribution: Singapore

This species is commonly planted for foliage effect along roadsides in Singapore. It is also used in herbal medicine, applied externally. Goh (1986) reported allergic contact dermatitis affecting the face and hands in a gardener who handled the plants. Patch tests were positive using a chrysanthemum oleoresin.

Goh C.L. (1986) Contact sensitivity to *Wedelia trilobata*. *Contact Dermatitis* **14**: 126.

XANTHIUM spp.

Common names: Clotbur. Cocklebur. Bathurst burr (*X. spinosum*)
Distribution: Probably USA. Widely naturalized in temperate regions

This genus of annual weeds has several members which are mechanical irritants. *Xanthium strumarium*, the cocklebur, is a greyish-green leafy weed. The fruit has spiny burs, about 1 cm long, with hooked spines, easily catching in fur and clothing. *Xanthium spinosum* has long three-pronged yellow spines. The flowers are inconspicuous. Shelmire (1940) and Burry *et al.* (1973) recorded positive reactions to oleoresins derived from *X. spinosum* and *strumarium*. Menz and Winkelmann (1987) obtained a high incidence of positive patch test reactions using *X. strumarium* oleoresin. It is not clear whether these findings are of clinical significance. However, two cases of allergic dermatitis due to *X. spinosum* were recorded by Rowe (1939): positive patch tests were obtained to the leaves and pollen.

Burry J.N., Kuchel R., Reid J.G. & Kirk J. (1973) Australian bush dermatitis. Compositae dermatitis in South Australia. *Medical Journal of Australia* **1**: 110–16.
Menz J. & Winkelmann R.K. (1987) Sensitivity to wild vegetation. *Contact Dermatitis* **16**: 169–73.
Rowe A.H. (1939) Contact allergy to cocklebur (*Xanthium spinosum*). *Archives of Dermatology and Syphilology* **39**: 149.
Shelmire B. (1940) Contact dermatitis from vegetation. *Southern Medical Journal* **33**: 337–46.

Ericaceae (including Pyrolaceae)

This family includes heather (*Erica*), *Rhododendron* and many other attractive shrubs. Agrup and Fregert (1968) report a positive patch test with *Rhododendron* '*indicum*', a dubious species of the *Azalea* section; cross-sensibility was noted with *Streptocarpus*. The sub-family Pyrolaceae includes wintergreen (*Pyrola*) as well as the North American genus *Chimaphila* (rheumatism weed or pipsissewa). Both these genera contain a yellow naphthaquinone, chimaphilin; this is irritant and probably contributes to the rubefacient effect of these plants. It is a moderate sensitizer in guinea pigs although there are no well-documented cases of allergic dermatitis in humans (Hausen & Schiedermair 1988).

Agrup G. & Fregert S. (1968) Patch test reactions to *Streptocarpus*. *Contact Dermatitis Newsletter* **4**: 72.

Hausen B.M. & Schiedermair (1988) The sensitizing capacity of chimaphilin, a naturally occurring quinone. *Contact Dermatitis* **19**: 180–3.

Primulaceae

PRIMULA obconica

Common name: Primula
Distribution: China. A popular flowering pot plant
Patch test: Primin 0.01% pet.

The greenhouse primula (Fig. 7.5.69) is a member of the Cortusoides section, bearing rounded, notched, hairy leaves and an umbel of lilac, pink, violet or purple flowers. It was introduced to Europe (by Charles Maries for Veitch Nurseries) from China in 1879. The modern *P. 'obconica'* cultivars are derived from hybrids between the species and the closely related *P. megasaefolia.*

Skin reactions to this species were recognized early in the horticultural literature. Subsequently, Oldacres (1889) described an 'obstinate rash' 'very much like urticaria', nearly always 'in well-to-do people who spent much time in greenhouses'. The rash affected hands, wrists and faces and in one case caused 'much oedema of the eyelids, so as to cause a horrible temporary disfigurement'. The eruption cleared after avoiding the plant (Oldacres 1889). Patch testing with the leaf was first described by Ferguson (1890) (one of the first applications of this technique).

Allergenicity
All parts of the plant are allergenic. Principally, the allergen is borne in and on the surface of microscopic glandular hairs, each composed of 2–6 cells. The density of these hairs is highest on the calyx (the bracts surrounding the flower head). The coarser long hairs, which impart roughness to the leaves, do not contain the allergen.

Although reasonably easy to cultivate in frost-free conditions, the plant may rot off if watered overhead. Because of this, the leaves are lifted up to permit watering around the edge of the plant. In addition, the plant requires frequent 'dead-heading', i.e. pulling off the highly allergenic calyces, as well as removal of dead leaves.

Prevalence of allergic contact dermatitis
Allergic sensitization occurs chiefly in individuals who have grown the plant. The true prevalence is not known, although it remains one of the commonest plants to cause allergic reactions in Britain. The prevalence may be under-estimated as the allergy is well recognized among gardeners and may not lead to referral, even to general practitioners. In routine patch testing clinics the allergen, primin, accounts for 1–1.8% of positive reactions (Logan & White 1988, Ingber & Menné 1990). There is a high female predominance, 85–96% (Hjorth 1966, Ingber & Menné 1990).

Although common in northern Europe, primula dermatitis is relatively rare in Spain, probably because it is more difficult to cultivate in the hot dry atmosphere (Fernández de Corres *et al.* 1987a). Cases have been reported from other countries including Japan (Nakamura 1983) and Australia (Apted 1988). Because of its allergenicity, it has been suggested that florists are reluctant to stock it, leading to a decreased prevalence in continental Europe (Roed-Petersen & Hjorth 1976). However, the production of plants by the Aalsmeer flower market increases each year (Ingber & Menné 1990) and it is still ubiquitous in garden centres.

Clinical features
These can be variable (Figs. 7.5.69–7.5.71). The typical pattern consists of linear streaks of erythema, of vesicles and bullae on the forearms, together with a vesicular eruption on the fingers. Sometimes the fingers only are

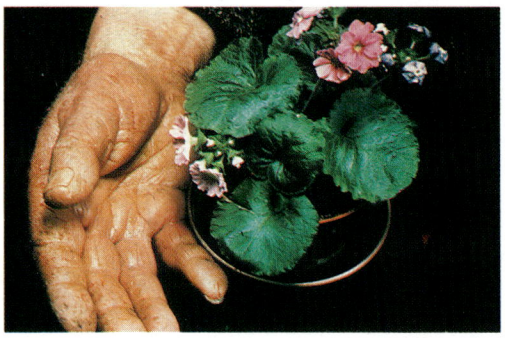

Fig. 7.5.69 *Primula obconica* causing hand dermatitis.

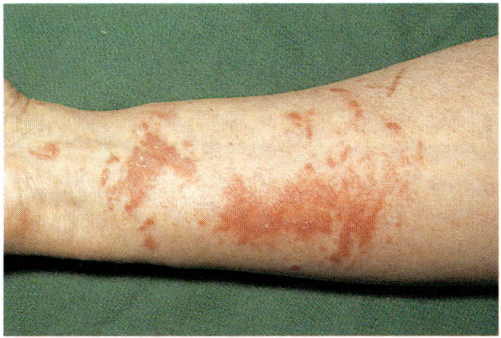

Fig. 7.5.70 Typical streaky dermatitis of the forearms caused by *Primula obconica*.

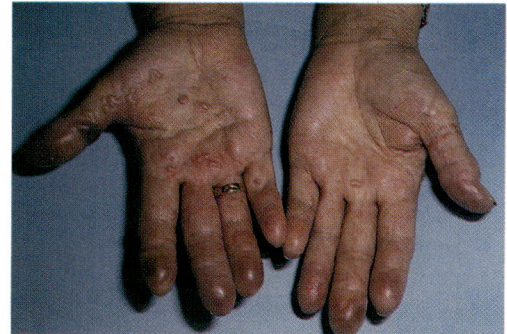

Fig. 7.5.72 Erythema multiforme-like eruption due to *Primula obconica*. (Courtesy of Dr M. Beck.)

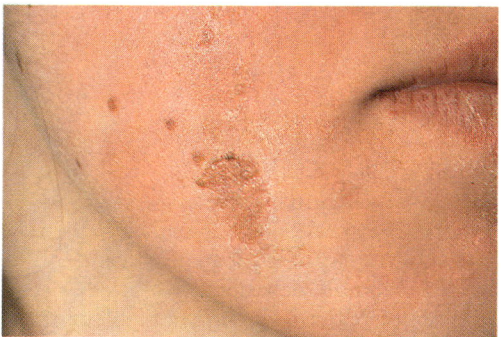

Fig. 7.5.71 Facial dermatitis after pricking out *Primula obconica* seedlings.

affected (Logan & White 1988). The face is commonly involved and palpebral oedema is sometimes the presenting feature (Hjorth 1966). A sensitized patient may develop facial erythema after entering a room containing a *Primula* plant. After handling the plant, the allergen is transferred by the finger to other sites, including the neck and external nares! Dermatitis may become generalized. In the detailed study by Hjorth (1966), only half of the cases had typical features and clinical diagnosis before patch testing included dyshidrotic eczema, seborrhoeic dermatitis of the scalp and scabies.

An eruption resembling erythema multiforme (Fig. 7.5.72) has been reported by several authors, including Rook and Wilson (1965) and Virgili and Corazza (1991).

The source of sensitization may be obscure. For example, one patient developed eczematous lesions after leaning on the balcony of her flat. It transpired that the balcony had been contaminated with material from a *Primula obconica* plant grown by the inhabitant of an upstairs flat! (Fernández de Corres *et al*. 1987b).

Avoidance of the plant should result in rapid clinical improvement although many patients deny the existence of the species in their home or workplace (Hjorth 1966).

Patch testing
Traditionally, *Primula obconica* leaf has been used. There are several drawbacks, including active sensitization. The allergenicity of the plant varies with season, being higher in summer and almost non-existent in winter. A healthy specimen, growing in a sunny window sill with abundant nitrogen, may be highly allergenic. Overwatering may quickly reduce its allergenicity and some cultivars are more allergenic than others (Hjorth 1966).

For routine screening, the allergen primin (**7.XXVIII**) is preferable (0.01% pet.). Sensitization is rare at this concentration (Ingber & Menné 1990) and its inclusion in a

Primin (2-methoxy-6-pentylbenzoquinone)

7.XXVIII

routine battery reveals a large number of clinically unsuspected cases (Logan & White 1988).

It is possible that primin is not the only allergen in *Primula obconica*. Using paper chromatography, Cairns (1964) obtained two components, each of which gave positive patch test reactions. However, Hausen (1978) suggests that the second band was an extraction artefact, being a quinhydrone oxidation product of primin. Dooms-Goossens *et al*. (1989) report two patients giving a history strongly suggestive of primula dermatitis; patch tests were positive using *P. obconica* but not with primin. Other quinones, including primetin, have been reported in another species of *Primula* (Hausen *et al*. 1983), *P. mistassinica*. (This is a North American member of the 'birds eye' primrose group, and not a known allergenic species.)

Where primula dermatitis is suspected and a primin patch test is negative, it is reasonable to patch test with material derived from the patient's own plant, either tested 'as is' or as an ether extract.

Cross-reaction
Although chemically similar quinones are ubiquitous in the plant kingdom, cross-reactions appear to be rare. Among four patients sensitive to dalbergione in rosewood, three reacted to *P. obconica* (Hjorth 1966) although 12 primula-sensitive patients failed to react to a battery of quinones derived from tropical trees (Fernández de Corrés *et al*. 1988).

Skin reactions to other Primula species
Irritant reactions are not uncommon in specialist growers of hardy primulas, including the popular *P. auricula* (Fig. 7.5.73). Allergic reactions to this species appear to be very rare (Alemany-Vall 1947) and the primin-sensitive patient can be reassured that currently available primroses and polyanthus cultures are also safe. Of the greenhouse species, *P. malacoides* appears innocuous. *Primula sinensis* 'rarely' causes contact dermatitis (Rook & Wilson 1965). A variant of the cowslip (*P. suaveolens* or *P. veris* spp. *columnae*) is a possible sensitizer (Argumosa

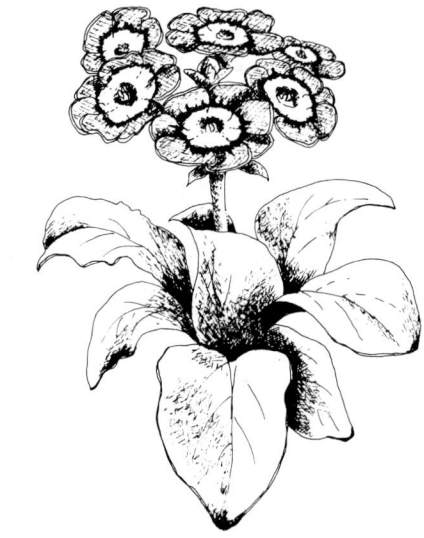

Fig. 7.5.73 *Primula auricula*.

1951). Although many hardy species contain primin (Hausen 1978), it is unlikely that the degree of exposure is adequate to cause sensitization. However, it is of note that some growers of *P. auricula* cultivars who develop dermatitis from the plants may achieve tolerance by handling them regularly; after a break of several days, further exposure causes recurrence of the eruption. This implies an allergic response to *P. auricula* (R. Archdale, personal communication).

Alemany-Vall R. (1947) Sensitilizacion a la *Primula auricula*: en reacciones y lesiones alergicas de la piel. *Medicina Clinica* **9**: 368–74.
Apted J. (1988) Contact dermatitis and *Primula obconica*. (Letter.) *Contact Dermatitis* **19**: 452.
Argumosa J.A. (1951) Sensibilizacion a la *Primula suaveolens*. *Revista Clinica Espanola* **41**: 261–3.
Cairns R.J. (1964) Plant dermatoses. *Transactions of the St John's Hospital Dermatological Society* **50**: 137–43.
Dooms-Goossens A., Biesmans G., Vandaele M. & Degreef H. (1989) *Primula* dermatitis: more than one allergen? *Contact Dermatitis* **21**: 122–4.
Ferguson J. (1890) The *Primula obconica*. *British Medical Journal* **ii**: 954–5.
Fernández de Corrés L., Leanizbarrutia I. & Muñoz D. (1987a) Contact dermatitis from *Primula obconica* Hance. *Contact Dermatitis* **16**: 195–7.
Fernández de Corrés L., Leanizbarrutia I., Muñoz D., Bernaola G. & Fernández E. (1987b) Contact dermatitis from neighbour's primula. *Contact Dermatitis* **16**: 234–5.
Fernández de Corrés L., Leanizbarrutia I. & Muñoz D.

(1988) Cross-reactivity between some naturally occurring quinones. *Contact Dermatitis* **18**: 186–7.

Hausen B.M. (1978) On the occurrence of the contact allergen primin and other quinoid compounds in species of the family Primulaceae. *Archives of Dermatological Research* **261**: 311–21.

Hausen B.M., Schmalle H.W., Marshall D. & Thomson R.H. (1983) 5,8-Dihydroxyflavone (primetin), the contact sensitizer of *Primula mistassinica* Michaux. *Archives of Dermatological Research* **275**: 365–70.

Hjorth N. (1966) *Primula* dermatitis. Sources of errors in patch testing and patch test sensitization. *Transactions of the St John's Hospital Dermatological Society* **52**: 207–19.

Ingber A. & Menné T. (1990) Primin standard patch testing: 5 years experience. *Contact Dermatitis* **2**: 15–19.

Logan R.A. & White I.R. (1988) *Primula* dermatitis: prevalence, detection and outcome. *Contact Dermatitis* **19**: 68–9.

Nakamura T. (1983) *Primula* dermatitis in Japan. *Contact Dermatitis* **9**: 328–9.

Oldacres E. (1889) Toxic symptoms produced by handling *Primula obconica*. *British Medical Journal* **ii**: 719.

Roed-Petersen J. & Hjorth N. (1976) Compositae sensitivity among patients with contact dermatitis. *Contact Dermatitis* **2**: 271–81.

Rook A. & Wilson H.T.H. (1965) *Primula* dermatitis. *British Medical Journal* **i**: 220–2.

Virgili A. & Corazza M. (1991) Unusual primin dermatitis. *Contact Dermatitis* **24**: 63–4.

CYCLAMEN persicum

Common name: Cyclamen
Distribution: Eastern Mediterranean. A common winter-flowering pot plant

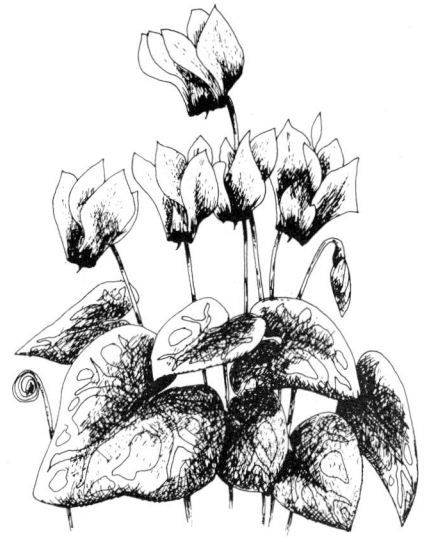

Fig. 7.5.74 *Cyclamen persicum.*

The florist's cyclamen is derived from *C. persicum* (Fig. 7.5.74), a common species in parts of Rhodes, Cyprus, Israel and Jordan. Agrup and Fregert (1968) describe a positive patch test to the leaf on a patient also allergic to *Streptocarpus* and Hjorth (reported in Mitchell & Rook 1979) has observed a positive reaction to an unidentified species.

Agrup G. & Fregert S. (1968) Patch test reactions to *Streptocarpus*. *Contact Dermatitis Newsletter* **4**: 72.

Mitchell T. & Rook A. (1979) *Botanical Dermatology*. Greengrass, Vancouver.

Styraceae

STYRAX

Common names: *S. tonkinensis*: Siam benzoin. *S. officinalis*: Storax (in part). Snowbell

Distribution: *S. tonkinensis* Tropical Asia. *S. officinalis* Greece and Asia Minor

Patch test: Balsam of Peru. Perfume series

Styrax tonkinensis is the source of an aromatic red-brown resin, Siam benzoin. This is an ingredient of compound tincture of benzoin (tinct. benz. co) (Fig. 7.5.75) which also contains balsams of Peru and Tolu, liquid storax, aloe, myrrh and angelica (Hjorth 1961). The name Friars' balsam is sometimes applied to this preparation, but the form used for inhalations is derived from the less allergenic Sumatra benzoin, obtained from other spp. including *S. benzoin* and *S. paralleoneurus* (Howes 1974). In ancient Greece and Egypt, the gum storax was obtained from the eastern Mediterranean species *Styrax officinalis*, by making cuts in the branches. According to Dioscorides it 'hath a warming, mollifying and concocting facultie' (Huxley & Taylor 1977). Most storax (liquid storax) is now derived from the Turkish species *Liquidambar orientalis*, a member of the witch hazel family (Hamamelidaceae) (q.v).

Sensitization follows exposure to compound tincture of benzoin which has been used topically for several years in the treatment of fissures and ulcers (Steiner & Leifer 1949). Today it is still used under plaster casts and other dressings (Spott & Shelley 1970), and it is a relatively common cause of allergic

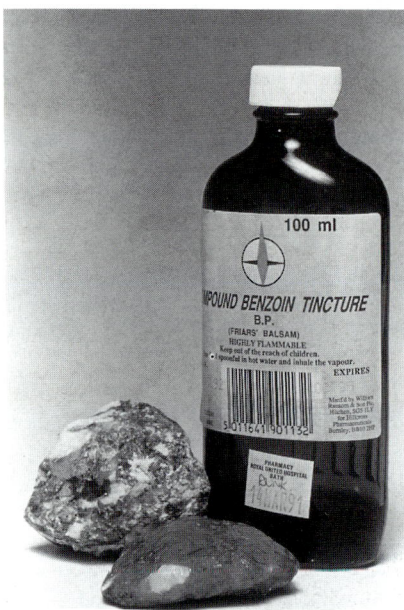

Fig. 7.5.75 Siam benzoin (red-brown) and Sumatra benzoin (multicoloured) used in compound tincture of benzoin. Resins kindly supplied by Margaret Hansen.

irritant dermatitis in children. Tillbury Fox in 1874 described widespread purpuric exanthem in a patient who inhaled the tincture (quoted in Hjorth 1961).

Active sensitization may occur following patch testing with the tincture (Steiner & Leifer 1949). As the allergens are similar to those in balsam of Peru (e.g. cinnamates), it is preferable to screen with the latter or a perfume series.

Hjorth (1961) Eczematous allergy to balsams. *Acta Dermato-Venereologica* **41** (suppl. 46): 1–211.
Howes F.N. (1974) *A Dictionary of Useful and Everyday Plants and Their Common Names.* Cambridge University Press, Cambridge.
Huxley A. & Taylor W. (1977) *Flowers of Greece and the Aegean.* Chatto & Windus, London.
Spott D.A. & Shelley W.B. (1970) Exanthem due to a contact allergen (benzoin) absorbed through skin. *JAMA* **214**: 1881–2.
Steiner K. & Leifer W. (1949) Investigations of contact-type dermatitis due to compound tincture of benzoin. *Journal of Investigative Dermatology* **13**: 351–9.

Oleaceae

JASMINUM officinale

Common name: Jasmine
Distribution: Asia. Widely naturalized in southern Europe and a popular garden plant
Patch test: Flower as is. Jasmine oil 20% pet. Jasmine absolute 2% pet. Perfume mix

The scented white flowers of this climbing shrub (Fig. 7.5.76) are irritant when handled or worn in garlands (Behl *et al.* 1979). The essential oil may be allergenic. Thirteen patients reacted to jasmine absolute 2% in a series of 1500 patch test patients (Santucci *et al.* 1987).

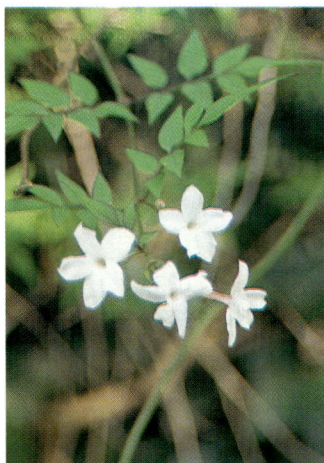

Fig. 7.5.76 *Jasminium officinale* (jasmine).

'Jasmine' perfume is often synthetically derived and allergic contact dermatitis is commonly caused by materials such as methylheptine carbonate or α-amyl cinnamaldehyde (Schorr 1975). *Trans*-jasmone, present in the oil itself, may be an allergen (Hausen 1988) (**7.XXIX**).

Trans-jasmone

7.XXIX

Behl P.N. & Captain R.H. (1979) *Skin Irritant and Sensitizing Plants Found in India*. S. Chand, Ram Naga, New Delhi.

Hausen B.M. (1988) *Allergiepflanzen Pflanzenallergene*. Ecomed Landsberg, Munchen.

Santucci B., Cristaudo A., Cannistraci C. & Picardo M. (1987) Contact dermatitis to fragrances. *Contact Dermatitis* **16**: 93–5.

Schorr W.F. (1975) Cinnamic aldehyde allergy. *Contact Dermatitis* **1**: 108.

OLEA europaea

Common name: Olive

Distribution: Mediterranean region, extensively cultivated in groves

Patch test: Scrapings of olive wood.
  Olive oil as is

The wild olive is a branched, spiny shrub found on rocky hillsides at low altitudes. Selected forms have been cultivated since the Minoan period (Fig. 7.5.77). The fruit, olives, are still a staple diet among peasant peoples. The oil is used in cookery and as an emollient. The hard wood is used to make souvenirs, including bowls, napkin rings, beads, crucifixes and musical pipes (Fisher 1989). According to Greek mythology, the goddess Athene created the olive tree, which is dedicated to her. The olive branch is a symbol of peace.

Allergic sensitization can be caused by wearing olive wood jewellery (Hausen & Rothenborg 1981, Fisher 1989). The allergens appear to be quinoid compounds, similar to those in teak and rosewood, although weaker sensitizers (Hausen *et al.* 1981). The oil itself may sensitize when applied topically (Sutton 1943, van Joost *et al.* 1981); it is an ingredient of some ointments (de Boer & van Ketel 1984). Malmkvist Padoan *et al.* (1990) report 13 cases of allergic contact dermatitis, particularly in patients with pre-existing gravitational eczema but also, occupationally, in pedicurists. These authors were unable to relate allergenicity to the known components, triolein, tripalmiton, squalene, tocopherol, etc. (Malmkvist Padoan *et al.* 1990).

De Boer E.M. & van Ketel W.G. (1984) Contact allergy to an olive oil containing ointment. *Contact Dermatitis* **11**: 128–9.

Fisher A.A. (1989) Allergic contact dermatitis from an olive wood necklace. *Cutis* **43**: 202–3.

Hausen B.M. & Rothenborg H.W. (1981) Allergic contact dermatitis caused by olive wood jewelry. *Archives of Dermatology* **117**: 732–4.

Malmkvist Padoan S., Pettersson A. & Svensson A. (1990) Olive oil as a cause of contact allergy in patients

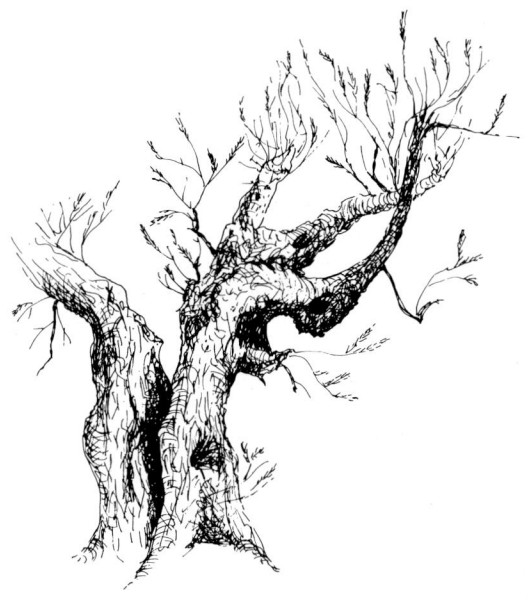
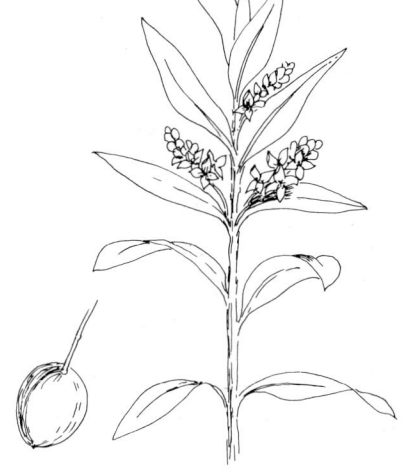

Fig. 7.5.77 *Olea europaea* (olive).

with venous eczema, and occupationally. *Contact Dermatitis* **23**: 73–6.
Sutton R.L. (1943) Contact dermatitis from olive oil. *JAMA* **122**: 34–5.
Van Joost T., Sillevis Smitt J.H. & van Ketel W.G. (1981) Sensitization to olive oil (*Olea europaea*). *Contact Dermatitis* **7**: 309–10.

Apocyanaceae

This family includes many decorative genera such as *Vinca* (periwinkle) and *Nerium* (oleander). Several species are of pharmacological importance, notably *Catharanthus roseus* (Madagascar periwinkle), the source of 'vinca' alkaloids such as vincristine and vinblastine. These are reported to cause allergic sensitization in workers extracting them (Valer 1965). *Nerium oleander* (Fig. 7.5.78) is a highly decorative shrub, native to Mediterranean regions (in damp areas) and Asia. It is grown as a pot plant for its scented pink, cream or white flowers and is widely planted in temperate areas by roadsides in the Mediterranean. It is highly poisonous.

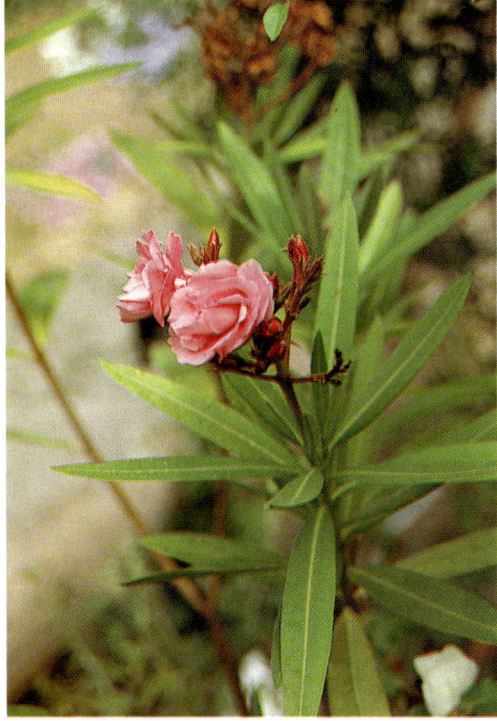

Fig. 7.5.78 *Nerium oleander.*

Dioscorides describes it as having 'a power destructive of dogs and of asses and of mules and of most four-footed creatures'. The reader should hesitate before using oleander twigs as barbecue skewers as 'three hundred soldiers were affected, some fatally, after eating meat so cooked' (Francis & Southcott 1967). Dermatitis has been reported in children (e.g. Dorsey 1962) although it may be irritant. Apted (1983) obtained a 'doubtful' positive patch test on an elderly woman who developed a papulovesicular eruption on the back after sunbathing under an oleander. Several other genera, *Acokanthera*, *Allamanda*, *Cryptostegia*, *Thevetia* and *Plumeria* (frangipani) are reported causes of dermatitis in Florida and Hawaii (Lampe 1986).

Apted J. (1983) Oleander dermatitis. *Contact Dermatitis* **9**: 321.
Dorsey C.S. (1962) Plant dermatitis in California. *California Medicine* **96**: 412–13.
Francis D.F. & Southcott R.V. (1967) *Plants Harmful to Man in Australia*. Miscellaneous Bulletin No. 1; Botanic Garden Adelaide, South Australia, p. 30.
Lampe K.F. (1986) Dermatitis-producing plants of south Florida and Hawaii. *Clinics in Dermatology* **4**: 83–93.
Valer M. (1965) Die bei der Erzengung van Devincan auf tretender Hautlasionen. *Berufsdermatosen* **13**: 96–110.

Asclepiadaceae

Several members of this mostly tropical family are cultivated as ornamentals, requiring greenhouse conditions in northern Europe and USA. Several species have an irritant milky latex and garlands (leis) made from the crown flower (*Calotropis gigantea*) cause irritant conjunctivitis in Hawaii (Wong 1949). Handa (1984) reports possible allergic contact dermatitis to *Calotropis procera*, the Sodom Apple. This plant is, however, known to be intensely irritant.

HOYA carnosa

Common name: Wax flower
Distribution: China, Australasia. A popular house plant
Patch test: ? Leaf as is

This climbing plant has green fleshy lance-shaped leaves. The flowers are white or very pale pink with a red star shape marking in the centre, long lasting and sweetly fragrant. An attractive form, *H. carnosa* cv *'variegata'*, has bluish–green leaves shaded with red and with creamy margins. Rothe (1986) reports a patient with strongly positive patch tests to this species and to *Philodendron scandens*. Repeat patch testing with *Hoya* alone gave a weaker reaction but the patient's dermatitis flared after handling the plant again. The allergen is unknown.

Handa F. (1984) Contact dermatitis due to the plant *Calotropis procera* (Vern : AK). A case report. *Indian Journal of Dermatology* **29**: 27–9.
Rothe A. (1986) *Hoya carnosa* — is it allergenic? *Contact Dermatitis* **14**: 250–2.
Wong W.W. (1949) Keratoconjunctivitis due to crown flower. *Hawaii Medical Journal* **8**: 339–41.

Hydrophyllaceae

PHACELIA

Common names: Desert heliotrope, scorpion weed, Californian bluebell

Distribution: USA, chiefly west and southwest, Mexico. Some species cultivated as ornamentals
Patch test material: Dried leaf (? false negative). Geranylhydroquinone (if available) 0.5% pet. — may sensitize

This large genus (about 200 species) (Fig. 7.5.79) contains many ornamental plants which are free-flowering and often fragrant. Most species are dwarf annuals or biennials; the whole plant is covered with fine trichomes ('hairs') which exude a sticky oil. The flowers are in various shades of blue and lavender. The following species are sometimes grown as hardy annuals:

Phacelia campanularia (upright gentian-blue flowers, a good 'bee plant'), *P. minor* (*P. whitlandia*) (common on coastal mountains in southern California; has numerous lilac flowers in a spike superficially resembling English bluebell), *P. tanacetifolia* (tansy-like leaves and upright heads of pale lavender flowers). All these species are reported to cause dermatitis in the USA (Munz 1932, Berry *et al.*

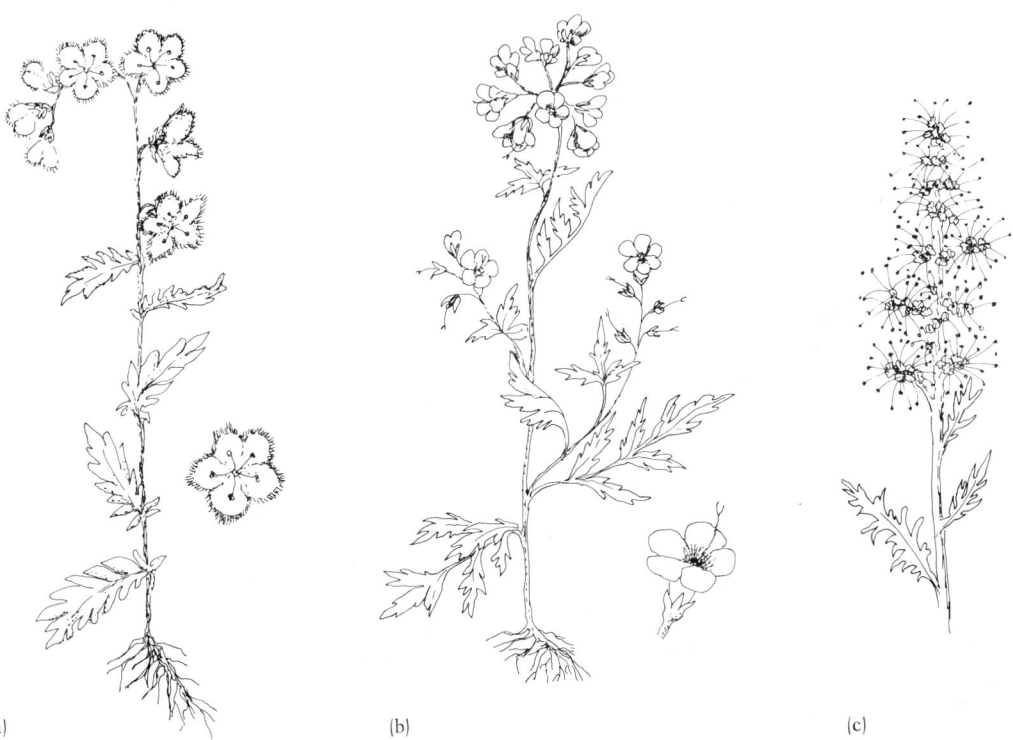

Fig. 7.5.79 *Phacelia* species; (a) *P. tanacetifolia*, (b) *P. minor*, (c) *P. sericea*.

1962). *Phacelia crenulata* and its var. *funerea* are common weeds of sandy, gravelly roadsides; hikers walking in desert areas or picking flowers during the spring may develop linear papules, vesicles or bullae on the legs, feet and hands superficially resembling poison ivy dermatitis (Berry et al. 1962).

The allergens include geranylhydroquinone (in *P. crenulata*) and geranylgeranylhydroquinone (in *P. minor* and *P. parryi*) (**7.XXX**), contained in the oil (Reynolds et al.

7.XXX Allergens in *Phacelia* spp.

n = 1 = geranylhydroquinone
n = 3 = geranyl geranylhydroquinone

1980, 1981, 1986). They decompose rapidly by oxidation, forming dark non-reactive compounds; these typically cause brown streaks on the skin (Munz 1932). Unfortunately, dried leaves may, therefore, give false negative patch test reactions (Reynolds et al. 1980). There is no cross-reaction with *Toxicodendron* spp. (Reynolds et al. 1980). Fourteen of 21 human volunteers were actively sensitized in a maximization test using 0.5% geranylhydroquinone (Reynolds et al. 1980).

Berry C.Z., Shapiro S.I. & Dahlen R.F. (1962) Dermatitis venenata from *Phacelia crenulata*. *Archives of Dermatology* **85**: 737–9.
Munz P.A. (1932) Dermatitis produced by *Phacelia* (Hydrophyllaceae). *Science* **76**: 194.
Reynolds G., Epstein W.L., Terry D. & Rodriguez E. (1980) A potent contact allergen of *Phacelia* (Hydrophyllaceae). *Contact Dermatitis* **6**: 272–4.
Reynolds G. & Rodriguez E. (1981) Prenylated hydroquinones: contact allergens from trichomes of *Phacelia minor* and *P. parryi*. *Phytochemistry* **20**: 1365–6.
Reynolds G.W. & Rodriguez E. (1986) Unusual contact allergens from plants in the family Hydrophyllaceae. *Contact Dermatitis* **14**: 39–44.

TURRICULA parryi

This aromatic shrub is native to the chaparral of southern California. According to Munz and Keck (1965) it causes severe dermatitis. Although recognized by botanists as a hazardous plant there are no reports of contact dermatitis in the dermatological literature. Reynolds et al. (1985), in a detailed study, derived numerous prenylated phenolic compounds from acetone washings of aerial surfaces of fresh plants. Two compounds, both derivatives of farnesyl hydroquinone (**7.XXXI**),

Farnesylhydroquinone

7.XXXI

elicited allergic skin reactions in guinea pigs. These chemicals are related to the more potent allergens in *Phacelia* spp.

Munz P.A. & Keck D.D. (1965) *A Californian Flora*. University of California Press, Berkeley.
Reynolds G.W., Proksch P. & Rodriguez E. (1985) Prenylated phenolics that cause contact dermatitis from glandular trichomes of *Turricula parryi*. *Planta Medica* **6**: 494–8.

WIGANDIA caracasana

Distribution: Central and tropical South America in mountains. Occasionally used as landscape ornamental in southwest USA. Rarely cultivated as half hardy annual or greenhouse perennial

This showy tree-like shrub (Fig. 7.5.80) is covered with stalked glandular trichomes. It grows to 3–4 m bearing oval, notched leaves up to 50 cm in length. The flowers are lilac, about 1.5 cm in diameter, with white tube. The type species has stinging hairs but var. *macrophylla* does not.

Allergic dermatitis to this species was described by Anderson and Ayres in 1931. Reynolds et al. (1989) refer to an outbreak of dermatitis in college students who were studying a planted stand of *Wigandia* as part of a plant identification exercise. Several quinones have been isolated from the glandular hairs (Reynolds et al. 1989). As in *Phacelia*, these oxidize on exposure to air giving the plant a sooty black appearance. The major potential allergen is 2,3-dimethoxygeranyl benzoquinone (Reynolds et al. 1989) (**7.XXXII**). Wigandol is a weaker allergen also found in the allied species, *W. kunthii* (Gomez et al. 1980).

Anderson N.P. & Ayres S., Jr. (1931) Dermatitis venenata due to *Wigandia caracasana*. *California and Western Medicine* **34**: 278–9.

Gomez F., Quijano L., Calderon J.S. & Rios T. (1980) New terpenoids isolated from *Wigandia kunthii*. *Phytochemistry* **19**: 2202–3.

Reynolds G.W., Gafner F. & Rodriguez E. (1989) Contact allergens of an urban shrub *Wigandia caracasana*. *Contact Dermatitis* **21**: 65–8.

Solanaceae

This large family (over 2000 species) includes common vegetables such as potato (*Solanum tuberosum*), tomato (*Lycopersicon lycopersicum*) and peppers (*Capsicum annuum* vars). The tobacco plant (*Nicotiana tabacum*) and deadly nightshade (*Atropa belladonna*) also belong to this family. Several members of the Solanaceae are poisonous and many are skin irritants.

ATROPA BELLADONNA

Common name: Deadly nightshade
Distribution: Alkaline soil in woods and thickets in southern England; not common. Also in continental Europe
Patch test: Atropine 1% : hyoscine 3%

This is a tall, straggling plant (Fig. 7.5.81) with dull-purple bell-shaped flowers and intense black berries surrounded by greenish bracts. Woody nightshade (a shrubby perennial with scarlet berries) and black nightshade (annual, small white flowers, small dull-black berries) are often mistakenly identified as this species. The berries are intensely poisonous, containing atropine and scopolamine (hyoscine). Culpeper wisely advised avoiding this plant. However, in ancient Rome, it was used to dilate the eyes (hence belladonna = beautiful lady). Belladonna alkaloids are toxic when applied topically to the skin, although allergic contact dermatitis is rare. Hyoscine has been reported to cause contact dermatitis

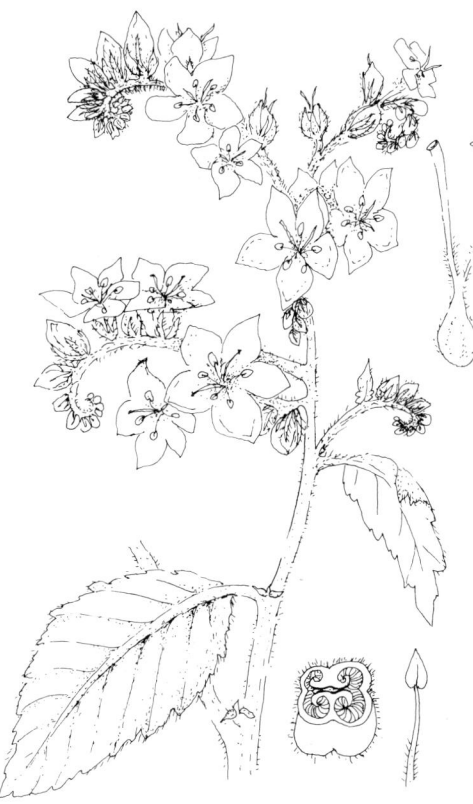

Fig. 7.5.80 *Wigandia caracasana*.

Wigandol

2,3-dimethoxygeranyl-benzoquinone

7.XXXII Allergens in *Wigandia*.

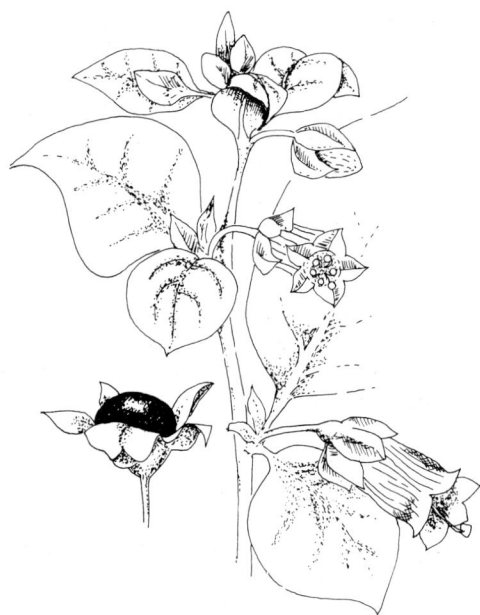

Fig. 7.5.81 *Atropa belladonna* (deadly nightshade).

when applied as transdermal patches in the treatment of travel sickness (Gordon et al. 1989). Atropine eyedrops have caused periocular dermatitis (van der Willigen et al. 1987). Williams and Du Vivier (1990) report an allergic reaction on the low back in a Ghanaian man who had applied proprietary belladonna plasters to the same site for 3 years; a patch test was positive to 1% atropine in petrolatum.

Gordon C.R., Shupak A., Doweck I. & Spitzer O. (1989) Allergic contact dermatitis caused by transdermal hyoscine. *British Medical Journal* **298**: 1220–1.
Van der Willigen A.H., de Graaf Y.P. & van Joost T. (1987) Periocular dermatitis from atropine. *Contact Dermatitis* **17**: 56–7.
Williams H.C. & Du Vivier A. (1990) Belladonna plaster — not as bella as it seems. *Contact Dermatitis* **23**: 119–20.

CAPSICUM annuum
(*C. frutescens*)

Common name: Pepper. Var. *abbreviatum*: Venetian pepper; var. *acuminatum*: cayenne; var. *cerasiforme*: cherry pepper; var. *conoides*: cane pepper; var. *fasciculatum*: red cluster pepper; var. *grossum*: sweet pepper; var. *longum*: paprika, cayenne, chilli
Distribution: Central America
Patch test: Capsicum oil 1% in ethanol. ?ether extract of paprika

The hot taste and irritancy of peppers are due to capsaicin (see p. 59). A vesicular dermatitis, presumably irritant, has been reported on operatives handling wet chilli beans, even when they were wearing rubber gloves (Behl & Captain 1973). The irritant effect of a capsaicin spray has been used by postal workers to deter dogs. The spray may have induced a true allergic reaction on the neck; the eruption relapsed after the patient ingested ginger ale (containing cayenne pepper) and a patch test was strongly positive to *C. annuum* (Fisher 1970). Allergic reactions appear to be unusual in food handlers, although reported by Cronin (1987). Paprika (*C. annuum* var. *longum*) caused 19% of positive reactions in patients tested for allergic contact dermatitis to spices. The incidence of fragrance mix sensitivity was increased in these patients (van den Akker et al. 1990). The allergen is unknown, although it may be capsaicin.

Behl P.N. & Captain R.H. (1973) *Skin Irritant and Sensitizing Plants Found in India*. S. Chad, Ram Nager, New Delhi.
Burnett J.W. (1989) Capsicum pepper dermatitis. *Cutis* **43**: 534.
Cronin E. (1987) Dermatitis of the hands in caterers. *Contact Dermatitis* **17**: 265–9.
Fisher A.A. (1970) Sechs gewürze aus dermatologischer sicht. *Hautarzt* **21**: 295–7.
van den Akker T.H.W., Roesyanto-Mahadi I.D., van Toorenenbergen A.W. & van Joost T.H. (1990) Contact allergy to spices. *Contact Dermatitis* **22**: 267–72.

LYCOPERSICON lycopersicum

Common name: Tomato
Distribution: Western South America. Cultivated worldwide
Patch test: Tomato skin and flesh as is

Minor degrees of irritation from tomato leaves and stems are probably very common in gardeners. Irritant effects may explain the older reports of dermatitis due to plants. Allergic dermatitis to tomatoes appears to be rare, although there are reports in the Hungarian literature (Szego in Mitchell &

Rook 1979). Allergy to tomato skin may occur in food handlers (Cronin 1987) and immediate hypersensitivity is recorded (Hjorth & Roed-Petersen 1976).

Cronin E. (1987) Dermatitis of the hands in caterers. *Contact Dermatitis* **17**: 265–9.
Hjorth N. & Roed-Petersen J. (1976) Occupational protein contact dermatitis in food handlers. *Contact Dermatitis* **2**: 28–42.
Mitchell J. & Rook A. (1989) *Botanical Dermatology*. Greengrass, Vancouver.

NICOTIANA tabacum

Common name: Tobacco
Distribution: Tropical and South America. Cultivated in temperate zones
Patch test: *Nicotiana tabacum* leaf (as is). 24-h ether extract of leaf (as is)

This species (Fig. 7.5.82) is widely cultivated, particularly in the Balkans, Turkey and parts of North America. Ornamental 'tobacco plants', grown for their sweetly fragrant flowers, are cultivars of *N. alata (affinis)*, *N. langsdorffii* and other species. Irritant reactions, such as erythema and urticaria, are common in operatives who handle *N. tabacum* leaves, particularly affecting harvesters, workers in cigarette factories and cigar salespersons (Rycroft *et al*. 1981). Allergic contact dermatitis is rare, affecting chiefly cigar rollers (e.g. Vero and Genovese 1941). Patch test-proven allergic dermatitis to tobacco leaf has been demonstrated in only three of over a thousand cases of hand eczema in a large cigar factory (Samitz *et al*. 1949). Since cigarette manufacture is more automated, skin reactions are even rarer in cigarette factory employees (Rycroft *et al*. 1981).

There are three reports of allergic contact dermatitis to tobacco smoke (Weary & Wood 1969, Neild 1981, Pecegueiro 1987). In the first two patients, positive patch tests were obtained using the smoked cigarette filter. In a subsequent case, a 26-year-old man presented with vesicular eczema at the sites of contact with the cigarette (Fig. 7.5.83) (Lovell & White 1985). Subsequently he developed facial eczema after exposure to tobacco smoke. On giving up smoking his eruption has cleared totally. Patch testing was positive using a 24-h ether extract of dried leaves of *N. tabacum* but further attempts to identify the allergen by thin layer chromatography were unsuccessful (Lovell & White 1987). The allergen is not nicotine (Silvette *et al*. 1957) and is present on green as well as cured leaves (Gonçalo *et al*. 1990). It should be stressed, however, that despite the regrettably great exposure to tobacco in society allergic contact dermatitis remains relatively rare. Other additives to tobacco should be considered, such as insecticides and fungicides, as well as curing agents and flavourings added to tobacco.

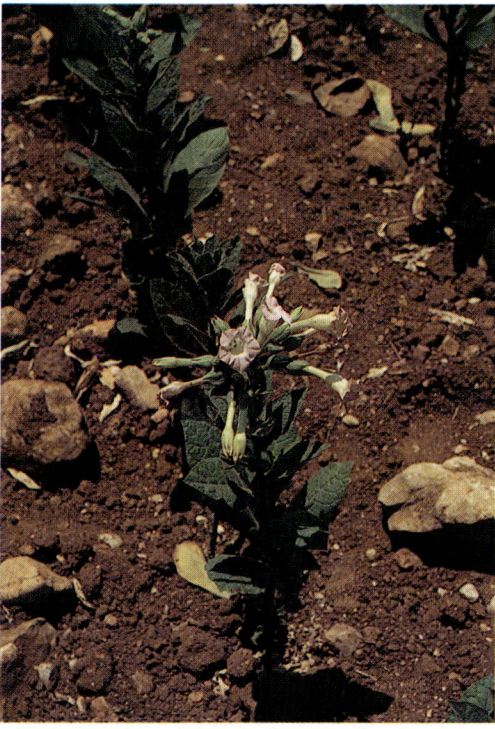

Fig. 7.5.82 *Nicotiana tabacum* (tobacco) in cultivation (Turkey).

Gonçalo M., Couto J. & Gonçalo C. (1990) Allergic contact dermatitis from *Nicotiana tabacum*. *Contact Dermatitis* **22**: 188–9.
Lovell C.R. & White I.R. (1985) Allergic contact dermatitis from tobacco in a consumer. *Journal of the Royal Society of Medicine* **78**: 409–10.
Neild V. (1981) Contact dermatitis from a cigarette constituent. *Contact Dermatitis* **7**: 153–4.
Pecegueiro M. (1987) Airborne contact dermatitis to

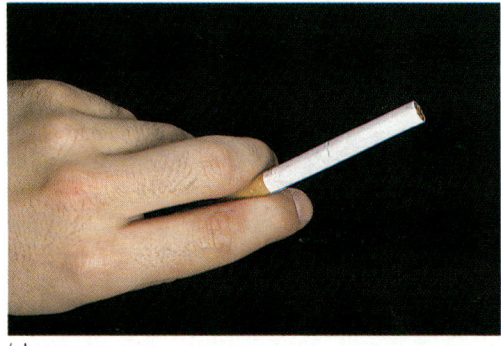
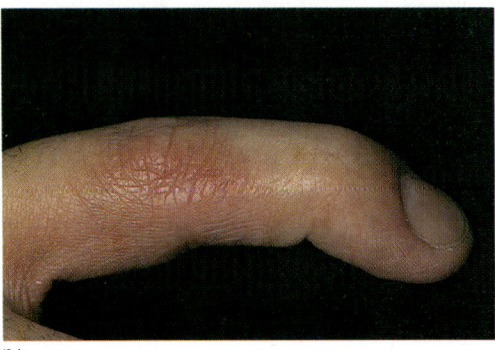
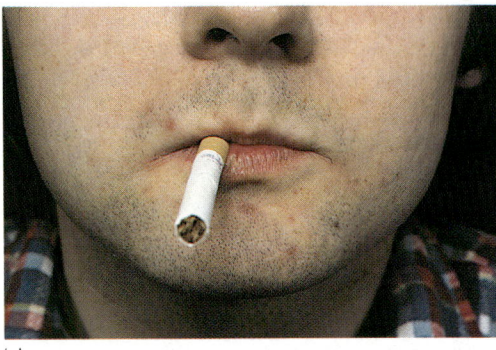
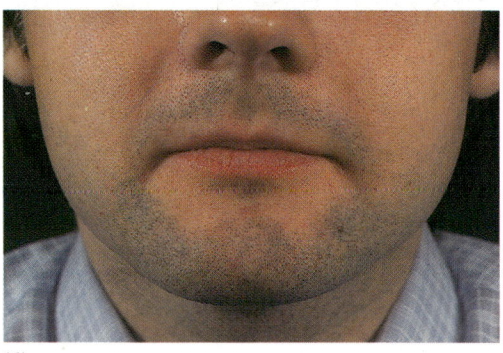

Fig. 7.5.83 Cigarette dermatitis in a consumer, occurring at four sites of exposure. A patch test with N. *tabacum* was positive.

tobacco. *Contact Dermatitis* **17**: 50–1.
Rycroft R.T.G., Smith N.P., Stok E.T. & Middleton K. (1981) Investigation of suspected contact sensitivity to tobacco in cigarette and cigar factory employees. *Contact Dermatitis* **7**: 32–8.
Samitz M.H., Mori P. & Long C.-F. (1949) Dermatological hazards in the cigar industry. *Industrial Medicine and Surgery* **18**: 434–9.
Silvette H., Larson P.S. & Haag H.B. (1957) Immunological aspects of tobacco and smoking. *American Journal of Medical Sciences* **234**: 561–82.
Vero F. & Genovese S. (1941) Occupational dermatitis in cigar makers due to contact with tobacco leaves. *Archives of Dermatology and Syphilology* **43**: 257–63.
Weary P.E. & Wood B.T. (1969) Allergic contact dermatitis from tobacco smoke residues. *JAMA* **208**: 1905–6.

Scrophulariaceae

VERBASCUM spp.

Common names: Mullein. Hightaper. Gordolobo (Italian)

Distribution: Europe, including Britain
Patch test: Dried leaf as is

Most members of this genus are biennial or short-lived perennials, with a large basal rosette of leaves and a tall single, or branched, spike of yellow flowers. In some species, notably *V. thapsus*, the moth mullein, the leaves are densely hairy and may cause irritant reactions on contact.

Mullein has been used in herbal medicine since antiquity. Gerard states that 'the country people ... do give their cattle the leaves to drink against the cough of the lungs'. Occupational dermatitis and bronchitis from gordolobo (a *Verbascum* species) was reported in a herbalist who reacted on patch testing with the dry leaf. Infusions of the flowers are still used for coughs, colds and tuberculosis (Romaguera *et al.* 1985).

Romaguera C., Grimault F. & Vilaplana J. (1985) Occupational dermatitis from gordolobo (mullein). *Contact Dermatitis* **12**: 176.

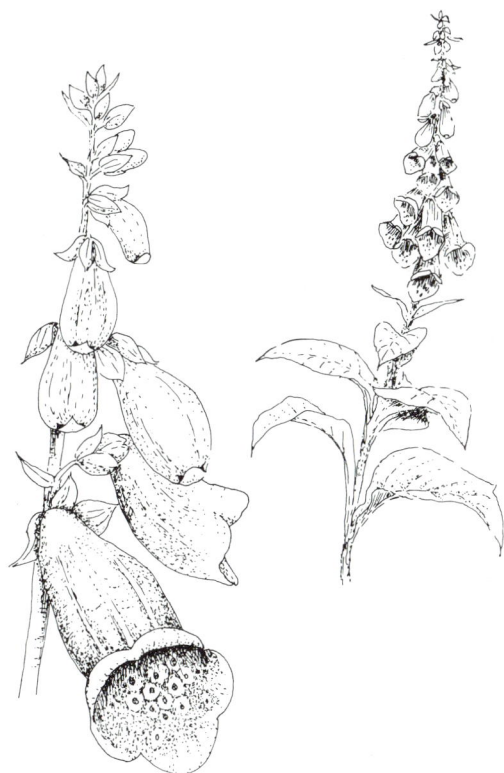

Fig. 7.5.84 *Digitalis purpurea* (foxglove).

DIGITALIS purpurea

Common name: Foxglove
Distribution: Europe, west Asia

This handsome biennial plant (Fig. 7.5.84) is of historical importance as the source of digitalis glycosides, now prepared synthetically. The plant is irritant, containing cardenolide (Hausen 1988). A vasculitic hypersensitivity to digoxin was reported by Brauner and Greene (1972).

Brauner G.J. & Greene M.H. (1972) Digitalis allergy: digoxin-induced vasculitis. *Cutis* **10**: 441.
Hausen B.M. (1988) *Allergrepflanzen-Pflanzenallergene*. Ecomed, Landsberg/Munchen.

Gesneriaceae

This family includes many popular ornamental house plants, such as *Saintpaulia*, the African violet, and *Sinningia* (gloxinia). Although the leaf hairs of many species may cause mechanical irritation, allergic contact dermatitis has only been attributed reliably to *Streptocarpus*. *Aeschynanthus* is a dubious sensitizer (van Ketel 1979).

STREPTOCARPUS cvs

Common name: Cape primrose
Distribution: Southern and tropical Africa
Patch test: Leaf or flower as is or ether extract.
  2,6-dimethoxy-1,4-benzoquinone 10% pet.
  (if available)

This attractive genus of herbaceous plants (Fig. 7.5.85) is justifiably popular: hybrids and cultivars derived from species such as *S. rexii* and *S. grandis* are ideal pot plants for

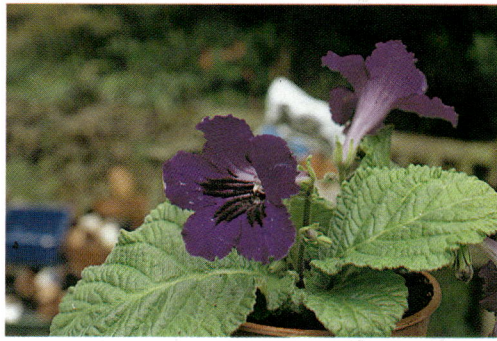

Fig. 7.5.85 *Streptocarpus* cultivar.

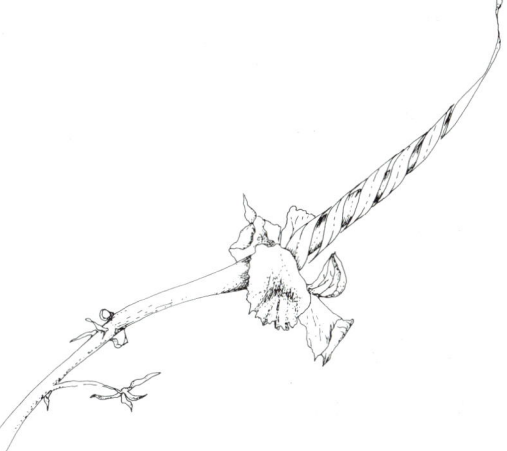

Fig. 7.5.86 Twisted seed pod of *Streptocarpus*.

greenhouse or windowsill culture. The bright-green, slightly hairy, tongue-shaped leaves are held in a rosette. In summer, the plants bear several showy tubular flowers, flared at the tips and brightly coloured. These are followed by twisted seed pods, hence the Greek name (6τρεπτος = twisted, καρπος = seed capsule) (Fig. 7.5.86).

Rook (1968) described contact dermatitis in two women working in a botanical garden. The leaves are reported as allergenic, cross-reacting with other Gesneriaceae (van Ketel 1973). However, patch testing with leaves may give false positive irritant reactions and an ether extract is preferable (Hjorth 1974). Hausen (1980) has isolated an allergenic quinone, 2,6-dimethoxy-1,4,-benzoquinone, also found in the important orchid genus, *Cymbidium*.

Hausen B.M. (1980) A new sensitizing quinone from *Streptocarpus* sp. (family Gesneriaceae). *Archives of Dermatological Research* **267**: 205.
Hjorth N. (1974) Irritant reactions from patch tests with *Streptocarpus*. *Contact Dermatitis Newsletter* **15**: 446.
Rook A. (1968) Contact dermatitis caused by *Streptocarpus*, a popular greenhouse plant. *Contact Dermatitis Newsletter* **3**: 52.
Van Ketel W.G. (1973) Allergic contact eczema from leaves of *Streptocarpus*. *Transactions of the St John's Hospital Dermatological Society* **59**: 73–7.
Van Ketel W.G. (1979) Occupational contact dermatitis due to *Codiaeum variegatum* and possibly to *Aeschynanthus pulcher*. *Dermatosen in Beruf und Umwelt* **27**: 141–2.

Pedaliaceae

SESAMUM indicum

Common name: Sesame
Distribution: ? India. Widely cultivated in India and other temperate areas
Patch test: Sesame oil 10% pet. Sesamolin 1% pet. (if available). Sesamin 1% pet. (if available)

The seeds of this annual herb are used extensively in cooking and baking; 'fast foods' such as burgers are often coated with them. The oil is valuable because it is slow to become rancid. It is used in Oriental cooking and in some margarines. It was a constituent of a proprietary zinc oxide plaster in the Netherlands. Allergic reactions to the ointment decreased when the oil was replaced by peanut oil (van Dijk *et al.* 1973). Allergic contact dermatitis has been recorded following the use of sesame oil in patients with leg ulcers (Malten 1972, Neering *et al.* 1975). It is added to lipsticks because of its 'non-sweating' effect (Hayakawa *et al.* 1987). Ground sesame seeds in the sweet delicacy, halva, have caused nausea and a widespread exanthem attributed to Type I hypersensitivity (Torsney 1964).

The allergens are sesamin and sesamolin (**7.XXXIII**), which are found in the unsaponifiable portion of the oil (Kubo *et al.* 1986). The oil does not contain sesamol (Hayakawa *et al.* 1987).

Sesamin

Sesamolin

7.XXXIII Allergens in sesame oil.

Hayakawa R., Matsunaga K., Suzuki M. *et al.* (1987) Is sesamol present in sesame oil? *Contact Dermatitis* **17**: 133–5.
Kubo Y., Nonaka S. & Yoshida H. (1986) Contact sensitivity to unsaponifiable substances in sesame oil. *Contact Dermatitis* **15**: 215–17.
Malten K.E. (1972) Sesame oil contact hypersensitivity in leg ulcer patients. *Contact Dermatitis Newsletter* **11**: 251.
Neering H., Vitanyi B.E.J., Malten K.E. & Van Dijk E. (1975) Allergens in sesame oil contact dermatitis. *Acta Dermato-Venereologica* **45**: 31–4.
Torsney P.J. (1964) Hypersensitivity to sesame seed. *Journal of Allergy* **35**: 514–19.
Van Dijk E., Neering H. & Vitanyi B.E.J. (1973) Contact hypersensitivity to sesame oil in patients with leg ulcers and eczema. *Acta Dermato-Venereologica* **53**: 133–5.

Labiatae (Lamiaceae)

This family contains many aromatic plants, including herbs used in medicine, perfumery and cooking. Essential oils are derived from several herbs and these are potential sources of allergic contact dermatitis.

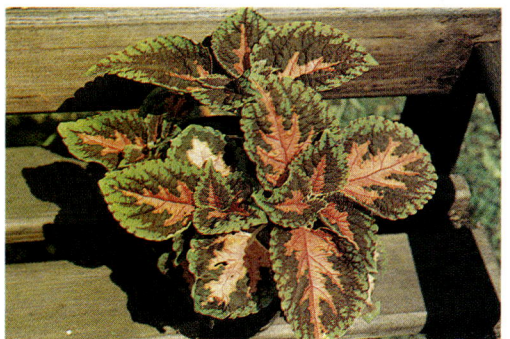

Fig. 7.5.87 *Coleus blumei* cultivar.

COLEUS blumei hybrids

Common name: Coleus
Distribution: Africa, tropical Asia. A popular foliage plant for pots and bedding
Patch test: Crushed leaf, ether extract 50%. Coleon O 0.01% in 94% ethanol

There are numerous cultivars of this attractive plant (Fig. 7.5.87). The leaves are oval, pointed at the tip and are in a bewildering variety of shades of green, red and brown. The flowers are small, blue-violet, held on a spike; however the flower stem is generally pinched out to encourage leaf development. The leaves have fine hairs which may be irritant; true allergic reactions are also recorded. A 40-year-old hospital gardener had been potting out *Coleus* over 20 years. After handling four cultivars of the plants more intensively for 1 year he developed facial and periorbital swelling and relapsed after subsequent exposure. Patch tests were positive with all four cultivars (Saihan & Harman 1978). Dooms-Goossens *et al.* (1987) reported airborne dermatitis in a young botanist who was researching for a thesis on the genus; he was specifically sensitive to *C. blumei* and *C. scutellarioides*. Patch tests were positive to coleon O 0.1% in 94% ethanol (**7.XXXIV**). This substance is a strong sensitizer in guinea pigs and may exceed 1% of the dry weight of the plant. It is structurally distinct from other plant allergens, having an abietane structure (Hausen *et al.* 1988). 0.1% may sensitize and 0.01% is preferable for patch testing (1990). The same allergen is found in the related genus *Plectranthus*, occasionally grown as a greenhouse plant. *Plectranthus barbatus* leaves are used as toilet paper in rural areas of Kenya; Owili (1977) reports perianal allergic reactions due to this practice.

Dooms-Goossens A., Borhijs A., Degreef H., Devriese E.G. & Geuns J.M.C. (1987) Airborne contact dermatitis to *Coleus*. *Contact Dermatitis* **17**: 109–10.
Hausen B.M., Devriese E.G. & Geuns J.M.C. (1988) Sensitizing potency of coleon O in *Coleus* species (Lamiaceae). *Contact Dermatitis* **19**: 217–18.
Owili D.M. (1977) Perianal dermatitis in Kenya due to *Plectranthus barbatus* leaves (Maigoya leaves). *East African Medical Journal* **54**: 571–3.
Saihan E.M. & Harman R.R.M. (1978) *Coleus* sensitivity in a gardener. *Contact Dermatitis* **4**: 234–5.

LAVANDULA spp.

Common name: Lavender
Distribution: Mediterranean, Atlantic Islands, Asia. Several species cultivated
Patch test: Lavender oil 5% pet.

Coleon O

7.XXXIV

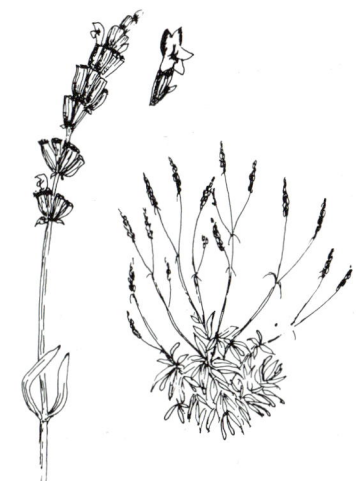

Fig. 7.5.88 *Lavandula spicata* (lavender).

Common lavender is *L. officinalis*
(*L. angustifolia*, *L. spicata* (Fig. 7.5.88),
L. vera), the major source of lavender oil and
water. Several cultivars are grown, including
dwarf forms and an albino. The grey leaves are
intensely fragrant, and the flowers are borne in
tight spikes. *Lavendula stoechas*, French
lavender, another source of lavender oil, is a
dwarf species with striking purple bracts
sticking up like ears at the top of the spike. Oil
of lavender has caused allergic hand eczema in
hairdressers (e.g. Brandao 1986) and individuals
have been sensitized after using proprietary
creams containing lavender oil, e.g.
Phenergan® cream (Zina & Bonu 1969, Rudzki
et al. 1976). Calnan (1970) recorded six positive
reactions to oil of lavender in 1147 patients
from several European patch test clinics.
Lavender oil contains geraniol, linalool and
linalylacetate (Windholz *et al.* 1983) (**7.XXXV**).
Hausen (1988) recommends patch testing with
30% linalool, 10% geraniol and 10%
linalylacetate. In Brandao's (1986) case, patch
testing with geraniol was negative.

7.XXXV Allergens in lavender oil.

Brandao F.M. (1986) Occupational allergy to lavender oil. *Contact Dermatitis* **15**: 249–50.
Calnan C.D. (1970) Oil of cloves, laurel, lavender, peppermint. *Contact Dermatitis Newsletter* **7**: 148.
Hausen B.M. (1988) *Allergiepflanzen Pflanzenellergene*. Ecomed Landsberg, Munchen.
Rudzki E., Grzywa Z. & Brno W.S. (1976) Sensitivity to 35 essential oils. *Contact Dermatitis* **2**: 196–200.
Windholz M., Budavari S., Blumetti R.F. & Otterbein E.S. (1983) *The Merck Index*. Merck & Co., Rahway, New Jersey, USA.
Zina G. & Bonu G. (1969) Phenergan cream (role of base constituents). *Contact Dermatitis Newsletter* **6**: 117.

MENTHA spp.

Common name: Mint. *Mentha aquatica*:
water mint; *M. X piperita*: peppermint;
M. X piperita var. *citrata*: bergamot mint;
M. pulegium: pennyroyal; *M. rotundifolia*:
apple mint; *M. spicata (viridis)* spearmint
Distribution: Europe, Asia. Many species cultivated
Patch test: Leaf as is, peppermint oil 2% pet.

Several species of mint (Fig. 7.5.89) are
cultivated as herbs or ornamental ground
covers. Oil of peppermint is derived from the
dried flower stems of *M. X piperita*, a hybrid
between *M. aquatica* and *M. spicata*. Dried
M. spicata leaves are used in mint sauce. Both
species are vigorous herbaceous plants with
oblong leaves and square stems. Numerous
small lilac or purple flowers are borne on leafy
spikes in late summer and autumn.
Peppermint oil is irritant but also causes
allergic contact dermatitis in food handlers
(Peltonen *et al.* 1985). Calnan (1970) reported
four positive patch tests in 1147 European
patch test patients. Peppermint leaf is used in

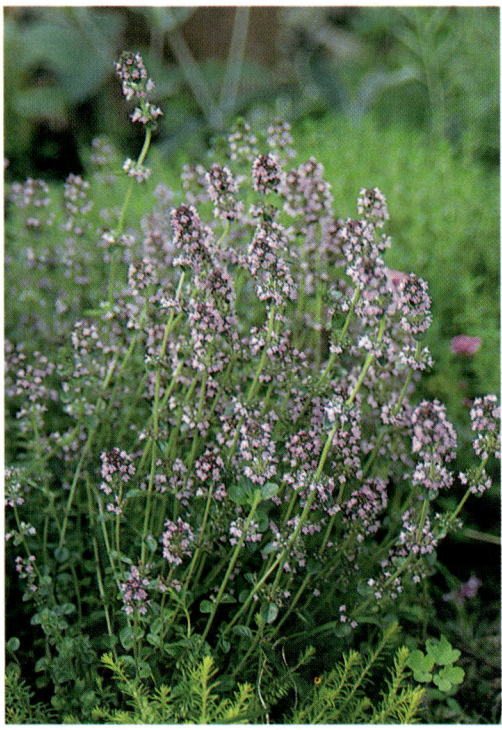

Fig. 7.5.89 *Mentha pulegium*, a species of mint commonly grown in herb gardens.

the cocktail mint julep, and has caused hand dermatitis in bartenders. Patch tests were positive to *M. X piperita* var. *citrata* but negative to *M. spicata* (Sams 1940). Menthol is possibly the allergen (7.XXXVI); menthol

7.XXXVI Allergens in *Mentha* spp.

crystals in cigarettes have caused perioral dermatitis (Camarasa & Alomar 1978). A patch test to spearmint flavouring (from *M. spicata*) was positive in a chewing gum finisher who also reacted to cassia (Morris 1954). The allergen may be L-carvone.

Calnan C.E.D. (1970) Oil of cloves, laurel, lavender and peppermint. *Contact Dermatitis Newsletter* **7**: 148.
Camarasa J.G. & Alomar A. (1978) Menthol dermatitis from cigarettes. *Contact Dermatitis* **4**: 169–70.
Morris G.E. (1954) Dermatoses among food handlers. *Industrial Medicine and Surgery* **23**: 343–4.
Peltonen L., Wickstrom G. & Vaahtoranta M. (1985) Occupational dermatoses in the food industry. *Dermatosen* **33**: 166–9.
Sams W.M. (1940) Occupational dermatitis due to mint. *Archives of Dermatology and Syphilology* **41**: 503–5.

MESONIA chinensis

Distribution: China, Japan

Goh (1988) reports sub-acute dermatitis on the hands of a Chinese male who worked in a soft drinks factory. A patch test was strongly positive to crushed leaves of this species, which he broke up and soaked in warm water to make a herbal tea. Fifteen controls were negative (Goh 1988).

Goh C.L. (1988) Occupational dermatitis from *Mesonia chinensis*. *Contact Dermatitis* **18**: 113.

SALVIA officinalis

Common name: Sage
Distribution: Central and eastern Mediterranean. Widely cultivated herb

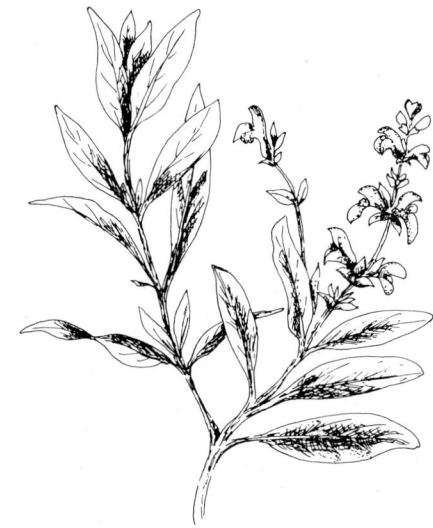

Fig. 7.5.90 *Salvia officinalis* (sage).

Patch test: Leaf as is, 10% ether extracts. ?Alantolactone

A tea made from sage (Fig. 7.5.90) has caused stomatitis and cheilitis (Zakon *et al.* 1947). Sertoli *et al.* (1978) report allergic dermatitis to *S. officinalis* but the patient otherwise reacted to compositae; these authors state that *S. officinalis* contains alantolactone. Clary oil, derived from *S. sclarea*, has caused dermatitis in perfumery workers (Gutman & Somov 1968).

Gutman S.G. & Somov B.A. (1968) [Allergic reactions caused by components of perfumery preparations.] *Vestnik Dermatologii i Venerologii* **42**: 62.
Sertoli A., Fabbri P., Campolmi P. & Panconesi E. (1978) Allergic dermatitis to *Salvia officinalis, Inula viscosa* and *Conyza bonariensis*. *Contact Dermatitis* **4**: 314.
Zakon S.J., Goldberg A.L. & Kahn J.B. (1947) Lipstick cheilitis: common dermatitis. Report of 32 cases. *Archives of Dermatology and Syphilology* **56**: 499.

THYMUS vulgaris

Common name: Thyme
Distribution: Europe, western Asia. Cultivated in herb gardens

Several species of thyme (Fig. 7.5.91) are cultivated in herb gardens; many are prostrate ground covers. *Thymus vulgaris*, the culinary thyme, is a low-growing, twiggy sub-shrub

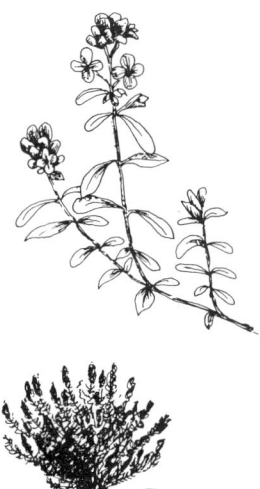

Fig. 7.5.91 *Thymus vulgaris* (thyme).

with small pale lilac flowers. It is the major source of oil of thyme, used as a rubefacient and in perfumes and toothpastes. Both preparations containing the oil have caused dermatitis, probably irritant (Greenberg & Lester 1954). Thyme oil contains thymol and its isomer, carvacrol. Thymol has caused dermatitis in dentists (Schwartz *et al.* 1957) and glossitis and cheilitis when used in toothpaste (Beinhauer 1940).

Beinhauer L.G. (1940) Cheilitis and glossitis from toothpaste. *Archives of Dermatology and Syphilology* **41**: 892.
Greenberg L.A. & Lester D. (1954) *Handbook of Cosmetic Materials*. Interscience, New York.
Schwartz L., Tulipan L. & Birmingham D.J. (1957) *Occupational Diseases of the Skin*, 3rd edn. Lea & Febiger, Philadelphia.

Polygonaceae

This family includes rhubarb (*Rheum rhaponticum*) and knotweed (*Polygonum* sp.) (Fig. 7.5.92). Both genera cause irritant contact dermatitis, chiefly due to calcium oxalate, although Moslein (1963) considered *Polygonum* sp. to cause true allergic, not irritant, reactions. Buckwheat flour (*Fagopyrum esculentum*) gave a positive patch test in a young atopic female baker who developed asthma and contact urticaria (Valdivieso *et al.* 1989). This may represent a

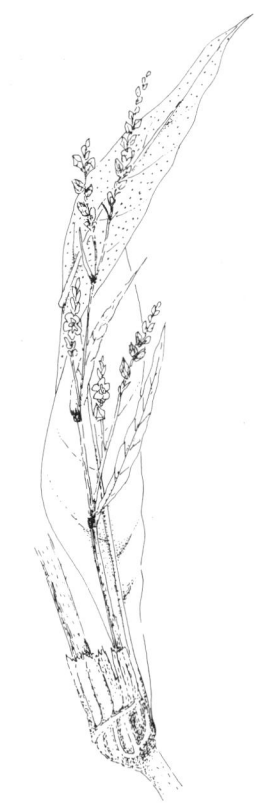

Fig. 7.5.92 *Polygonum nodosum* (knotweed).

'hybrid' type of sensitivity as postulated by Malten (1968).

Malten K.E. (1968) The occurrence of hybrids between contact allergic eczema and atopic dermatitis (and vice versa) and their significance. *Dermatologica* **136**: 404–6.
Moslein P. (1963) Pflanzen als Kontakt-Allergene. *Berufsdermatosen* **11**: 24–32.
Valdivieso R., Moneo I., Pola J. *et al.* (1989) Occupational asthma and contact urticaria caused by buckwheat flour. *Annals of Allergy* **63**: 149–52.

Myristicaceae

MYRISTICA fragrans

Common names: Nutmeg, mace
Distribution: Moluccas, cultivated in tropics
Patch test: Powdered nutmeg as is. Ether extract 1% pet. Eugenol 2% pet. ? Isopropyl myristate 5% pet.

The seed of this evergreen tree is the nutmeg of commerce (Fig. 7.5.93). Mace is the fleshy

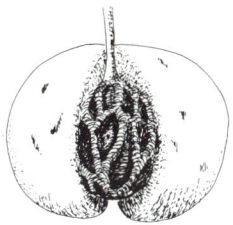

Fig. 7.5.93 Nutmeg and mace. Mace is the fleshy pericarp around the nutmeg seed.

aril which surrounds the seed. In a recent study of contact allergy to spices, nutmeg was the commonest allergen, accounting for 28% of positive reactions in a group selected for suspected 'indicators' of spice sensitivity (van den Akker *et al.* 1990). Nutmeg contains at least two potential sensitizers. Eugenol is a major component (Bennett *et al.* 1988); this may explain the association with sensitivity for fragrance mix (van den Akker *et al.* 1990). Another component is a triglyceride of myristic acid; isopropyl myristate is a recognized, if rare, cosmetic allergen (Calnan 1968, Wilkinson 1969) and myristates appear to have been responsible for allergic stomatitis due to nutmeg (Morrien 1979). Ether extraction of nutmeg may yield more positive reactions that patch testing with the dry powder, perhaps due to exposure of hidden antigens (van den Akker *et al.* 1990).

Bennett A., Stamford I.F., Tavares I.A. *et al.* (1988) The biological activity of eugenol, a major constituent of nutmeg (*Myristica fragrans*). Studies on prostaglandins, the intestine and other tissues. *Phytotherapy Research* **2**: 124–30.
Calnan C.D. (1968) Isopropyl myristate sensitivity. *Contact Dermatitis Newsletter* **3**: 41.
Morrien J.J. (1979) Allergische stomatitis met ernstige ulceratie door gebruik van een smaakstof (*Myristica*). *Nederlands Tijschrift voor Geneeskunde* **124**: 243–4.
Van den Akker T.H.W., Roesyanto-Mahadi I.D., Van Toorenenbergen A.W. & Van Joost T.H. (1990) Contact allergy to spices. *Contact Dermatitis* **22**: 267–72.
Wilkinson D.S. (1969) Isopropyl myristate. *Contact Dermatitis Newsletter* **6**: 144.

Lauraceae

CINNAMOMUM cassia

Common names: Cassia. Chinese cinnamon
Distribution: China, naturalized in Malaysia

CINNAMOMUM zeylanicum

Common name: Cinnamon
Distribution: Sri Lanka, cultivated
Patch test: Cinnamon or cassis oil 0.5% pet. Cinnamic aldehyde 1% pet.

Cinnamomum is a genus of small tropical evergreen trees or shrubs with oval glossy leaves (Fig. 7.5.94). The spice cinnamon is derived chiefly from the bark of *C. zeylanicum*, although other species can be used (Calnan 1976), including *C. tamala* (from India), *C. loureirii* (Vietnam), and *C. olivieri* (Australia). *Cinnamomum cassia* is the source of oil of cassia, sometimes termed 'oil of cinnamon' in the USA (Laubach *et al.* 1953).

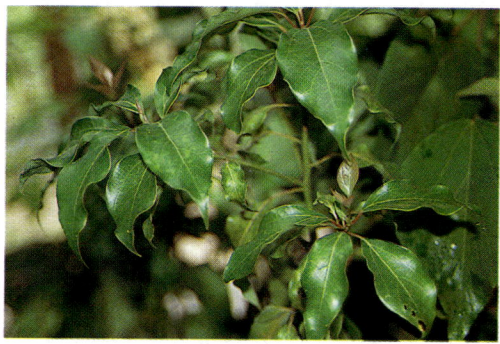

Fig. 7.5.94 *Cinnamomum zeylanicum*.

Both cassia and cinnamon are irritants and sensitizers although they do not necessarily cross-react (Laubach *et al.* 1953). The major constituent is cinnamic aldehyde (cinnamaldehyde) (**7.XXXVII**). The essential oil from cassia bark contains up to 90% cinnamic aldehyde, whereas the concentration in cinnamon leaf is rarely more than 7% (Fisher 1975). Cinnamic aldehyde can cause contact urticaria, through histamine release by a pharmacological mechanism (Nater *et al.* 1977). It is also a potent allergen. Sensitization may occur following occupational exposure to

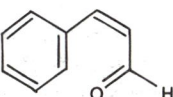

Cinnamic aldehyde

7.XXXVII

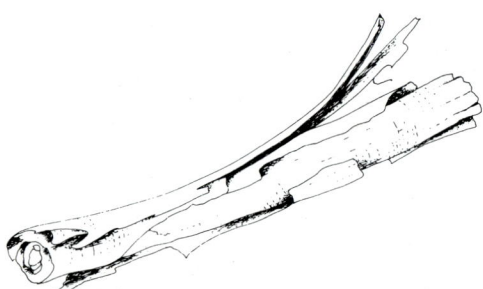

Fig. 7.5.95 Cinnamon stick.

cassis oil, e.g. candy makers (Kern 1960), bakers or confectioners (Malten 1979); it is used in perfumes and in pharmaceutical products (Schwartz *et al.* 1957). Affected patients may present with a persistent and intensely pruritic eruption of the hands. True cinnamon oil is also used in cosmetics and toothpastes (Calnan 1976). Cinnamon bark can sensitize when used as a culinary spice (Fig. 7.5.95) (Niinimäki 1984) and perioral dermatitis has been reported from a hot punch containing it (Farkas 1981). Allergic reactions may be severe; Goh and Ng (1988) reported multiple tense bullae resembling pemphigoid in a young Malay female who rubbed ground cinnamon stick on her scars.

Allergy to cassia or cinnamon can usually be deduced from the history and a positive patch test with cinnamic aldehyde. Cross-reactions can occur between cinnamon/cassia and other aromatic oils and balsams (Calnan 1976).

Calnan C.D. (1976) Cinnamon dermatitis from an ointment. *Contact Dermatitis* **2**: 167–70.
Farkas J. (1981) Perioral dermatitis from marjoram, bay leaf and cinnamon. *Contact Dermatitis* **7**: 121.
Fisher A.A. (1975) Allergic eczematous contact dermatitis due to foods. *Cutis* **16**: 603.
Goh C.L. & Ng S.K. (1988) Bullous contact allergy from cinnamon. *Dermatosen in Beruf und Umwelt* **36**: 186–7.
Kern A.B. (1960) Contact dermatitis from cinnamon. *Archives of Dermatology* **81**: 599–600.
Laubach J.L., Malkinson F.D. & Ringrose E.J. (1953) Chelitis caused by cinnamon (*cassia*) oil in toothpaste. *JAMA* **152**: 404.
Malten K.E. (1979) Four bakers showing positive patch tests to a number of fragrance materials which can also be used as flavours. *Acta Dermato-Venereologica* **59** (Suppl. 85): 117–21.
Nater J.P., De Jong M.C.J.M., Baar A.J.M. & Bluemink E. (1977) Contact urticarial responses to cinnamaldehyde. *Contact Dermatitis* **3**: 151.
Niinimäki A. (1984) Delayed-type allergy to spices. *Contact Dermatitis* **11**: 34–40.
Schwartz L., Tulipan L. & Birmingham D.J. (1957) *Occupational Diseases of the Skin*, 3rd edn. Lea & Febiger, Philadelphia.

LAURUS nobilis

Common names: Sweet bay. Laurel (in part)
Distribution: Mediterranean. Commonly grown as a culinary herb (usually as a container plant)
Patch test: Leaf as is. Laurel oil 2–5% pet. or in ether

An aromatic shrub or tree (Fig. 7.5.96), growing up to 15 m with a dark green-brown bark and glossy, leathery lance-shaped leaves. The clusters of flowers are small and yellowish, followed by black cherry-like fruits. In ancient Greece, it was sacred to the god Apollo. Its leaves were chewed by his priestesses at Delphi, enabling them to pronounce oracles. A

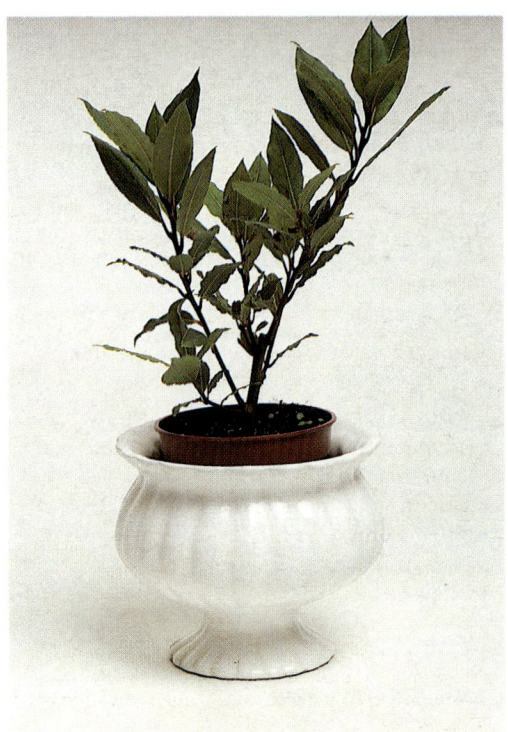

Fig. 7.5.96 *Laurus nobilis* (sweet bay).

laurel wreath was awarded to Greek and Roman poets and athletes. The word 'baccalaureate' (corrupted to 'bachelor') derives from the berried crown of laurel placed on the heads of newly qualified doctors (Huxley & Taylor 1977). The common 'cherry' laurel of English shrubberies is an unrelated species, *Prunus laurocerasus*.

The leaves are used extensively in cooking soups and casseroles; they are the source of 'oil of bay' which has a reputation as a soothing herb. Culpeper recommends it for 'the itch, scabs and weals in the skin' and it is an ingredient of Vegebom® ointment, used in France and Germany to treat insect bites. This is the major source of sensitization in continental Europe (e.g. Hausen 1985). The oil was also in hat bands and was the cause of 90% of cases of hat dermatitis. Rarely, sensitization occurs from handling bay leaves in cooking (Fousserean et al. 1967). *Laurus nobilis* is reported to cause 17.8% of cases of plant dermatitis in Strasbourg (Asakawa et al. 1974). The potential allergens vary in different parts of the plant (Foussereau et al. 1975). The leaf contains several sesquiterpene lactones, including costunolide, desacetyl laurenobiolide (**7.XXXVIII**) and tulipinolide, which have been

Costunolide   Laurenobiolide

7.XXXVIII Allergens in *Laurus nobilis*.

shown to act as haptens in sensitized guinea pigs (Cheminat et al. 1984). These substances are chemically similar to the sesquiterpene lactones found in members of the unrelated families Compositae, liverworts (*Frullania*) and Magnoliaceae. Cross-reactions can occur (Asakawa et al. 1974, Foussereau et al. 1975).

Asakawa Y., Benezra C., Ducombs G., Foussereau J., Muller J.C. & Ourisson G. (1974) Cross-sensitization between *Frullania* and *Laurus nobilis*. *Archives of Dermatology* **110**: 957.
Cheminat A., Stampf J.L. & Benezra C. (1984) Allergic contact dermatitis to laurel *Laurus nobilis* L: isolation and identification of haptens. *Archives of Dermatological Research* **276**: 178–81.
Foussereau J., Benezra C. & Ourisson G. (1967) Contact dermatitis from laurel. I. Clinical aspects. *Transactions of the St John's Hospital Dermatological Society* **53**: 141, 147.
Foussereau J., Muller J.C. & Benezra C. (1975) Contact allergy to *Frullania* and *Laurus*: cross-sensitization and chemical structure of the allergens. *Contact Dermatitis* **1**: 223.
Hausen B.M. (1985) Lorbeer-Allergie. Ursache, Wirkung und Folgen der ausserlicher. Anwendung eines sogenannten Nuturheilmittels. *Deutsche Medizinische Wochenschrift* **110**: 634–8.
Huxley A. & Taylor W. (1977) *Flowers of Greece and the Aegean*. Chatto & Windus, London.

Proteaceae

GREVILLEA spp.

Common names: Silk Oak. Spider Flower. Kahili Flower (Hawaii)
Distribution: Mostly Australia. Cultivated extensively in parks and gardens in Australia and southern USA (California and Hawaii)
Skin reactions: Allergic contact dermatitis. Urticaria
Patch test: 0.1% ethanol extract of flower in petrolatum
Allergens: Pentadecylresorcinol. Tridecylresorcinol
Cross-sensitivity: *Toxicodendron*

The genus *Grevillea* contains 250 species, mostly Australian, ranging from low shrublets to forest trees (Lothian 1989). The important allergenic species belong to the section *Eugrevillea*. Most have pinnate or pinnatisect leaves and the heads of toothbrush-like flowers range in colour from red to yellow, cream and white.

In 1847, Leichhardt, an explorer who led an expedition to Queensland, described a member of his party who developed a blistering eruption after carrying *Grevillea* pods near the skin. Traditionally, natives of northwest Australia use a secretion from a tree species to scarify their bodies (Lothian 1989). More recently dermatitis has been reported from garlands (leis) made with the flowers (Arnold 1942) and eye irritation has occurred in Californian linesmen exposed to sawdust from *Grevillea robusta* (quoted in Menz et al. 1986).

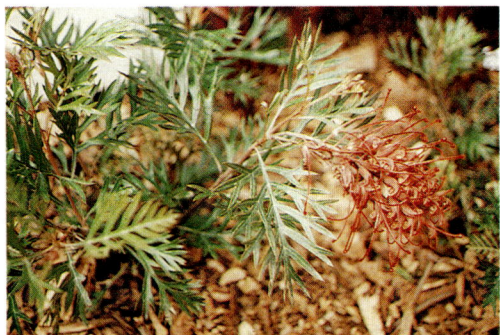

Fig. 7.5.97 *Grevillea* cultivar 'Robyn Gordon.' (Courtesy of Mr T.R.N. Lothian.)

Acute contact urticaria has been described due to *G. juniperina* (Apted 1988).

Although several species cause allergic contact dermatitis, the hybrid X 'Robyn Gordon' has been implicated most frequently (Menz 1985, Menz *et al.* 1986). This vigorous shrub (Fig. 7.5.97) is a natural hybrid between *G. bipinnatifida* and the red form of *G. banksii* and grows to a height of approximately 1.5 m. Because it is attractive, having a long flowering season, is easily propagated and tolerant of a wide range of soil types, it is popularly grown in Australian gardens and also in the frost-free southern states of the USA.

Contact with the plant, especially the flower, induces a bullous eruption similar to that caused by poison ivy and poison oak (*Toxicodendron* spp.). Menz *et al.* (1986) obtained positive patch tests with fresh flowers. There was no photopotentiation of patch tests by UVA. A 0.01% ether extract of flowers gave positive reactions in all clinically affected patients, although a 0.1% ethanol extract dispersed in petrolatum is more stable and convenient. Positive reactions were observed to *Toxicodendron succedaneum* (Japanese wax tree) leaf, even in individuals who gave no history of previous exposure. This suggests true cross-sensitivity. Patch tests using tridecylresorcinol (0.1%) were positive but using resorcinol (2%) were negative, indicating that the long carbon side chain is a necessary part of the hapten. Both tridecylresorcinol and pentadecylresorcinol have been isolated from the wood of *G. banksii* and *G. robusta*; these are structurally similar to pentadecylcatechol

(a major hapten in *Toxicodendron* spp.) (Menz *et al.* 1986) (**7.XXXIX**).

5-pentadecylresorcinol ($C_{15}H_{31}$)
(*G. banksii*)

5-pentadecenylresorcinol ($C_{15}H_{27}$)
(*G. banksii*)

3-pentadecylcatechol ($C_{15}H_{31}$)
(hydrourushiol)

Tridecylresorcinol ($C_{15}C_{27}$)
(*G. robusta*)

7.XXXIX Allergens in *Grevillea* spp., compared with pentadecylcatechol.

Apted J. (1988) Acute contact urticaria from *Grevillea juniperina*. (Letter.) *Contact Dermatitis* **18**: 126.
Arnold H.L. (1942) Dermatitis due to the blossom of *Grevillea banksii*. *Archives of Dermatology and Syphilology* **45**: 1037–51.
Lothian N. (1989) *Grevillea* species and hybrids causing contact dermatitis. *Australasian Journal of Dermatology* **30**: 111–13.
Menz J. (1985) Contact dermatitis from plants of the *Grevillea* family — two case reports. *Australasian Journal of Dermatology* **26**: 74–6.
Menz J., Rossi R.E., Taylor W.C. & Wall L. (1986) Contact dermatitis from *Grevillea* 'Robyn Gordon'. *Contact Dermatitis* **15**: 126–31.

Santalaceae

SANTALUM album

Common name: Sandalwood
Distribution: Malaysia, India. Cultivated in India
Patch test: Sandalwood oil 10% pet. Santalol 2% pet.

The pale-yellow heartwood of this tree yields oil of sandalwood (santal) used in perfumery. A report of photoallergy to the oil, leading to persistent light reactivity (Starke 1967), may have been due to contaminants. Sandalwood powder and oil in incense were found to be sensitizers in a patient who developed depigmented contact dermatitis. The allergen is santalol, a sesquiterpene alcohol (Hayakawa et al. 1987). No cases of allergic dermatitis have been attributed to the wood, which is used to make furniture and trinkets (Woods & Calnan 1976).

Hayakawa R., Matsunaga K. & Arima Y. (1987) Depigmented contact dermatitis due to incense. *Contact Dermatitis* **16**: 272–4.
Starke J.C. (1967) Photoallergy to sandalwood oil. *Archives of Dermatology and Syphilology* **96**: 62–3.
Woods B. & Calnan C.D. (1976) Toxic woods. *British Journal of Dermatology* **94** (Suppl. 13): 1–97.

Euphorbiaceae

Several members of this important family (the spurges) possess a highly irritant milky latex (see pp. 59–62). Allergic reactions are rare, with two probable exceptions.

CODIAEUM variegatum var. pictum

Common name: Croton of florists (*not* true Croton)
Distribution: Tropical Asia. Widely grown as a foliage house plant
Patch test: Leaf as is or water extract

This sub-shrub is popularly grown for its alternatively variegated leaves, which often change from green and yellow to red (Fig. 7.5.98). Contact dermatitis occurs in nursery gardeners. Although chiefly irritant, allergic reactions are also reported (Hausen & Schultz 1977, Schmidt & Olholm-Larsen 1977, van Ketel 1979, Cleenewerck & Martin 1989). Irritant reactions, which may be delayed, are attributed to diterpene (phorbol) esters (Hausen & Schulz 1977) but the allergen has not been determined. It is water-soluble (Van Ketel 1979) but not ether-extractable (Schmidt & Olholm-Larsen 1977).

Cleenewerck M.-B. & Martin P. (1989) Occupational contact dermatitis due to *Codiaeum variegatum* L., *Chrysanthemum indicum* L., *Chrysanthemum* X *hortorum* and *Frullania dilatata* L. In Frosch P.J. *et al.* (eds) *Current Topics in Contact Dermatitis*. Springer-Verlag, Berlin, pp. 149–57.
Hausen B.M. & Schultz K.H. (1977) Occupational contact dermatitis due to croton (*Codiaeum variegatum* (L.) A. Juss. var *pictum* (Lodd.) Muell Arg.). *Contact Dermatitis* **3**: 289–92.
Schmidt H. & Olholm-Larsen P. (1977) Allergic contact dermatitis from croton (*Codiaeum*). *Contact Dermatitis* **3**: 100.
Van Ketel W.G. (1979) Occupational contact dermatitis due to *Codiaeum variegatum* and possibly to *Aeschynanthus pulcher*. *Dermatosen in Beruf und Umwelt* **27**: 141–2.

EUPHORBIA pulcherrima

Common name: Poinsettia
Distribution: Central America. A common house plant
Patch test: Leaf as is. 10% water or methanol extract (Hausen 1988)

The brilliant red bracts of this plant (Fig. 7.5.99) make it a popular Christmas present, although plants seldom survive after the

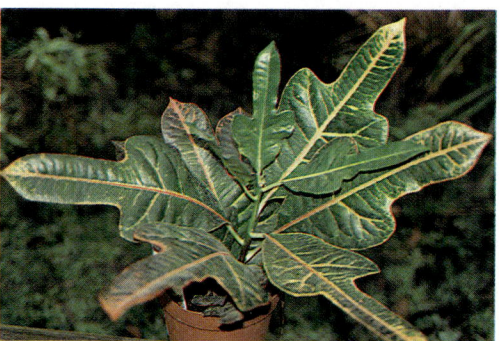

Fig. 7.5.98 *Codiaeum* cultivar (florist's 'Croton').

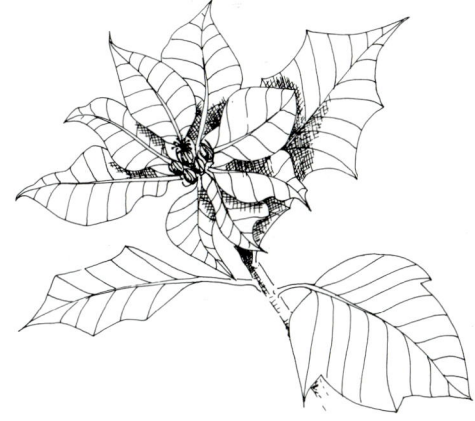

Fig. 7.5.99 Poinsettia.

festive season. It appears to be considerably less irritant than other *Euphorbia* species. Santucci *et al.* (1985) obtained positive patch tests in two individuals with a history suggesting allergic contact dermatitis; however allergy appears to be rare. The allergen is unknown.

Hausen B.M. (1988) *Allergiepflanzen-Pflanzenallergene.* Ecomed, Landsberg/Munchen.
Santucci B., Picardo M. & Cristando A. (1985) Contact dermatitis from *Euphorbia pulcherrima. Contact Dermatitis* **12**: 285–6.

RICINUS communis

Common name: Castor oil plant
Distribution: Tropical Africa and Asia. Naturalized in Mediterranean region

This is a rapidly growing, tall annual (Fig. 7.5.100). It is reported to have grown up to provide shade above the prophet Jonah's head while he awaited the destruction of Nineveh (Jonah 4:6, *Jerusalem Bible* 1971). It has red-brown palm-like leaves and spikes of flowers composed either of red pistils or creamy stamens; petals are absent. The seeds are highly ornamental, oval, brown or black marbled with white, brown or grey. Castor oil is derived from the seeds. It causes Type I reactions, although allergic contact dermatitis has been reported following exposure to cosmetics, such as lipsticks containing castor oil (Sai 1983a, b, Andersen 1984). Castor oil contains a triglyceride of ricinoleic acid. The free acid, which appears to be the allergen, is released on hydrolysis when the oil becomes rancid (Andersen *et al.* 1984).

Andersen K.E. (1984) Lipstick dermatitis related to castor oil. *Contact Dermatitis* **11**: 253–4.
Sai S. (1983a) Lipstick dermatitis caused by castor oil. *Contact Dermatitis* **9**: 75.

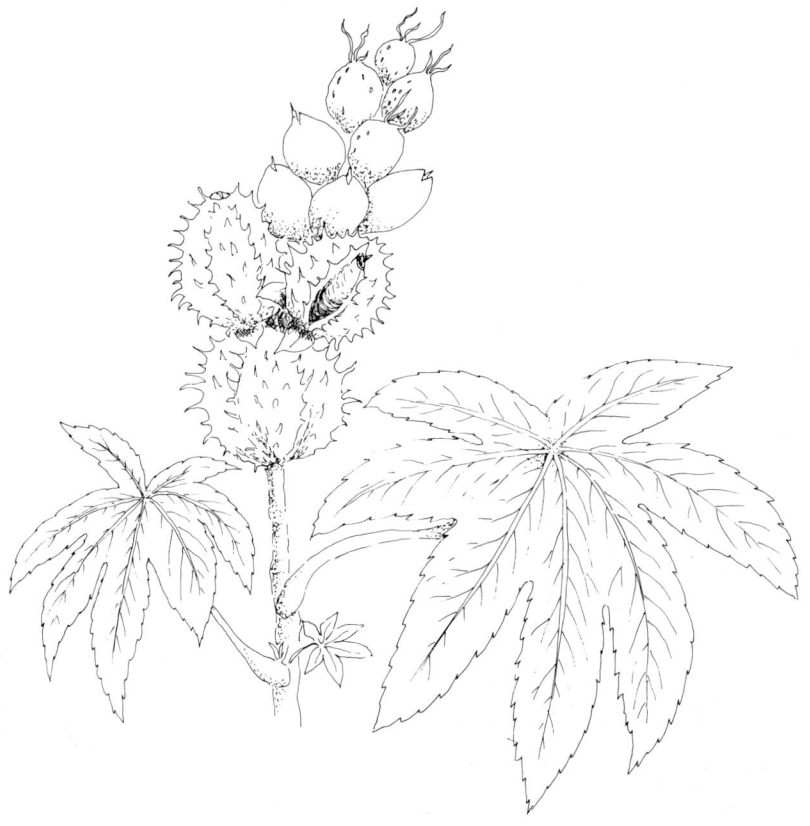

Fig. 7.5.100 *Ricinus communis* (castor oil plant).

Sai S. (1983b) Lipstick dermatitis caused by ricinoleic acid. *Contact Dermatitis* **9**: 524.

Buxaceae

SIMMONDSIA

Simmondsia chinensis and *S. californica* are desert shrubs native to Arizona, California and New Mexico. Jojoba oil is a liquid wax ester mixture derived from the ground or crushed seeds (Windholz *et al.* 1983). In the past the oil has been derived from the edible fruit of *Ziziphus jujuba* and *Z. lotus*, spiny shrublets both native to the eastern Mediterranean. Jojoba oil is used as a moisturizer and has potential as an industrial lubricant. Scott and Scott (1982) report allergic contact dermatitis to the oil in six individuals.

Scott M.J. & Scott M.J., Jr. (1982) Jojoba oil. (Letter.) *Journal of the American Academy of Dermatology* **6**: 545.
Windholz Z.M., Budavari S., Blumetti R.F. & Otterbein E.S. (1983) *The Merck Index: An Encyclopedia of Chemicals, Drugs and Biologicals.* Merck & Co. Inc., Rahway, NJ, USA.

Cannabaceae

This family includes the infamous *Cannabis* (Indian hemp) (Fig. 7.5.101), which is irritant and may be allergenic (Behl *et al.* 1979). Hop (*Humulus lupulus*) (Fig. 7.5.102) is naturalized throughout northern temperate areas and is probably native to eastern Europe and Asia. Irritant reactions occur in hop pickers (Cookson & Laughton 1953). A 43-year-old female working in a laboratory investigating hops, developed conjunctivitis, rhinitis and facial dermatitis. A positive patch test was obtained to the dust of pulverized hops. The authors postulate allergy as well as irritant dermatitis (Raith & Jager 1984). Possible allergens are oxidation products of myrcene, humulone and iupulone.

Behl P.N. & Captain R.M. (1979) *Skin Irritant and Sensitizing Plants Found in India.* S. Chand, Ram Naga, New Delhi.
Cookson T.S. & Laughton S. (1953) Hop dermatitis in Herefordshire. *British Medical Journal* **2**: 376–9.
Raith L. & Jager K. (1984) Hop allergy. *Contact Dermatitis* **11**: 53.

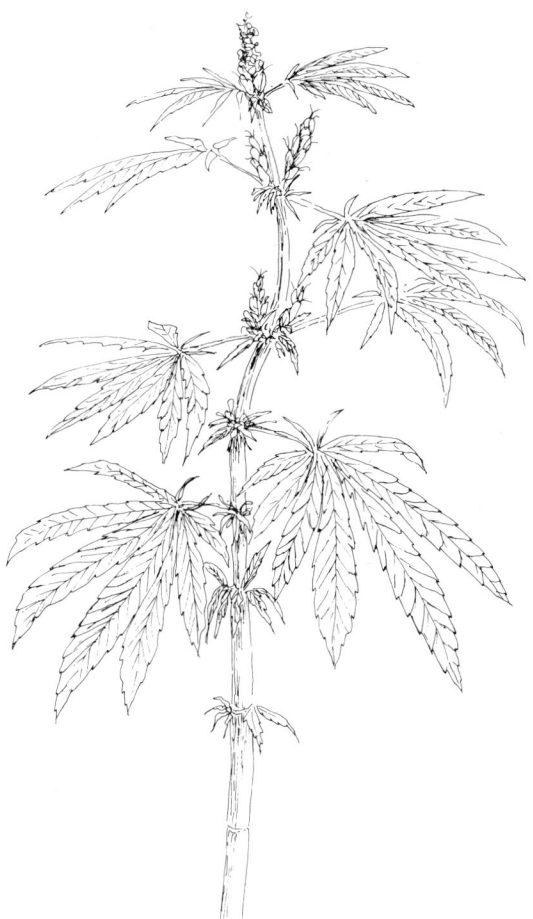

Fig. 7.5.101 *Cannabis indica* (Indian hemp).

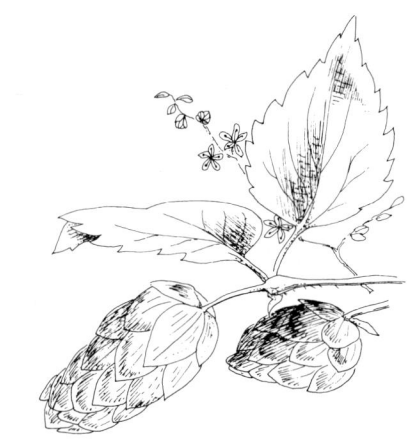

Fig. 7.5.102 *Humulus lupulus* (hop).

Juglandaceae

JUGLANS spp.

Common names: Walnuts. *J. nigra*: black walnut. *J. regia*: walnut
Distribution: *J. nigra* North America. *J. regia* Himalayas and west Asia. Both spp. widely cultivated especially in town gardens
Patch test: Wood shavings

The walnuts are handsome deciduous trees up to 20 m in height. The bark is greyish and the leaves yellowish-green with 7–9 oval, pointed leaflets. The male catkins are greenish. The timber is used in furniture and for veneering. Walnut juice and oil are used as dyes. The wood of both species appears to be irritant, although *J. regia* wood may sensitize (Schleicher 1974). It has caused apparent allergic contact reactions in a cabinet maker with multiple sensitivities (Woods & Calnan 1976). Juglone may be a sensitizer.

Schleicher H. (1974) Uber phytogene allergische Kontaktekzeme. *Dermatologische Monatsschrift* **160**: 433.
Woods B. & Calnan C.D. (1976) Toxic woods. *British Journal of Dermatology* **94** (Suppl. 13).

Fagaceae (Cupuliferae)

QUERCUS spp.

Common name: Oak
Distribution: Widespread, mostly northern hemisphere
Patch test: Ethanol extract of bark

Several species of oak (Fig. 7.5.103) are native to Europe. Woods and Calnan (1976) describe dermatitis in a joiner who was allergic to oak and also to the conifer *Thuja plicata*. Campolmi *et al.* (1986) report three patients who developed acute eczema or a prurigo-like eruption after country pursuits (hunting, wood-cutting and walking in the woods). Patch tests were positive to usnic acid and to tannins derived from the bark, leaves and branches. Plant material was washed with 95% ethanol (10 ml/g) for 16 h in a shaking water bath at 20°C and the extraction repeated twice. The substrates were then pooled (Campolmi *et al.*

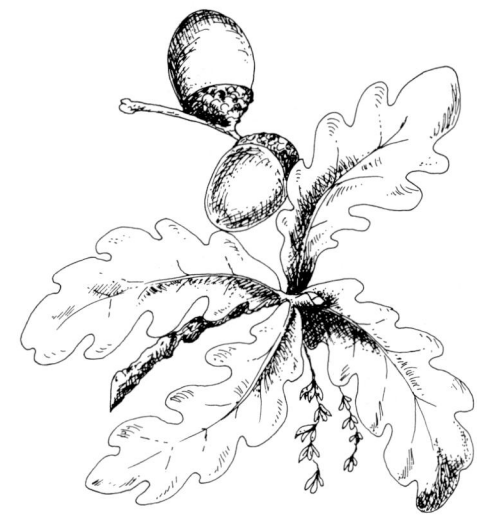

Fig. 7.5.103 *Quercus robur* (oak).

1986). Tannins are produced in trees, notably oaks, in galls (excrescences on the twigs and branches often due to parasitic wasps). Contact dermatitis is rare (Lewis 1944).

Campolmi P., Lotti T., Francalanci S. & Sertoli A. (1986) Contact sensitivity to oak. *Contact Dermatitis* **14**: 314.
Lewis G.M. (1944) Dermatitis venenata due to tannins. *Archives of Dermatology and Syphilology* **50**: 138.
Woods B. & Calnan C.D. (1976) Toxic woods. *British Journal of Dermatology* **94** (Suppl. 13).

Salicaceae

POPULUS spp.

Common name: Poplar
Distribution: Northern temperate areas. Widely planted

Several species of this rapidly growing tree (Fig. 7.5.104) are grown as screens or by roadsides. The sawdust from poplar trees has caused a severe exfoliative dermatitis (Weber 1953). However, most cases of allergic contact dermatitis are due to propolis (bee glue). This is a transformation product derived from *Populus* species. It is used by bees to seal holes in honeycombs, smooth out internal walls of the hive and protect the entrance against intruders (Bunney 1968). It was used in ancient Egypt to embalm the dead (Hausen *et al.* 1987a).

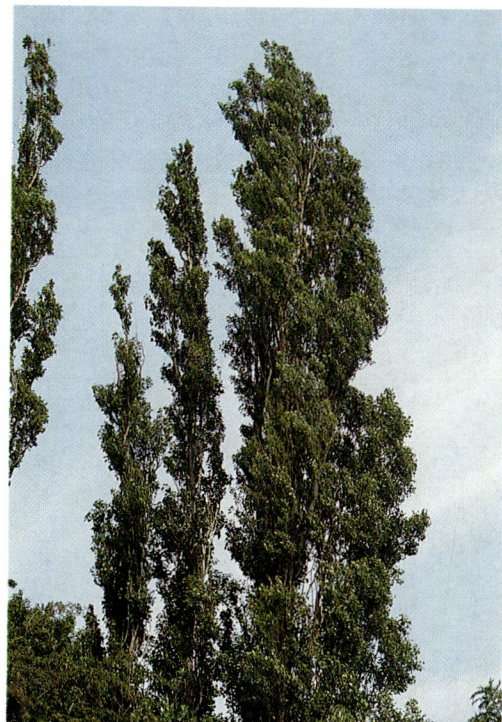

Fig. 7.5.104 Poplar trees.

Propolis is a dark brown or greenish resinous material with a faint, pleasant smell resembling cinnamon. Crude preparations may contain insect corpses (Raton 1990). Allergic dermatitis was well reviewed by Bunney (1968). It has been reported from central Europe (Rudzki & Grzywa 1983, Macháčkova 1985, 1988) and Japan (Nakamura 1988). Bee keepers are classically affected, although propolis has been used by manufacturers of stringed instruments; it is claimed to enhance the tone of violins made by old masters and is still used in Cremona. It is an ingredient of polishes and varnishes (Monti *et al.* 1983). Ointments containing propolis are used particularly in eastern Europe, and cause allergic reactions (Raton *et al.* 1990). With the increasing trend to 'natural' products, propolis is more frequently incorporated in moisturizing and other creams (Hausen *et al.* 1987a). Oral ingestion of propolis has caused cheilitis and perioral eczema (Kokel & Trevisan 1983), as well as exacerbating hand dermatitis (Trevisan & Kokel 1987).

Patients allergic to propolis frequently show cross-sensitivity to balsam of Peru (e.g. Cirasino *et al.* 1987, Young 1987), although not always (Rudzki & Grzywa 1983). Recently, a major allergen of propolis has been identified as 1,1-dimethylallyl caffeic acid ester (Hausen *et al.* 1987b) (**7.XL**). A 1% synthetic

1,1-dimethylallyl-caffeic acid ester

7.XL

preparation of this substance produced an allergic reaction in eight out of nine patients with propolis allergy (Ginanneschi *et al.* 1989).

Bunney M.H. (1968) Contact dermatitis in beekeepers due to propolis (bee glue). *British Journal of Dermatology* **86**: 17–23.
Cirasino L., Pisata A. & Fasani F. (1987) Contact dermatitis from propolis. *Contact Dermatitis* **16**: 110–11.
Ginanneschi M., Acciai M.C., Sertoli A. & Bracci S. (1989) Propolis allergy: synthesis and patch testing of 1,1-dimethylallyl caffeic acid ester and its O-methyl derivatives. *Contact Dermatitis* **21**: 267–9.
Hausen B.M., Wollenweber E., Sennff H. & Post B. (1987a) Propolis allergy (I). Origin, properties, usage and literature review. *Contact Dermatitis* **17**: 163–70.
Hausen B.M., Wollenweber E., Sennff H. & Post B. (1987b) Propolis allergy (II). The sensitizing properties of 1,1-dimethylallyl caffeic acid ester. *Contact Dermatitis* **17**: 171–7.
Kokel J.F. & Trevisan G. (1983) Contact dermatitis from propolis. *Contact Dermatitis* **9**: 518.
Macháčkova J. (1985) Contact dermatitis to propolis. *Contact Dermatitis* **13**: 43–4.
Macháčkova J. (1988) The incidence of allergy to propolis in 605 consecutive patients patch tested in Prague. *Contact Dermatitis* **18**: 210–12.
Monti M., Berti E., Carminati G. & Cusini M. (1983) Occupational and cosmetic dermatitis from propolis. *Contact Dermatitis* **9**: 163.
Nakamura T. (1988) Sensitivity to propolis in Japan. *Contact Dermatitis* **18**: 313.
Raton J.A., Aguirre A. & Diaz-Perez J.L. (1990) Contact dermatitis from propolis. *Contact Dermatitis* **22**: 183–4.
Rudzki E. & Grzywa Z. (1983) Dermatitis from propolis. *Contact Dermatitis* **9**: 40–5.
Trevisan G. & Kokel J.F. (1987) Contact dermatitis from propolis: role of gastrointestinal absorption. *Contact Dermatitis* **16**: 48.

Weber L.F. (1953) Dermatitis venenata due to native woods. *Archives of Dermatology and Syphilology* **67**: 388.

Young E. (1987) Sensitivity to propolis. *Contact Dermatitis* **16**: 49–50.

Orchidaceae

The orchid family is one of the largest in the plant kingdom and the highly complex flowers are often of extreme beauty. One of the inner segments (petals) is modified to form an elaborate 'lip'. The name 'orchid' derives from the paired tubers of many European terrestrial species, which resemble testicles. Not surprisingly, the tubers have gained a reputation for aphrodisiac qualities. Culpeper warns that orchid tubers 'provoke lust exceedingly'. Dioscorides states that if the larger tuber is eaten by a man, he will beget a male child. In several Mediterranean countries the tubers were, until recently, ground up and made into a thin gruel ('salep'). An increasing number of hardy terrestrial orchids is being grown by enthusiasts (Cribb & Bailes 1989) and an extensive research programme is currently being undertaken at the Royal Botanic Gardens, Kew, to understand their cultivation requirements and techniques of raising from seed. Of the hardy genera, only *Cypripedium* spp. have been reported to cause allergic contact dermatitis.

Several tropical and sub-tropical genera are in cultivation. Although traditionally the province of the well-to-do, many of these genera are proving amenable to cultivation as windowsill and house plants. A few are terrestrial or lithophytic (growing on rocks), such as *Cymbidium* and *Paphiopedilum*. Most are epiphytic (growing in trees). Allergic contact dermatitis appears to be very rare in most ornamental genera (Rasmussen 1986), although minor and transient episodes of hand dermatitis were observed in a large orchid farm in Singapore (Hardie & Ragan 1981). The one exception is *Vanilla*, which was of considerable economic importance. Much vanilla flavouring is now prepared synthetically, although vanilla pods are still available. Hausen (1984) has found quinonoid constituents in many ornamental orchids, including *Dendrobium nobile* and *Phalaenopsis* (increasingly grown as a house plant).

CYPRIPEDIUM

Common name: Lady's slipper
Distribution: Europe, Asia, North and Central America

This genus of fibrous-rooted terrestrial orchids (Fig. 7.5.105) is found throughout the northern

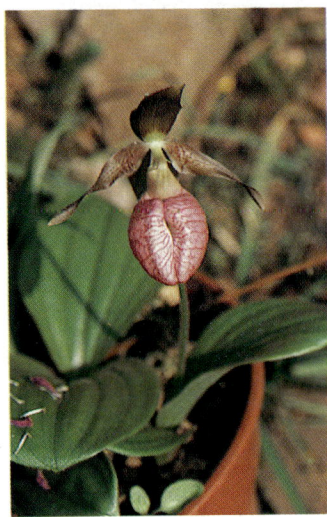

Fig. 7.5.105 *Cypripedium acaule.*

hemisphere in temperate parts of North America, Europe and Asia. *Cypripedium calceolus* has the distinction of being the rarest British native, being reduced to one station through over-collection. Its American relatives var. *parviflorum* and var. *pubescens* are relatively abundant in the eastern states and are in cultivation. Contact dermatitis to *Cypripedium* spp. has been reported since 1875 (Schmalle & Hausen 1979). The hairy leaves and stems cause irritant dermatitis (Woods 1962). Delayed irritant reactions may occur (McCord 1962). Four American spp. are reported to cause dermatitis, *C. acaule, calceolus, candidium,* and *reginae* (Beierlein 1957, Ulbrich 1965). *Cypripedium calceolus* contains an allergenic quinone, cypripedin (Schmalle & Hausen 1979) (**7.XLI**).

Cypripedin

7.XLI

PAPHIOPEDILUM

Common name: Lady's slipper
Distribution: Tropical and sub-tropical Asia

This tropical genus (Fig. 7.5.106) is closely related to *Cypripedium* and some species,

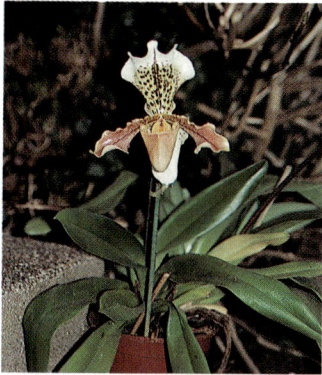

Fig. 7.5.106 *Paphiopedilum insigne*.

notably *P. insigne*, are not uncommon house plants. The leaves are held in fans and are typically thick and spotted or marbled. The genus has been reviewed recently by Cribb (1987). Hausen (1980) reported an eczematous eruption in an amateur grower who was repotting 500 plants. Patch tests were positive to leaf, stem and petal, together with quinoids obtained from an ether extract of
P. haynaldianum. Paphiopedilum fairreanum is also allergenic (Hausen 1980), and it seems likely that the allergen is found in other species.

CYMBIDIUM

Distribution: Tropical and sub-tropical Asia

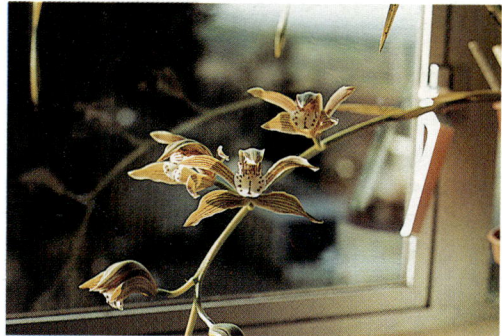

Fig. 7.5.107 *Cymbidium longifolium*.

Members of this Asiatic genus and their hybrids (Fig. 7.5.107) are grown as house plants and extensively for the cut flower market. Pre-packed solitary blooms are freely available from florists. A Japanese office worker who handled *Cymbidium* cultivars for several years, and also handled *Primula obconica*, developed a bullous eruption on the palms and fingers (Hausen *et al.* 1984). Positive patch tests were obtained with *P. obconica*, stem juice of *Cymbidium* spp. and, subsequently, a quinone isolated from *Cymbidium* spp., 2,6-dimethoxy-1,4-benzoquinone (**7.XLII**). This quinone elicited strong reactions in guinea pigs sensitized to *Cymbidium* leaf. It is found in at least 50 plant and wood species, where it is recognized as a sensitizer (Hausen 1978).

2,6-dimethoxy-1,
4-benzoquinone
(in Cymbidium spp.)

7.XLII

VANILLA

Distribution: Tropical, Central and South America. Widely cultivated in tropical Africa

Vanilla planifolia (Fig. 7.5.108) is the major source of vanilla flavouring and is still grown

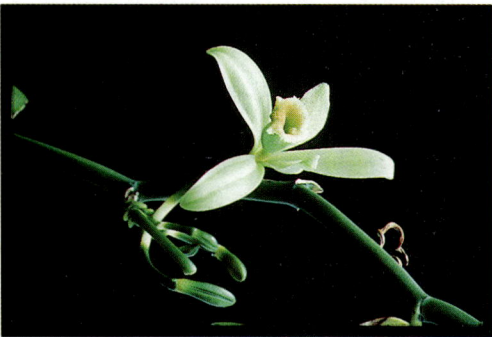

Fig. 7.5.108 *Vanilla planifolia*. (Courtesy of R. McKenzie.)

in plantations in Mexico, Madagascar and Tahiti. The plants are vine-like, reaching many feet in length, and mature specimens produce many large, fugaceous greenish flowers. The mite *Tyroglyphus farinae* lives on the pods and can produce an urticated papular eruption. Allergic contact dermatitis occurs, not only in individuals who cultivate and harvest the plants, but also in those who handle vanilla pods (Fig. 7.5.109) in the sweet and perfume industry (Wang 1987). Hjorth and Weismann (1972) reported allergic contact dermatitis, with a positive patch test to vanilla, in a sandwich maker. The syndrome 'vanillaism' or 'vanillism' is comprised of dermatitis, rhinitis, bronchospasm and even vertigo. Vanillin (**7.XLIII**) is a crystalline benzaldehyde derived from glycosides such as glucovanillic alcohol, which occur in the plant. Cross-reaction occurs between vanilla and balsam of Peru (Rudzki 1976).

Vanillin (in Vanilla spp.)

7.XLIII

Beierlein H. (1957) Allergischer Hautausschlag verursacht durch den amerikanischen Prachtfrauenschuh *Cypripedium reginae*). *Orchidee* **8**: 95.
Cribb P. (1987) *The Genus Paphiopedilum*. Royal Botanic Gardens, Kew; Collingridge Books, London.
Cribb P. & Bailes C. (1989) *Hardy Orchids*. Christopher Helm, London.
Hardie R.A. & Ragan V.S. (1981) A survey of orchid growers. *Contact Dermatitis* **7**: 47–8.
Hausen B.M. (1978) Sensitising capacity of naturally occurring quinones. V. 2, 6-Dimethoxy-p-benzoquinone. *Contact Dermatitis* **4**: 204–13.
Hausen B.M. (1979) New allergenic quinones in orchids. *Archives of Dermatological Research* **264**: 102–3.
Hausen B.M. (1980) Allergic contact dermatitis to quinones in *Paphiopedilum haynaldianum* (Orchidaceae). *Archives of Dermatology* **116**: 327–8.
Hausen B.M. (1984) Toxic and allergenic orchids. In Arditti J. (ed.) *Orchid Biology*. Cornell University Press, Ithaca, NY, pp. 262–82.
Hausen B.M., Schoji A. & Jarchow O. (1984) Orchid allergy. *Archives of Dermatology* **120**: 1206–8.
Hjorth N. & Weismann K. (1972) Occupational dermatitis in chefs and sandwich makers. *Contact Dermatitis Newsletter* **11**: 301.
McCord C.P. (1962) The occupational toxicity of cultivated flowers. *Industrial Medicine and Surgery* **31**: 365.
Rasmussen J.E. (1986) Contact dermatitis from orchids. *Clinics in Dermatology* **4**: 31–5.
Rudzki E. (1976) Immediate reactions to balsam of Peru, cassia oil and ethyl vanillin. *Contact Dermatitis* **2**: 360–1.

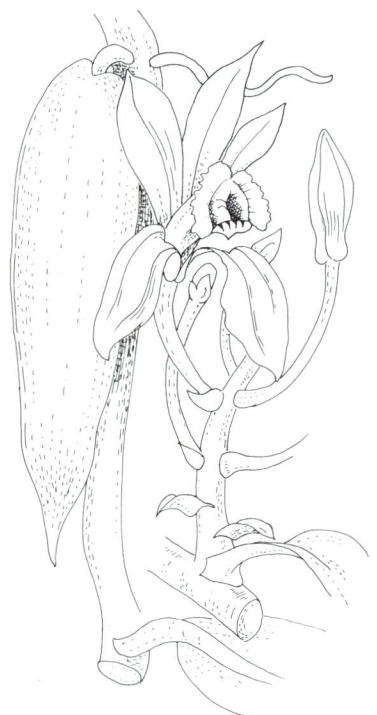

Fig. 7.5.109 Vanilla pod.

Schmalle H. & Hausen B.M. (1979) A new sensitising quinone from lady slipper (*Cypripedium calceolus*). *Naturwissenschaften* **66**: 527–8.

Ulbrich A.P. (1965) Contact dermatitis caused by plants. *Journal of the American Osteopathic Association* **64**: 1023.

Wang X.S. (1987) Occupational contact dermatitis in manufacture of vanillin. *Chinese Medical Journal* **100**: 250–4.

Woods B. (1962) Irritant plants. *Transactions of the St John's Hospital Dermatological Society* **48**: 75–82.

Zingiberaceae

A large family of herbaceous perennials with tuberous roots, mostly native to tropical India and Malaysia. Several members are used as culinary spices and many are irritants.

ALPINIA spp.

Common name: Galangal
Distribution: Tropical Asia

The dried root of *A. officinarum*, galangal, is an important spice in Thai cooking, imparting a delicate gingery flavour to meat dishes, especially satays. Laos powder, the ground root of *A. galanga*, is used especially in poultry dishes. Neering and van Ketel (1974) reported a positive patch test with *A. galanga* in a cook who handled this powder; the patient also reacted to other Zingiberaceae.

Neering H. & van Ketel W.G. (1974) *Allergy From Some Spices Used in Indonesian Cooking.* Symposium on contact dermatitis. Gentofte, Denmark.

CURCUMA longa

Common name: Turmeric
Distribution: India, Malaysia
Patch test: Turmeric powder ?as is

Turmeric powder, which imparts a yellow colour and spicy flavour to curries, is obtained by grinding the rhizomes of this species. The active principle is curcumin, allied to zingerone found in ginger. Allergic contact dermatitis to turmeric powder was described in an Indian spice miller (Goh & Ng 1987).

Goh C.L. Ng S.K. (1987) Allergic contact dermatitis to *Curcuma longa* (turmeric). *Contact Dermatitis* **17**: 186.

ELLETARIA cardamom

Common name: Green cardamom
Distribution: India, Sri Lanka. Cultivated in all tropical areas (including West Indies)
Patch test: Cardamom powder as is. Oil of cardamom 2% pet.

The green (true cardamom) seeds (Fig. 7.5.110) are used in oriental cooking. Oil of cardamom is distilled from the ripe seeds. It is used in curry sauces, liqueurs and in perfumery.

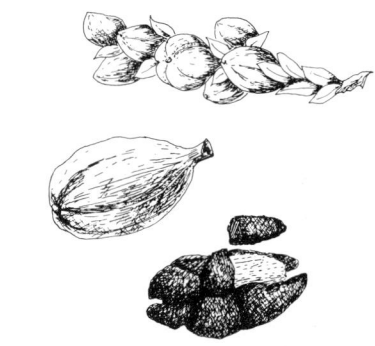

Fig. 7.5.110 *Elletaria cardamom* seeds (green and black cardamoms).

Allergic dermatitis is rare, although it has been reported in a confectioner (Mobacken & Fregert 1975). Potential allergens include several terpenoids, including citral and citronellal (Bernhard *et al.* 1971) as well as borneol (Mobacken & Fregert 1975) (**7.XLIV**).

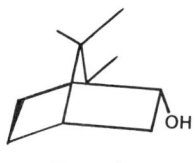

Borneol

7.XLIV

Borneol is found also in coriander (Ziegler 1982). There are no reports of allergic sensitization through the use of oil of cardamom in perfumery (Greenberg & Lester 1954).

Bernhard R.A., Wijesekera R.O.B. & Chichester C.O. (1971) Terpenoids of cardamom oil and their comparative distribution among varieties. *Phytochemistry* **10**: 177.

Greenberg L.A. & Lester D. (1954) *Handbook of Cosmetic Materials*. Interscience, New York.

Mobacken H. & Fregert S. (1975) Allergic contact dermatitis from cardamom. *Contact Dermatitis* **1**: 175–6.

Ziegler E. (1982) *Die Natürlichen und Kunstlichen Aromen*. A Hüthig, Heidelberg.

ZINGIBER officinale

Common name: Ginger

Distribution: India, Australasia. Cultivated throughout tropics

Patch test: Ginger powder 5% in ethanol (Hjorth & Roed-Petersen 1976)

The rhizomes of this pungent herb (Fig. 7.5.111) are used widely in cooking, chiefly in a powdered form. Ginger and its oil are irritant but allergic reactions are also recorded (Greenberg & Lester 1954, Hjorth 1961). Positive patch tests were obtained in food handlers with fingertip dermatitis, although irritancy was not fully excluded (Sinha *et al.* 1977). Possible allergens include zingerone and gingerol (**7.XLV**), as well as borneol and citral (Behl & Captain 1979).

Zingerone

Gingerol

7.XLV Allergens in ginger.

Behl P.N. & Captain R.M. (1979) *Skin Irritant and Sensitizing Plants Found in India*. S. Chand, Ram Naga, New Delhi.

Greenberg L.A. & Lester D. (1954) *Handbook of Cosmetic Materials*. Interscience, New York.

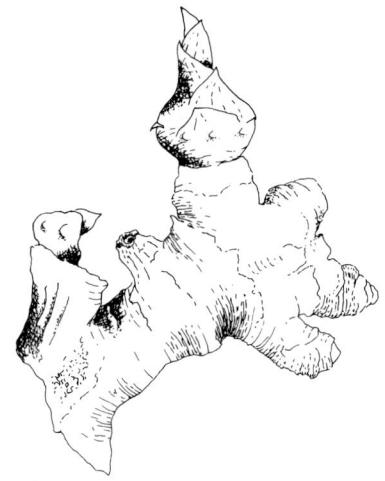

Fig. 7.5.111 *Zingiber officinale* (ginger root).

Hjorth N. (1961) *Eczematous Allergy to Balsams*. Munksgaard, Copenhagen.

Hjorth N. & Roed-Petersen J. (1976) Occupational protein contact dermatitis in food handlers. *Contact Dermatitis* **2**: 28–42.

Sinha S.M., Pasricha J.S., Sharma R.C. & Kandhari K.C. (1977) Vegetables responsible for contact dermatitis of the hands. *Archives of Dermatology* **113**: 776–9.

Dioscoraceae

DIOSCOREA batatas

Common name: Chinese yam

Distribution: Philippines, cultivated in tropics and some temperate regions

The tubers of several *Dioscorea* spp. (yams) (Fig. 7.5.112) are edible when cooked, although irritant when handled raw, due to calcium oxalate raphides (crystals). A 9-year-old girl is reported who developed dermatitis after being accidentally hit on the cheek with a spoon containing grated raw *D. batatas* tuber. Patch tests were positive using 1%, 10% and 20% grated tuber in water. Normal controls were negative (Kubo *et al.* 1988). The allergen is unknown.

Kubo Y., Nonaka S. & Yoshida H. (1988) Allergic contact dermatitis from *Dioscorea batatas* Decaisne. *Contact Dermatitis* **18**: 111–12.

ALOEACEAE

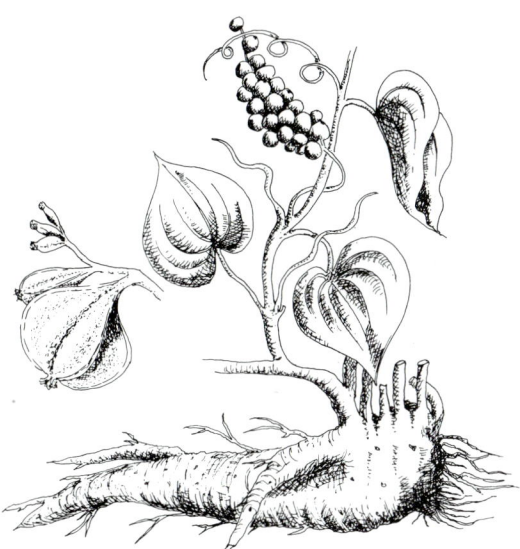

Fig. 7.5.112 *Dioscorea batatas*.

TAMUS communis

Common name: Black bryony
Distribution: Euromediterranean area including southern Britain, in woods and hedgerows

This twining plant has a large tuber, yellow green flowers in spikes and red berries. The leaves are often asymmetrical, heart shaped. White bryony (*Bryonia*) has five-lobed leaves and larger greenish white flowers; it is botanically unrelated, belonging to the Cucurbitaceae (cucumber family). The root is known to be rubefacient. The berries are also used as a counter-irritant and may cause delayed hypersensitivity (Miliavskiĭ 1979, Schmidt 1983, Schmidt & Fernandez de Corres 1990). The allergen is water-extractable but not extractable using organic solvents. No controls were reported (Schmidt & Fernandez de Corres 1990).

Miliavskiĭ A.I. (1979) [Contact dermatitis caused by black bryony.] *Vestnik Dermatologii i Venerologii* **7**: 49–50.
Schmidt R.J. (1983) The dermatitic properties of black bryony. *Contact Dermatitis* **9**: 390–6.
Schmidt R.J. & Fernandez de Corres L. (1990) An unusual case of delayed contact sensitivity to black bryony berries (*Tamus communis* L). (Abstr.) *Contact Dermatitis* **23**: 260–1.

Aloeaceae

ALOE spp.

Common name: Aloe
Distribution: Mostly South and tropical Africa, extending to Yemen and India
Patch test: Leaf as is, medicaments

Several species of this succulent genus are grown as pot plants (Fig. 7.5.113) on windowsills or in greenhouses. Aloes have been used in medicine for several millennia. *Aloe vera* (*barbadensis*) in particular is still used to treat pruritus, ringworm and burns, even as a hair tonic. The drug 'bitter aloes' is obtained from the dried sap from sliced *Aloe* leaves (Noble 1976). Several proprietary ointments, including homoeopathic remedies, and cosmetics contain bitter aloes. Allergic contact dermatitis has followed topical application of a jelly derived from *A. arborescens* (Schoji 1982, Nakamura & Kotajima 1984) and *A. vera* (Morrow *et al.* 1980). A positive patch test to tincture of aloes

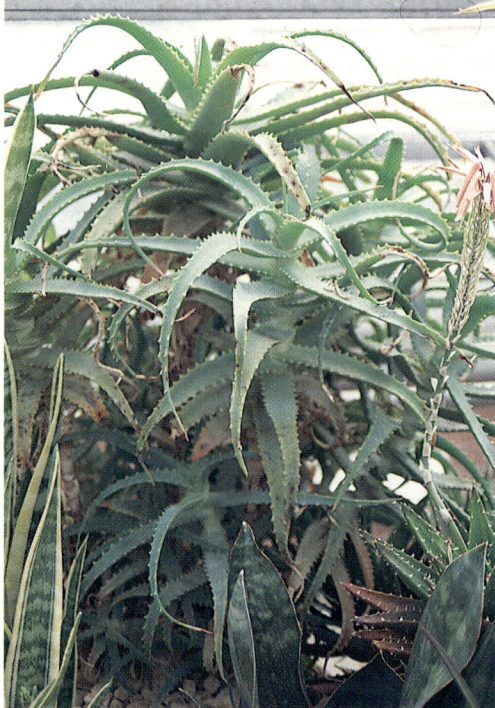

Fig. 7.5.113 *Aloe arborescens*.

was obtained in two patients with contact dermatitis caused by compound tincture of benzoin (Steiner & Leifer 1949). The allergen may be an anthraquinone, aloin or emodin (Mitchell & Rook 1979).

Mitchell J. & Rook A. (1979) *Botanical Dermatology.* Greengrass, Vancouver.
Morrow D.M., Rapaport M.J. & Strick R.A. (1980) Hypersensitivity to aloe. *Archives of Dermatology* **116**: 1064–5.
Nakamura T. & Kotajima S. (1984) Contact dermatitis from *Aloe arborescens. Contact Dermatitis* **11**: 51.
Noble W.C. (1976) *Aloes for Greenhouse and Indoor Cultivation.* National Cactus and Succulent Society, Oxford.
Shoji, A. (1982) Contact dermatitis to *Aloe arborescens. Contact Dermatitis* **8**: 164–7.
Steiner K. & Leifer W. (1949) Investigations of contact-type dermatitis due to compound tincture of benzoin. *Journal of Investigative Dermatology* **13**: 351–9.

Asparagaceae

ASPARAGUS officinalis

Common name: Asparagus
Distribution: Central Europe, Mediterranean region, widely cultivated
Patch test: 10% ether extract (MEK or pet.), 10% water extract

The soft young leaf shoots of this plant (Fig. 7.5.114) are a gastronomic delicacy. Dermatitis due to asparagus was first recorded in 1880 by Guntz (Mitchell & Rook 1979). It is mostly irritant, although some case histories suggest the development of allergic sensitization in cooks, gardeners and canners. It appears that only the young shoots cause dermatitis (Stewart 1972, quoted in Mitchell & Rook 1979). The allergen is unknown and Hausen (1988) recommends patch testing with 10% ether and water extracts.

Hausen B.M. (1988) *Allergiepflanzen-Pflanzenallergene.* Ecomed, Landsberg/München.
Mitchell J.C. & Rook A. (1979) *Botanical Dermatology.* Greengrass, Vancouver.

Agavaceae

AGAVE spp.

Common name: *A. americana*: century plant. *A. sisalana*: sisal

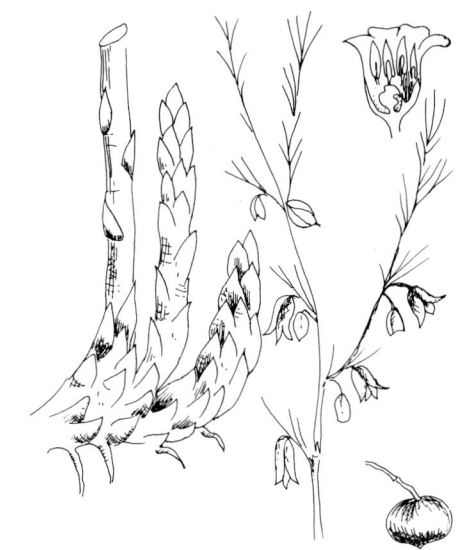

Fig. 7.5.114 *Asparagus officinalis.*

Distribution: Central America, esp. Mexico and southern USA. Widely planted, esp. Mediterranean seaboard

Many members of this genus are spectacular succulent plants. *Agave americana*, the century plant, forms large rosettes of leaves (over 1 m diameter) and a tall (3 m or more) stem with numerous plantlets (Fig. 7.5.115). The main rosette dies after 'flowering'. *Agave sisalana* has been grown commercially for its tough fibres.

Many species are highly irritant (Kerner et al. 1973) but it is possible that they are also sensitizers (Dorsey 1962). *Agave americana* leaf has been applied topically as a rubefacient, and is reported to cause allergic contact dermatitis when used therapeutically (Shatoian & Golomozenko 1987). Open, rather than closed, patch tests are recommended because of the irritancy of these plants (Kerner et al. 1973).

Dorsey C.S. (1962) Plant dermatitis in California. *California Medicine* **96**: 412.
Kerner J., Mitchell J.C. & Maibach H.I. (1973) Irritant contact dermatitis from *Agave americana. Archives of Dermatology* **108**: 102.
Shatoian I. & Golomozenko V.F. (1987) Contact dermatitis caused by *Agave* used for therapeutic purposes. *Vestnik Dermatologii i Venerologii* **2**: 63–4.

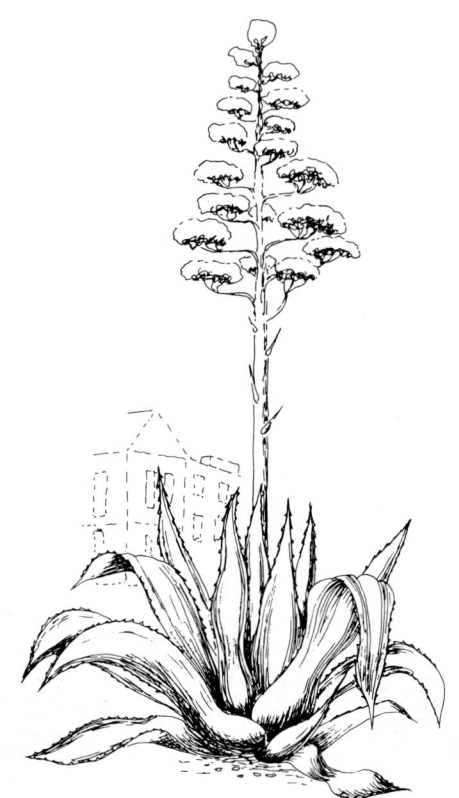

Fig. 7.5.115 *Agave americana* (century plant).

Hyacinthaceae

HYACINTHUS orientalis cvs

Common name: Hyacinth
Distribution: Eastern Mediterranean, widely grown
Patch test: Leaf as is

The garden hyacinth (Fig. 7.5.116) is derived from the more graceful species *H. orientalis*. Several colour variations and even double-flowered forms are grown, either 'forced' in pots for Christmas or outdoors for spring flowering. The red spherical bulbs are an important cause of irritant dermatitis in bulb planters and sorters (Chapter 2.1). Hyacinth oil derived from the scented flowers has caused allergic contact dermatitis (Varga 1936). It contains eugenol and other potential sensitizers. Patch testing with the bulb may cause irritant reactions. Munoz *et al.* (1989)

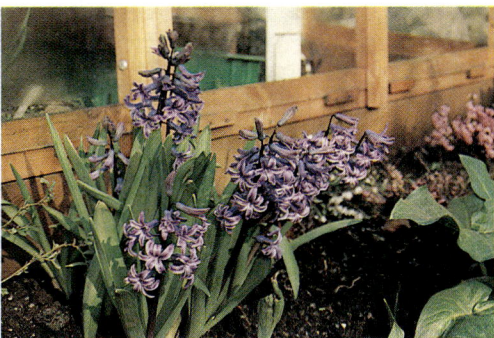

Fig. 7.5.116 Garden hyacinth.

obtained a positive patch test reaction to hyacinth leaf in a nurse with multiple plant sensitivities.

Muñoz D., Urrutia I., Leanizbarrutia I. & Fernández de Corres L. (1989) Contact dermatitis from plants in a geriatric nurse. *Contact Dermatitis* **20**: 227–8.
Varga A.V. (1936) Durch Hyazinthenöle verursachtes. Ekzema generalisation acutum. *Dermatologische Wochenschrift* **102**: 104–6.

Alliaceae

ALLIUM

Common names: Onion, garlic, chives, etc.
Distribution: Worldwide
Patch test: 50% garlic/onion in arachis oil. Diallyldisulphide 5% (0.1%) pet.

The genus *Allium* contains many important vegetables; in addition, several species are grown as ornamental plants. Wild species of *Allium* are found in all temperate regions in the northern hemisphere, extending to Central America and South Africa. Some ornamental species have become naturalized weeds in Australia and New Zealand. The important culinary species are listed in Table 7.5.10. Most species are bulbous: the bulb of garlic (*A. sativum*) is made up of a cluster of small bulblets (cloves), whereas onion (*A. cepa*) has a more typical bulb made up of concentric rings of leaf bases. In leek (*A. porrum*) the 'bulb' is often merely a continuation of the leaf stalk. The flowers of *Allium* species are held in an umbel (several flowers arising from a single plant). This may be globular as in onion, or

Table 7.5.10 Edible allium species.

Species	Common name	Origin	Features
A. cepa	Onion	West Asia	Hollow leaves. Stem swollen at middle. Off-white flowers in globular umbel
v. *aggregatum*	Potato onion		
v. *ascalonicum*	Shallot	? Syria	
	Spring onion		
v. *perutile*	Everlasting onion		
viviparum	Tree onion	? Egypt	
A. fistulosum	Welsh onion	East Asia	Smaller plant with hollow leaves
A. porrum	Leek	Mediterranean	Greenish white flowers. Strap-like leaves sheathing the stem
A. sativum	Garlic	Central Asia	Narrow, keeled leaves. Delicate pale purple flowers, sometimes with bulbils, on 30 cm stems
A. schoenoprasum	Chives	Europe (including Britain)	Forms a light clump of grass-like leaves. Showy tight umbels of purple flowers
A. tuberosum	Chinese chives	East Asia	Larger, whitish flowers

loose, with the flower stalks (pedicels) at different lengths (e.g. *A. triquetrum*, Fig. 7.5.119). The leaves always arise at ground level, although they may sheathe the stem, creating a 'false stem'.

Garlic, in particular, has a long history of use in folk medicine, as a stimulant, expectorant and vampire repellent! However, as Culpeper remarks, 'the offensiveness of the breath of him that hath eaten Garlick will lead you by the nose to the knowledge hereof'.

Irritant contact dermatitis to onion and garlic is common in housewives and food handlers, although rare in gardeners, greengrocers and nursery gardeners who handle the irritant bulbs.

Allergic contact dermatitis to garlic was first reported in a meat grinder (Edelstein 1950). Garlic is the most frequent cause of fingertip dermatitis in housewives (Sinha *et al.* 1977) and caterers (Cronin 1987) (Fig. 7.5.117). Burks (1954) described the typical 'occupational gesture'; the garlic clove is held between the thumb and first/second finger of the non-dominant hand, whilst a knife is held in the dominant hand (Fig. 7.5.118). This leads to a characteristic distribution of hyperkeratotic eczema on the tips of the first two or three fingers of the non-dominant hand. The lesions may persist for many years and

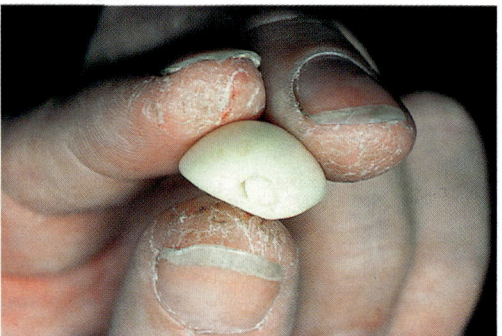

Fig. 7.5.117 Fingertip dermatitis from garlic.

can resemble psoriasis. A garlic crusher or tube of garlic paste may effect a rapid cure.

Less typically, patterns may occur reflecting a different pattern of exposure. A meat grinder developed an eruption on the forearm he used to wipe meat, contaminated with garlic, from his machine (Edelstein 1950). A 78-year-old major developed a generalized eczema after his wife applied crushed garlic in wet dressings to a wound (Bojs & Svensson 1988). A bullous eruption on the shins due to application of garlic was reported in a malingerer (Pirogova & Katyukhina 1970).

Allergic contact dermatitis to onion is less well documented, although patch tests to

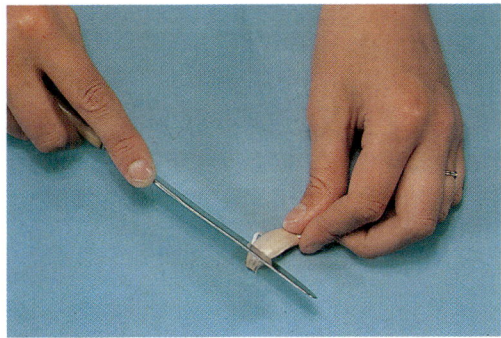

Fig. 7.5.118 Cutting a garlic clove, the occupational gesture.

onion may be positive in garlic-sensitive individuals (Bleumink et al. 1972).

Allium triquetrum, an ornamental species with loose umbels of white flowers (Fig. 7.5.119), caused an extensive dermatitis with pronounced oedema within 1 h of exposure, later followed by exfoliation. Subsequently, the patient developed wheezing and tightness of the throat after eating pickled onions (Black 1972).

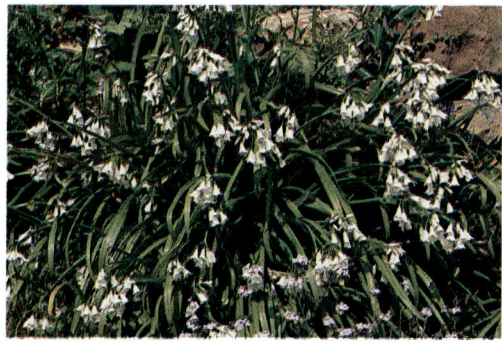

Fig. 7.5.119 *Allium triquetrum*.

The allergens in garlic are diallyldisulphide and allicin (Papageorgiou et al. 1983) (**7.XLVI**). Allicin, in particular, contributes to the pungent smell and taste. Diallyldisulphide is probably also the major allergen in leeks and chives (Hjorth & Roed-Petersen 1976). The allergens in onion are unknown: although cross-reaction between onion and garlic was noted by Burks (1954), onion extracts and

Diallyldisulphide
$CH_2=CH-CH_2-S-S-CH_2-CH=CH_2$

Allicin
$CH_2=CH-CH_2-S(O)SCH_2-CH=CH_2$

7.XLVI

tulipalin A (the allergen in tulip) were negative on patch testing in three garlic-sensitive individuals (van Ketel & de Haan 1978).

Because of their irritancy, garlic and onion should never be used 'neat' in patch testing. A chemical burn and subsequent keloid reaction may result. Pasricha and Guru (1979) recommend crushing peeled chives with an equal weight of distilled water, keeping overnight at room temperature and patch testing with the filtrate. Cronin (1987) found 50% garlic or onion in arachis oil to be non-irritant. Patch test results correlated well with 5% diallyldisulphide in petrolatum. This concentration was also used by Hjorth and Roed-Petersen (1976) and Papageorgiou et al. (1983). However, Bojs and Svensson (1988) obtained 19 irritant reactions in 76 controls at this concentration, and recommended 0.1%! Diallyldisulphide is not generally available.

Black H. (1972) Contact dermatitis from onion weed plant. *Contact Dermatitis Newsletter* **11**: 282.
Bleumink E., Doeglas H.M.G., Klokke A.H. & Nater J.P. (1972) Allergic contact dermatitis due to garlic. *British Journal of Dermatology* **87**: 6–9.
Bojs G. & Svensson A. (1988) Contact allergy to garlic used for wound healing. *Contact Dermatitis* **18**: 179–81.
Burks J.W. (1954) Classic aspects of onion and garlic dermatitis in housewives. *Annals of Allergy* **12**: 592–6.
Cronin E. (1987) Dermatitis of the hands in caterers. *Contact Dermatitis* **17**: 265–9.
Edelstein A.J. (1950) Dermatitis caused by garlic. *Archives of Dermatology and Syphilology* **61**: 111.
Hjorth N. & Roed-Petersen J. (1976) Occupational protein contact dermatitis in food handlers. *Contact Dermatitis* **2**: 28–42.
Papageorgiou C., Corbet J.-P., Menezes-Brandao F., Pecegueiro M. & Benezra C. (1983) Allergic contact dermatitis to garlic (*Allium sativum* L.). Identification of the allergens: the role of mono-, di- and trisulphides present in garlic. *Annals of Dermatological Research* **275**: 229–34.
Pasricha J.S. & Guru B. (1979) Preparation of an appropriate antigen extract for patch tests with garlic. *Archives of Dermatology* **115**: 230.

Pirogova E.P. & Katyukhina Z.D. (1970) Artificial dermatitis caused by garlic. *Vestnik Dermatologii i Venerologii* **44**: 53.

Sinha S.M., Pasricha J.S., Sharma R.L. et al. (1977) Vegetables responsible for contact dermatitis of the hands. *Archives of Dermatology* **113**: 776–9.

Van Ketel W.G. & Haan P. (1978) Occupational eczema from garlic and onion. *Contact Dermatitis* **4**: 53.

Amaryllidaceae

NARCISSUS spp. and hybrids

Common names: Daffodil, narcissus, jonquil, hoop-petticoat

Distribution: Europe, Meditteranean region, north Africa. Popular cut flowers, pot and garden plants. ? Naturalized in South-East Asia

Patch test: Leaf, stem and flower of suspected plant. NB irritancy

This very popular genus of spring-flowering bulbous plants (Fig. 7.5.120) includes many attractive species and a bewildering range of hybrids. Traditionally, the genus derives its name from a legendary Greek youth who fell in love with his own reflection in a pool (hence 'narcissism'): quite rightly, the gods turned him into a flower. Probably, however, the name is derived from 'narkao' (fall stiff), because of its narcotic properties. The horticulturally important sections of the genus are listed in Table 7.5.11. In addition, there are several other attractive species grown in specialist collections (see Blanchard 1990). The flowers of all species have a central inner ring (corona or crown) which may be very prominent, forming a cup or trumpet.

All *Narcissus* bulbs (Fig. 7.5.121) can be irritant when handled in bulk, because of their content of calcium oxalate crystals (Hjorth & Wilkinson 1968). Flower pickers, bunchers and packers are chiefly affected; bulb planting was a major cause of fingertip dermatitis (Palmer & Freeman 1934), but many larger growers now use a mechanical process. Minor degrees of irritant dermatitis (daffodil itch) are common; as well as the fingertips, the hands, forearms and occasionally face, neck and genitalia are affected. Allergic dermatitis to *Narcissus* is relatively uncommon (Hausen & Oestmann 1988). There appear to be well documented cases of allergy to *N. poeticus* (Agrup 1969), *N. jonquilla* (Fig. 7.5.122)

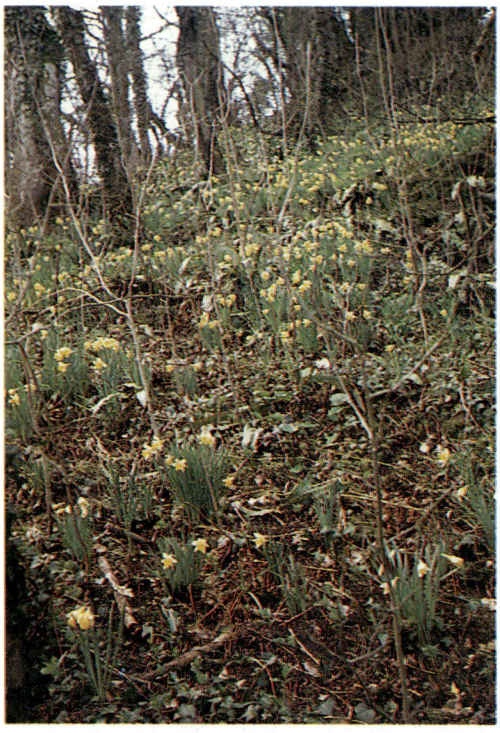

Fig. 7.5.120 *Narcissus pseudonarcissus* (Lent lily) naturalized in the Mendips.

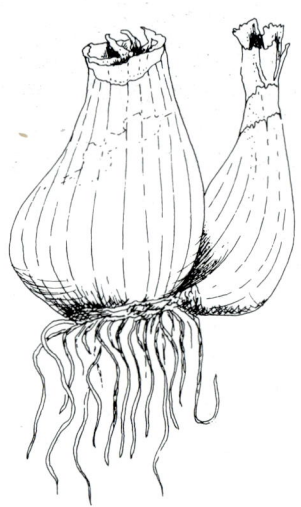

Fig. 7.5.121 Daffodil bulb.

Table 7.5.11 Important species of narcissus.

Section	Typical species	Common names	Notes
Tazettae	N. tazetta	Roman n., bunch-flowered n.	Multi-flowered, often scented, flowering in winter. Often grown as pot plants for Christmas
	N. papyraceus	Paper white	
	N. bertolonii	Soleil d'or	
Narcissus	N. poeticus	Pheasant's eye, florist's narcissus	Large, scented white flowers with small orange or red corona. Grown in gardens and as cut flowers
Jonquillae	N. jonquilla	Jonquil	Dwarf (about 20 cm) with small bright-yellow, intensely scented flowers. A parent of many dwarf hybrids, grown as rock plants
Ganymedes	N. triandus	Angel's tears	Dwarf. Grown in rock gardens
Bulbocodium	N. bulbocodium	Hoop petticoat	Dwarf. Grown in rock gardens
Pseudo-narcissus (trumpet daffodils)	N. pseudo-narcissus	Wild daffodil Lent lily	Members of this group are the parents of the popular yellow daffodils, grown extensively in gardens and for cut flowers
	N. obvallaris	Tenby daffodil	

(Stryker 1936), *N. pseudonarcissus* (Gonçalo et al. 1987) and *N. tazetta* (Agrup 1969). In several studies, the species or cultivar was not specified. Although daffodil dermatitis is typically occupational in origin, a positive patch test using daffodil leaves was obtained in a geriatic nurse (Muñoz et al. 1989).

The allergens have not been precisely determined in humans. In a detailed study (involving 100 kg of bulbs and 30 kg of cut flowers!), Gude et al. (1988) isolated two alkaloids, masonin and homolycorin, which are weak sensitizers in guinea pigs (**7.XLVII**). Both these alkaloids are found in other members of the Amaryllidaceae family. Cross-reaction has been noted with snowdrop (*Galanthus nivalis*) (Bleumink & Nater 1974). Because of the irritancy of the plant, patch tests should be carried out with caution, using gently bruised leaf, stem and flower. A 10–20% water or ethanol extract may be less irritant (Bleumink & Nater 1974). Test controls for irritancy.

Agrup G. (1969) Hand eczema and other hand dermatoses in south Sweden. *Acta Dermato-Venereologica* **49** (Suppl. 61): 1–91.

7.XVLVII Alkaloids derived from *Narcissus*.

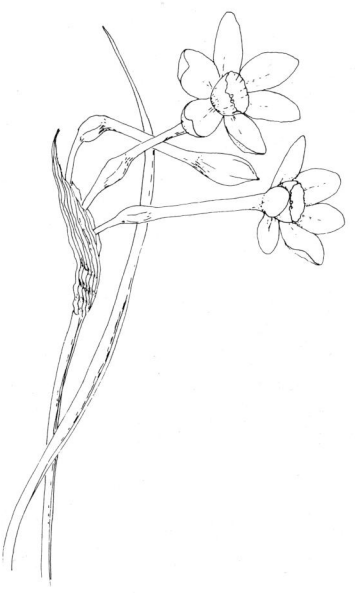

Fig. 7.5.122 *Narcissus jonquilla* (jonquil).

Blanchard J.W. (1990) *Narcissus: A Guide to Wild Daffodils*. Alpine Garden Society, Surrey.

Bleumink E. & Nater J.P. (1974) Contact dermatitis in a gardener caused by daffodil. *Berufsdermatosen* **22**: 123.

Gonçalo S., Freitas J.D. & Sousa I. (1987) Contact dermatitis and respiratory symptoms from *Narcissus pseudonarcissus*. *Contact Dermatitis* **16**: 115–16.

Gude M., Hausen B.M., Heitsch H. & Konig W.A. (1988) An investigation of the irritant and allergenic properties of daffodils (*Narcissus pseudonarcissus* L.) Amaryllidaceae. *Contact Dermatitis* **19**: 1–10.

Hausen B.M. & Oestmann G. (1988) Untersuchungen über die Häufigkeit berufsbedingter allergischer Hauterkrankungen auf einem Blumengrossmarkt. *Dermatosen in Beruf und Umwelt* **36**: 117–24.

Hjorth N. & Wilkinson D.S. (1968) Contact dermatitis IV Tulip fingers, hyacinth itch and lily rash. *British Journal of Dermatology* **80**: 696–8.

Muñoz D., Urrutia I., Leanizbarrutia I. & Fernandez de Corres L. (1989) Contact dermatitis from plants in a geriatric nurse. *Contact Dermatitis* **20**: 227–8.

Palmer W.H. & Freeman J. (1934) 'Lily rash': an occupational dermatitis. *Lancet* **ii**: 755–6.

Stryker G.V. (1936) Contact dermatitis caused by the jonquil (*Narcissus jonquilla*). *Journal of Industrial Hygiene and Toxicology* **18**: 462–5.

Alstroemeriaceae

ALSTROMERIA

Common name: Peruvian lily

Distribution: Andean foothills, esp. Chile and Peru. Widely grown as a border perennial and for cut flowers

Patch test: ? Petal, leaf as is (NB may sensitize) or tulip bulb or tuliposide, 0.01% pet.

This genus of beautiful plants was first introduced to cultivation in Europe by Klas Alstroemer in 1754. The largest concentration of species (31) is found in Chile (Bayer 1987). All species have a cluster of tuberous roots and produce leafy stems, bearing one to several brightly coloured flowers. Although several species are found in specialist collections, only two are widely grown. *Alstroemeria aurantiaca*, with orange flowers, is grown as a border plant, particularly in cottage gardens. *Alstroemeria ligtu* has given rise to numerous colour varieties, mostly in shades of lilac and pink, with darker veins and mottling on the petals (Fig. 7.5.123). The flowers are long-lasting and *Alstroemeria* cultivars are grown extensively for the cut-flower market. Plants are grown for this purpose in Holland, South America, USA and Australia. Since 1963 the Dutch have bred varieties which bloom all the year round (Marks 1988).

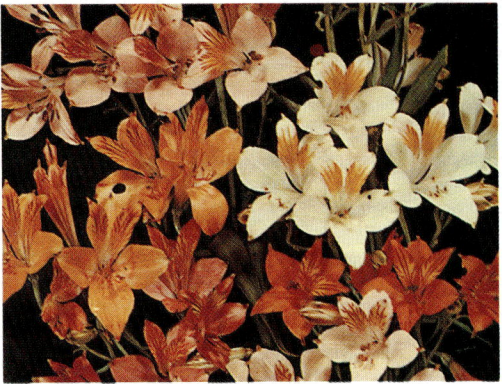

Fig. 7.5.123 *Alstroemeria ligtu* cultivars.

Cases of allergic contact dermatitis to *Alstroemeria* were first reported by Rook (1961) and Cronin (1972). Because of the increasing popularity of the genus, there is also an increased risk of exposure (Rook 1981). *Alstroemeria* and tulips are now the commonest causes of allergic reactions in wholesale and retail florists (Hausen & Oestmann 1988, Thibutot 1990).

The leafy stems are a major disadvantage to florists, who strip off the leaves manually (Fig. 7.5.124). Individual flowers are detached and used in wreaths and corsages. The florist, therefore, has considerable exposure to the broken plant, encouraging sensitization. Dermatitis affects typically the fingertips, as in 'tulip finger' (Rook 1961, Cronin 1972, Rycroft & Calnan 1981), although the eruption can be more extreme. *Alstroemeria* may have contributed to an airborne pattern of contact dermatitis in a florist (Illuminati *et al.* 1988). Post-inflammatory depigmentation may occur (Bjorkner 1982).

The major allergen is tuliposide A, which on hydrolysis is converted to tulipalin A (**7.XLVIII**). This allergen is found also in tulip, as well as in other members of the lily family, such as *Erythronium* (Slob 1973, Slob *et al.* 1975). This explains the apparent cross-reaction with tulip found on patch testing (Cronin 1972, van Ketel 1975, Santucci *et al.*

7.XLVIII Allergens in *Alstroemeria* and *Tulipa*.

Tuliposide A

Tupalin A
(α methylene-Y-butyrolactone + glucose)

1985). The allergen is found in greatest concentration in the flowers (Slob 1973).

Patch tests are positive using the flower and leaf, but there is the risk of active sensitization (Hausen *et al.* 1982). One patient patch tested with *Alstroemeria* developed well-demarcated areas of depigmentation at the patch test sites (Bjorkner 1982). Van Ketel *et al.* (1975) found that all *Alstroemeria*-sensitive patients reacted to tulip bulb, and this may be a safer material to use for patch testing. Patch testing with the purified allergen is ideal. Tulipalin A is unstable, but the glucosidic form, tuliposide A, can be extracted from flower petals using methanol, and can be stored at room temperature. A concentration of 0.01% is recommended (Hausen *et al.* 1982).

The allergen penetrates vinyl (PVC) but not nitrile gloves (Marks 1988). Thiboutot *et al.* (1990) suggest that a barrier cream containing cysteine may be protective.

Bayer E. (1987) Die gattung *Alstroemeria* in Chile. *Mitteilungen der Botanischen Staatssammlung Munchen* **24**: 1–362.
Bjorkner B.E. (1982) Contact allergy and depigmentation from *Alstroemeria*. *Contact Dermatitis* **8**: 178–84.
Cronin E. (1972) Sensitivity to tulip and *Alstroemeria*. *Contact Dermatitis Newsletter* **11**: 286.
Hausen B.M. & Oestmann G. (1988) Untersuchungen uber die Haufigkeit berufsbedingter allergischer Hauterkrankungen auf einem Blumengrossmarkt. *Dermatosen in Beruf und Umwelt* **36**: 117–24.
Hausen B.M., Prater E. & Schubert H. (1982) The sensitizing capacity of *Alstroemeria* cultivars in man and guinea pig. *Contact Dermatitis* **9**: 46–54.

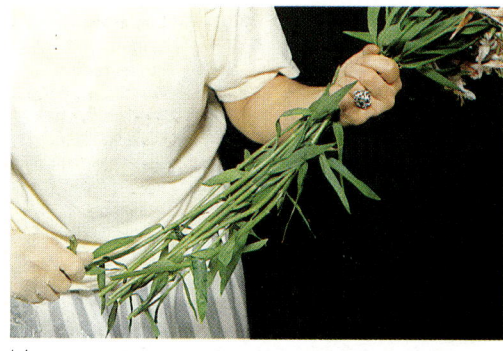

(a)

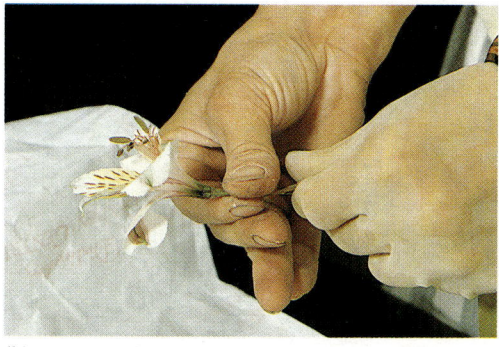

(b)

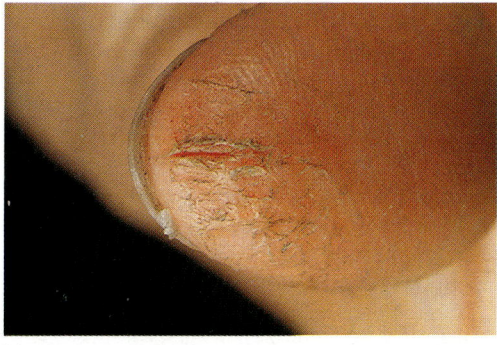

(c)

Fig. 7.5.124 Handling *Alstroemeria* flowers, the occupatonal gestures; (a) stripping leaves from stems; (b) wiring flower; (c) fissured fingertip dermatitis. (Courtesy of Dr M. Beck.)

Illuminati R., Russo R., Guerra L. & Melino M. (1988) Occupational airborne contact dermatitis in a florist. *Contact Dermatitis* **18**: 246.
Marks J.G., Jr. (1988) Allergic contact dermatitis to *Alstroemeria*. *Archives of Dermatology* **124**: 914–16.
Rook A.J. (1961) Plant dermatitis. The significance of variety-specific sensitization. *British Journal of Dermatology* **73**: 283–7.

Rook A.J. (1981) Dermatitis from *Alstroemeria*. *Contact Dermatitis* **7**: 355–6.
Rycroft R.J.G. & Calnan C.D. (1981) *Alstroemeria* dermatitis. *Contact Dermatitis* **7**: 284.
Santucci B., Picardo M., Iavarone C. *et al.* (1985) Contact dermatitis to *Alstroemeria*. *Contact Dermatitis* **12**: 215–19.
Slob A. (1973) Tulip allergens in *Alstroemeria* and some other Liliiflorae. *Phytochemistry* **12**: 811–15.
Slob A., Jekel B., de Jong B. & Schlatmann C. (1975) On the occurrence of tuliposides in the Liliiflorae. *Phytochemistry* **14**: 1997–2005.
Thibutot D.M., Hamory B.H. & Marks J.G. (1990) Dermatoses in floral shop workers. *Journal of the American Academy of Dermatology* **22**: 54–8.
Van Ketel W.G., Verspyck Mijnssen G.A.W. & Neering H. (1975) Contact eczema from *Alstroemeria*. *Contact Dermatitis* **1**: 323–4.

Liliaceae

TULIPA spp. and hybrids

Common name: Tulip
Distribution: Europe, Mediterranean region; Asia, extending from Turkey to India
Patch test: Portion of leaf as is; acetone extract of bulb in 70% ethanol

Most of the tulips (Fig. 7.5.125) grown in gardens are hybrids or cultivars derived from the dubious species *Tulipa gesnerana* which is naturalized in southwest Europe and cultivated areas of southern Asia (*Flora Europaea* 1980). 'Foster' tulips are derived from *T. fosteriana* and 'water lily' tulips from *T. kaufmanniana*. Several smaller and more graceful species are grown as rock garden plants. Dutch bulb growers have produced a bewildering variety of cultivars.

Professional bulb growers are particularly at risk of contact dermatitis which is mostly allergic (Rook 1961). Irritant reactions are due to the abrasive bulb coat (tecta) (Fig. 7.5.126). Unlike other bulbs, tulips do not contain significant amounts of calcium oxalate crystals. Allergic contact dermatitis is common, especially in the Netherlands; since 'tulip fingers' is seasonal and sometimes mild it is probably under-reported (Hjorth & Wilkinson 1968). In Denmark it accounts for 4% of plant dermatitis (Hjorth 1969). Cultivars appear to differ in allergenicity. The cultivars 'Rose Copeland' and '*praeludium*' are notorious among bulb handlers and florists

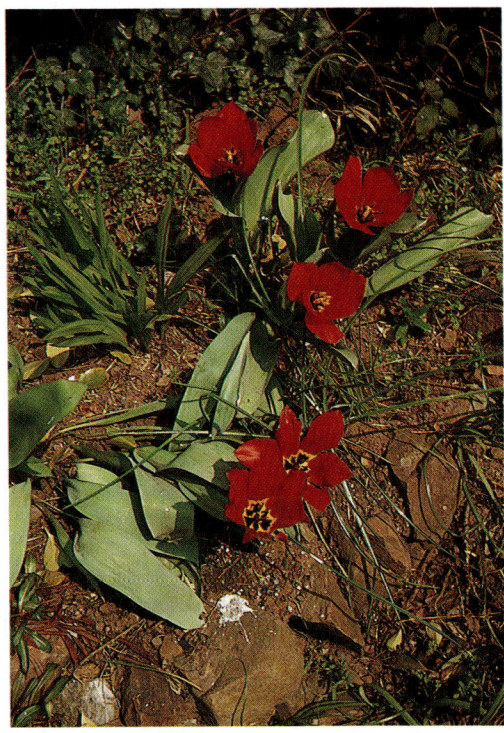

Fig. 7.5.125 *Tulipa schrenkii*, one of the origins of the modern hybrids.

(Rook 1961, van der Werff 1959). 'Red Emperor', a cultivar of *T. fosteriana*, possesses less antigen than other cultivars (Verspyck Mijnssen 1969). The sensitizing power of the bulb varies according to the season (Hjorth & Wilkinson 1968). The technique of harvesting the flowers also affects the risk of contact sensitization. In Sweden and Germany the bulb is split with a knife, yielding a longer

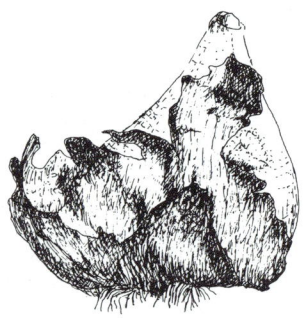

Fig. 7.5.126 Tulip bulb.

stem and the risk of dermatitis is 60% in operatives (Hjorth & Wilkinson 1968). 'Tulip fingers' may occur among bulb diggers, sorters and packers after several years' safe handling of the bulbs. Severe tingling and erythema of the fingertips ('tulip fire') occurs particularly around fingernails within 24 h of handling the bulbs. Later, granulation tissue develops under the nails, with onycholysis and transverse splitting of the nail plate and even subungual abscesses (Bertwistle 1935). These changes may be chiefly irritant in origin. In sensitized individuals a hyperkeratotic fissuring eczema develops under the distal nail plate, spreading to the periungual region and the fingertips (Hjorth & Wilkinson 1968). Secondary spread to the arms, face and genitalia is seen particularly in flower pickers (van der Werff 1959, Verspyck Mijnssen 1969).

Type I reactions have been reported, including rhinitis, conjunctivitis, asthma and urticaria (van der Werff 1959, Lahti 1986).

Tulip bulbs contain several glucosides, including tuliposides A and B (see **7.XLVIII**). These are weakly allergenic but are rapidly hydrolysed to tulipalin A and B. Tulipalin A appears to be the sensitizer in clinical practice (Bergmann et al. 1967, Verspyck Mijnssen 1969) although tulipalin B also causes sensitization in guinea pigs (Benezra et al. 1985). Lesser amounts of the allergen are found in the leaf and least of all in the petals. Tulipalin A also occurs in the dog's tooth violet, *Erythronium* (Fig. 7.5.127), and in *Alstroemeria* spp. (q.v.) (Slob 1973). As the allergens are not freely available, patch testing should be performed with either a portion of tulip leaf or crushed bulb epidermis after removal of the bulb coat. To reduce false positive reactions, and to avoid seasonal variation of the allergen concentration, an extract of the bulb is preferable. Crushed fresh bulbs are shaken with 4:1 acetone:water for 90 min and the extract dried, then taken up in 70% ethanol to a 1% dilution (Hjorth & Wilkinson 1968).

Secondary prevention may reduce the prevalence and severity of tulip dermatitis. Operatives should be encouraged to keep their fingernails trimmed and to apply emollients; finger stalls (cots) may help (Schwartz et al. 1957).

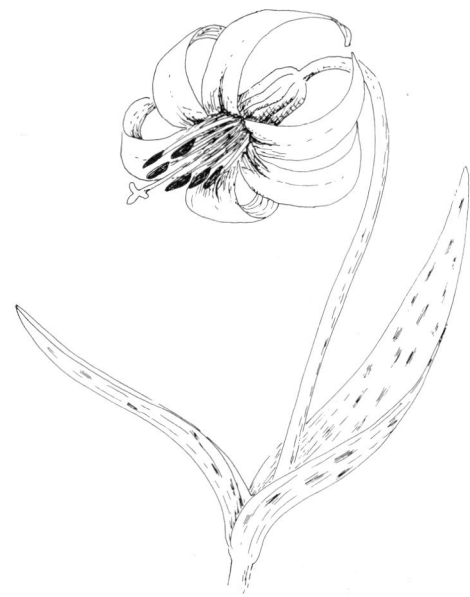

Fig. 7.5.127 *Erythronium dens-canis* (dog's tooth violet).

Benezra C., Ducombs G., Sell Y. & Foussereau J. (1985) *Plant Contact Dermatitis*. B.C. Decker, Toronto.

Bergmann H.H., Beijersbergen J.C.M., Overeem J.C. & Sijpesteijn A.K. (1967) Isolation and identification of α-methylene-γ-butyrolactone, a fungitoxic substance from tulips. *Recueil des Travaux Chimiques des Pays-Bas* **86**: 709–13.

Bertwistle A.P. (1935) Tulip fingers. *British Medical Journal* **2**: 255–6.

Flora Europaea, Vol. 5. (1980) Cambridge University Press, Cambridge.

Hjorth N. (1969) Plant dermatitis. *Contact Dermatitis Newsletter* **6**: 126.

Hjorth N. & Wilkinson D.S. (1968) Tulip fingers, hyacinth itch and lily rash. *British Journal of Dermatology* **80**: 696–8.

Lahti A. (1986) Contact urticaria and respiratory symptoms from tulips and lilies. *Contact Dermatitis* **14**: 317–19.

Rook A.J. (1961) Plant dermatitis. The significance of variety-specific sensitization. *British Journal of Dermatology* **73**: 283.

Schwartz L., Tulipan L. & Birmingham D.J. (1957) *Occupational Diseases of the Skin*, 3rd edn. Lea & Febiger, Philadelphia.

Slob A. (1973) Tulip allergens in *Alstroemeria* and other Liliiflorae. *Phytochemistry* **12**: 811–15.

Verspyck Mijnssen G.A.W. (1969) Pathogenesis and causative agent of 'tulip fingers'. *British Journal of Dermatology* **81**: 737–45.

Van der Werff P.T. (1959) Occupational diseases among workers in bulb industries. *Acta Allergologica* **14**: 338–55.

Iridaceae

The genus *Iris* includes many highly ornamental garden plants, ranging from the bearded iris hybrids to delicate spring-flowering bulbous species. Orris root of perfumery is extracted from the dried rhizome of *Iris 'florentina'* (Figs 7.5.128, 7.5.129) which is probably an ancient albino cultivar of *Iris germanica* (Mathew 1981). Orris root has been used as a cheaper substitute for violet perfume and has caused irritant reactions. It contains calcium oxalate. Crude orris root may also be allergenic (Ramirez & Eller 1930, Greenberg & Lester 1954).

Iris pseudacorus (yellow flag) has been used medicinally as a strong purgative. The

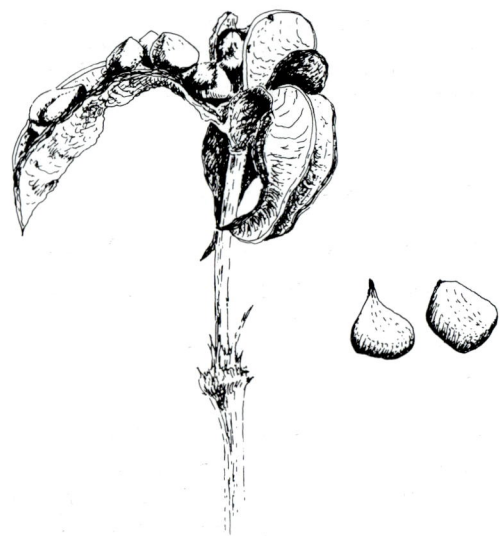

Fig. 7.5.130 *Iris pseudacorus* seeds.

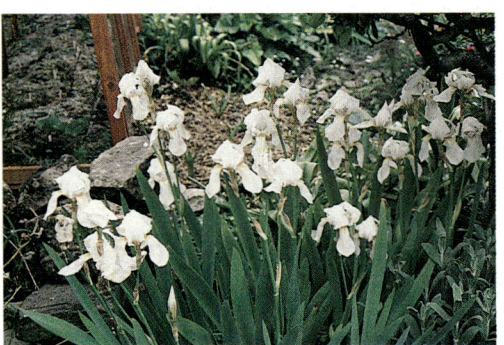

Fig. 7.5.128 *Iris florentina*, source of Orris root.

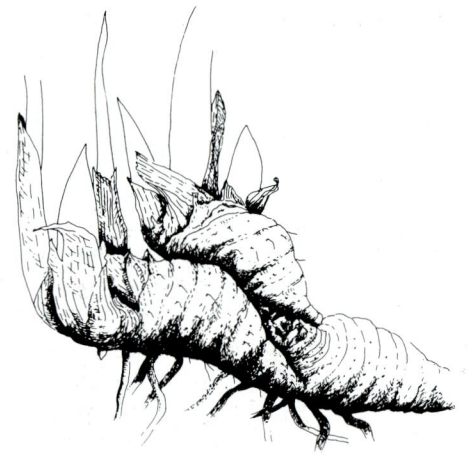

Fig. 7.5.129 Rhizome of *Iris florentina*.

herbalist, Meyrick, warned that it has been found to procure plentiful evacuations from the bowels when all other means have proved ineffectual' (Mathew 1981). It is a tall, vigorous plant with large yellow flowers with or without a dark blotch. It grows in marshy areas throughout Europe and much of Asia. The seeds are large and shiny (Fig. 7.5.130). Calnan (1970) reported dermatitis of the wrists, arms and face, caused by a bracelet made from the seeds. Patch tests were positive to the leaf and seed (Calnan 1970).

Shelmire (1940) reported *Iris* (?species) to be a 'minor sensitizer'. Hjorth (1961) recorded a positive patch test on a petal of blue iris (? perhaps a Dutch iris — *Iris xiphium* cv.) and van der Willigen *et al.* (1987) also reported a positive patch test to an unspecified iris flower in a florist who was also allergic to safflower.

Calnan C.D. (1970) *Iris pseudacorus* L. Contact Dermatitis Newsletter **8**: 171.
Greenberg L.A. & Lester D. (1954) *Handbook of Cosmetic Materials*. Interscience, New York.
Hjorth N. (1961) *Eczematous Allergy to Balsams, Allied Perfumes and Flavouring Agents*. Musksgaard, Copenhagen.
Mathew B. (1981) *The Iris*. Batsford, London.
Ramirez M.A. & Eller J.J. (1930) The 'patch test' in 'contact dermatitis' (dermatitis venenata). *Journal of Allergy* **1**: 489–95.

Shelmire B. (1940) Contact dermatitis from vegetation. *Southern Medical Journal* **33**: 337–46.
Van der Willigen A.H., van Joost T.H., Stolz E. & van der Hoek J.C.S. (1987) Contact dermatitis to safflower. *Contact Dermatitis* **17**: 184–6.

Kaalund-Jørgensen O. (1951) Eczema perioculare (dermatitis of the eyelids). *Acta Dermato-Venereologica* **31**: 83.
Lampe K.F. (1986) Dermatitis-producing plants of south Florida and Hawaii. *Clinics in Dermatology* **4**: 83–93.

Commelinaceae

ZEBRINA pendula (TRADESCANTIA)

Common names: Tradescantia. Wandering Jew
Distribution: Mexico, South America. A common foliage house plant
Patch test: ?Leaf as is

The common 'tradescantia' (Fig. 7.5.131) has creeping reddish stems with striped, oval, hairy leaves. Several cultivars are grown. It is used as a windowsill plant or in hanging baskets. True *Tradescantia* is a genus of herbaceous perennials, native mostly to North America and commonly grown as garden plants. Reports of contact dermatitis to *Zebrina* are scanty and mostly anecdotal, and may chiefly reflect irritancy. Kaalund-Jørgensen (1951) reported a positive patch test reaction in a woman with eyelid dermatitis. *Setcreasea purpurea* (purple queen) is another popular house plant with rich purple leaves. It is recorded as a cause of dermatitis in Florida and Hawaii (Lampe 1986).

Palmae (Arecaceae)

COCOS nucifera

Common name: Coconut
Distribution: ? Tropical Asia. Widely cultivated in tropics
Patch test: Bark as is

The coconut is an important economic tree (Fig. 7.5.132). It is a major source of vegetable fat; it is a staple item of diet in tropical Asia and the 'hairs' on the nuts are used for matting (coir) as well as an environmentally acceptable substitute for peat in horticulture. Coconut oil contains several saturated fatty acids and is the basis of scalp pomades used in psoriasis and seborrhoeic dermatitis. Falling coconuts are a cause of death during hurricanes. Most dermatitis associated with coconuts is due to a mite infestation (Nasution *et al.* 1973) and may mimic scabies. Coconut tree climbers, who tap a liquor from coconut palms in India (toddy tappers), frequently develop frictional lichenification on the hands, legs and feet. One male toddy tapper developed a widespread excoriated eruption and was patch test positive to coconut bark and fibrous leaf sheath (Srinivas *et al.* 1987). Two further patients with positive patch tests were reported by Balachandran *et al.* (1990).

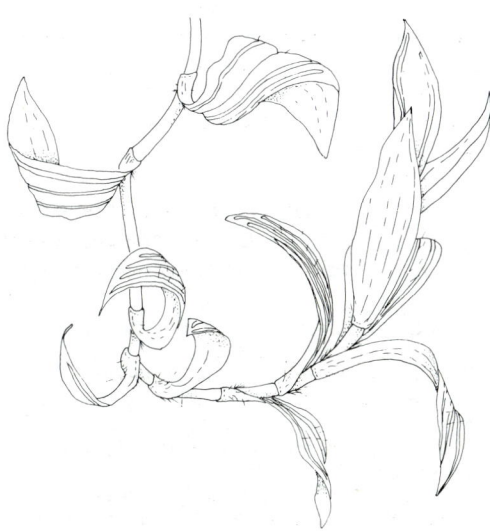

Fig. 7.5.131 *Zebrina pendula*.

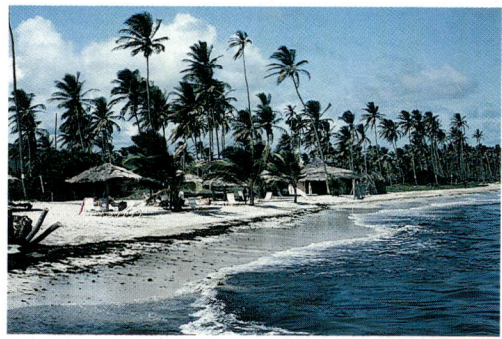

Fig. 7.5.132 Coconut palms fringing the beach (Fiji). (Courtesy of S. Young.)

Balachandran C., Srinivas C.R., Shenoy S.D. & Edison K.P. (1992) Occupational dermatosis in coconut palm climbers. *Contact Dermatitis* **26**: 143.

Nasution D., Klokke A.H. & Nater J.P. (1973) A survey of occupational dermatoses in Indonesia. *Berufsdermatosen* **21**: 215–222.

Srinivas C.R., Balachandran N. & Singh K.K. (1987) Occupational dermatosis and allergic contact dermatitis in a toddy tapper. *Contact Dermatitis* **16**: 294–5.

Araceae

This large and diverse family (aroids) contains many economically important and decorative plants, which share a unique floral structure. The male and female flowers are small, borne separately on a club-like, often phallic, stem (spadix) surrounded by a modified petal-like leaf (spathe). The arum lily (*Zantedeschia aethiopica*) is a good example. Members of the family range in size from the small, aquatic weed, *Pistia stratiotes*, the water lettuce, to *Amorphophallus titanum*, one of the largest flowering plants known, with a spathe 2–3 m tall. *Colocasia* species (taro, eddo) are widely cultivated in the tropics for their edible tubers. Many species have strikingly blotched and patterned inflorescences, sometimes emanating a foul smell of dung, wet fish or rotten meat. The monarch of the East (*Sauromatum*) is a typical example and several other species are cultivated by more or less eccentric enthusiasts. Bown (1988) is strongly recommended for an informative and very readable account of this family.

A few species are widely cultivated as house or greenhouse plants for their ornamental foliage. These are listed in Table 7.5.12. Most species are intensely irritant. Routine patch testing with common house plant genera such as *Dieffenbachia* should be avoided as the plant material may cause chemical burns. Two species appear to cause allergic contact dermatitis and are discussed below. The irritant properties of the other species are reviewed in Chapter 5.2 and Table 7.5.12 (pp. 230–31) (q.v.).

Bown D. (1988) *Aroids*. Timber Press, Portland, Oregon.

Drach G. & Maloney W.H. (1963) Toxicity of the common house plant *Dieffenbachia*. *JAMA* **184**: 1047–8.

Francis D.F. & Southcott R.N. (1967) *Plants Harmful to Man in Australia*. Miscellaneous Bulletin No. 1, Botanic Garden, Adelaide, South Australia.

Ippen H., Wereta-Kubek M. & Rose U. (1986) Schleimhautreaktionen durch Zimmerpflanzen der Gattung *Dieffenbachia*. *Dermatosen in Beruf und Umwelt* **34**: 93–101.

Klarmann E.G. (1958) Perfume dermatitis. *Annals of Allergy* **16**: 425.

Yoshizawa K. (1971) Ocular injury caused by bulbs of *Amorphophallus konjac* K. Koch. *Acta Societa Ophthalmologica Japonica* **75** (Suppl. 1): 50–8.

EPIPREMNUM pinnatum cv. 'areum' (SCINDAPSUS aureus, POTHOS aureus, RAPHIDOPHORA aurea)

Common names: Devil's ivy. Pothos. Taro vine. Hunter's robe

Distribution: Solomon Islands. Naturalized in tropics. A popular foliage house plant

Patch test: ? Leaf as is. 1% ether extract of leaf

This attractive variegated climbing/scrambling plant (Fig. 7.5.133) has oval leaves when juvenile. As the plant grows, the leaves become larger and sometimes slashed. It flowers rarely in cultivation. In tropical areas it becomes a rampant, but attractive, ground cover. Dermatitis has been recorded in Hawaii and Florida (Morton 1962, Lampe 1986). It is mostly irritant although Mobacken (1975) demonstrated patch test positivity in a florist who developed a papulovesicular dermatitis after handling the plant on two occasions. Negative patch tests were obtained in 21 controls (Mobacken 1975). The allergen is unknown. Hausen (1988) recommends patch

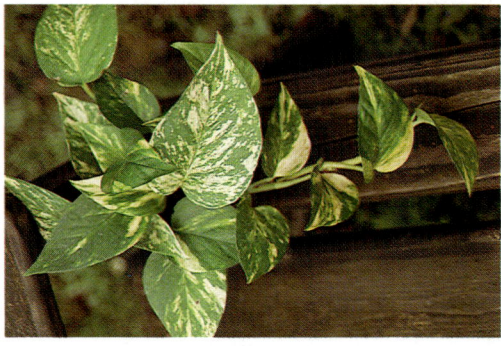

Fig. 7.5.133 *Epipremnum pinnatum*.

testing with a 1% ether extract. It would appear to be a rare sensitizer.

Hausen B.M. (1988) *Allergiepflanzen-Pflanzenallergie*. Ecomed, Landsberg/München.
Lampe K.F. (1986) Dermatitis-producing plants of south Florida and Hawaii. *Clinics in Dermatology* **4**: 83–93.
Mobacken H. (1975) Allergic plant dermatitis from *Scindapsus aureus*. *Contact Dermatitis* **1**: 60–1.
Morton J.F. (1962) Ornamental plants with poisonous properties II. *Proceedings of the Florida State Horticultural Society* **78**: 484–91.

PHILODENDRON scandens ssp. oxycardium (cordatum)

Common name: Sweetheart vine
Distribution: Tropical and sub-tropical America
Patch test: ? Leaf as is. 1% ether extract of leaf (pet.)

This species, which is often grown under a variety of pseudonyms, is an important foliage houseplant (Fig. 7.5.134). Together with *Monstera*, it is an almost essential article of office furniture. As its Greek botanical name suggests, it 'loves trees', climbing through tropical rain forests. Even in cultivation, it may climb several feet. Most contact dermatitis is irritant, although allergic reactions have been described by Ayres and Ayres (1958), Zina and Bonu (1960), Rothe (1986) and Hammershøy and Verdich (1980) and the allergenic potential of the plant may be underestimated (Ayres 1983). Hammershøy and Verdich (1980) obtained positive patch tests using the leaves, stems and ether extracts. The allergen is believed to be 5-heptadecatri-8(Z), 11(Z), 14(Z)-enylresorcinol (Reefstrup *et al.* 1982) (**7.XLIX**).

5-heptadecatri-8(Z), 11(Z), 14(Z), enylresorcinol

7.XLIX

Ayres S., Jr. (1983) *Philodendron* vine as a cause of plant dermatitis. (Letter.) *Journal of the American Academy of Dermatology* **9**: 962.
Ayres S. & Ayres S., III. (1958) *Philodendron* as a cause of contact dermatitis. *Archives of Dermatology* **78**: 330–3.
Hammershøy C. & Verdich J. (1980) Allergic contact dermatitis from *Philodendron scandens* Koch et Sello subsp *oxycardium* (Schott) Bunting. *Contact Dermatitis* **6**: 95–9.
Reefstrup T., Hammershøy O., Boll R.M. & Schmidt H. (1982) *Philodendron scandens* Koch et Sello subsp *oxycardium* (Schott) Bunting, a new source of allergenic alkyl resorcinols. *Acta Chemica Scandinavica* **B36**: 291–4.
Rothe A. (1986) Hoya carnosa — is it allergenic? *Contact Dermatitis* **14**: 250–2.
Zina G. & Bonu G. (1960) Eruzione allergica de contatto con *Philodendron*. *Minerva Dermatologica* **35**: 157–8.

Gramineae (Poaceae)

The grass family is one of the largest and most successful. It includes cereals and many food plants. Mechanical irritation is commonly caused by awns and dust during harvesting. Several species induce contact urticaria (Chapter 4). Allergic contact dermatitis appears to be uncommon and perhaps difficult

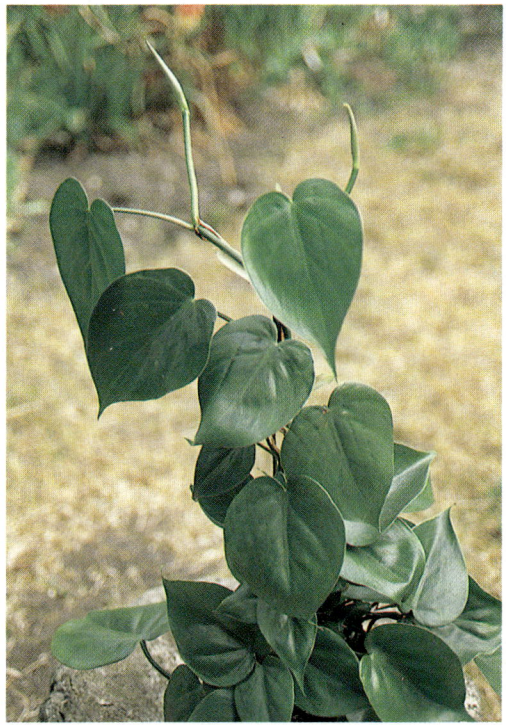

Fig. 7.5.134 *Philodendron scandens*.

Table 7.5.12 Aroids grown as house or greenhouse plants.

Genus	Species	Common names	Distinctive features	Dermatological importance
Acorus	gramineus	Sweet flag	Grass-like leaves, often variegated. Dwarf	Oil of calamus (from Acorus calamus). Rhizomes were used in perfumery and may sensitize (Klarmann 1958)
Alocasia	macrorhiza, sanderiana, etc.	Elephant's ears, Cunjevoi	Glossy, often metallic-looking leaves, arrow-shaped, often lobed on the margins	Irritant (Francis & Southcott 1967). May cause severe lip burning and swelling
Amorphophallus	esp. konjac (rivieri)	Ol, Moyu	Spectacular palm-like leaves on tall mottled stalks. Inflorescence massive, hideous, borne before the leaves. Grown as a tropical bedding plant and, in Hawaii, for edible tubers	Irritant, especially to eyes (Yoshizawa 1971)
Anthurium	esp. scherzerianum	Flamingo plant	Dull green leathery leaves. Spathe large, flattened, glossy, scarlet-red	Irritant
Caladium	bicolor, hybrids	Caladium	Arrow-shaped, often multi-coloured leaves. Sometimes used in sub-tropical bedding. Popular house plants	Irritant
Dieffenbachia	picta, seguine	Dumbcane, leopard lily	Erect, green woody stems, resembling sugar cane. Oblong leaves, often mottled with white, pale green or yellow	Intensely irritant (Drach & Maloney 1963, Ippen et al. 1986)

Epipremnum (Scindapsus)	pinnatum cv. 'aureum'	Devil's ivy, Pothos	Oval, yellow and green marbled leaves	Irritant. Allergenic (see below)
Monstera	deliciosa	Swiss cheese plant, fruit salad plant	Climbing glossy green leaves with slashes and perforations. A common office plant	Irritant. Possibly allergenic. Unripe fruit acrid; ingestion of (edible) ripe fruit causes urticaria (Francis & Southcott 1967). It rarely fruits in Britain!
Philodendron	scandens (cordatum)	Sweetheart vine	Climbing, heart-shaped leaves. A common office plant	Irritant. Allergenic (see below)
Sauromatum	venosum	Monarch of the East, Voodoo lily	Purchased as tubers in the spring. A malodorous yellow red-blotched spathe with red spadix erupts rapidly from the dry tuber. If planted, a palm-like leaf follows	? Irritant
Scindapsus	See Epipremnum			
Spathiphyllum	wallisii (esp. cv. 'Mauna Loa')	Peace lily, white sail	Elliptic leaves, thin texture, wavy margins. Pure white fragrant inflorescence with a green midrib on underside. Spiky spadix	Irritant
Zantedeschia (Richardia)	aethiopica	Arum lily, Calla lily	Glossy heart-shaped leaves and large white spathe with yellow spadix. Popular in floristry because of long-lasting flowers. Also grown in sheltered areas as a border, waterside or aquatic plant. Naturalized in parts of Australia and Mediterranean	Irritant and poisonous (Francis & Southcott 1967)

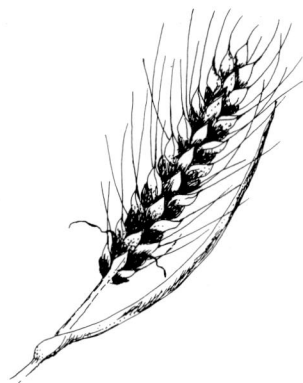

Fig. 7.5.135 *Triticium vulgare* (wheat).

to distinguish from irritant reactions. However, there are cases of apparent allergic reactions to barley (Solomons 1971), wheat (Fig. 7.5.135) (Pigatto *et al.* 1987), oat bran (Fig. 7.5.136) (Dempster 1981) and to an oatmeal bath in a child with atopic dermatitis (Riboldi *et al.* 1988).

These cases may reflect the phenomenon of a 'hybrid eczema' between allergic contact dermatitis and atopic eczema, as postulated by Malten (1968). The last case was associated with a strongly positive RAST (radioallergosorbent test) to oats (Riboldi *et al.* 1988).

Dempster J.G. (1981) Contact dermatitis from bran and oats. *Contact Dermatitis* **7**: 122.
Malten K.E. (1968) The occurrence of hybrids between contact allergic eczema and atopic dermatitis (and vice versa) and their significance. *Dermatologica* **136**: 404–406.
Pigatto P.D., Polenghi M.M. & Altomare G.F. (1987) Occupational dermatitis in bakers. A clue for atopic dermatitis. *Contact Dermatitis* **16**: 263–71.
Riboldi A., Pigatto PD., Altomare G.F. & Gibelli E. (1988) Contact allergic dermatitis from oatmeal. *Contact Dermatitis* **18**: 316–17.
Solomons B. (1971) Sensitization to oats and barley. *Contact Dermatitis Newsletter* **10**: 231.

BAMBUSA spp.

Common name: Bamboo
Distribution: Tropical and sub-tropical regions
Patch test: Tip of bamboo shoot as is

Bamboo stems are used in the manufacture of furniture; natural bamboo is covered with a rough hairy bark which can cause mechanical irritation and has been used in criminal poisoning (Mitchell & Rook 1979). Schiff (1951) described hyperpigmented contact dermatitis in workers sanding bamboo stems for tennis racquets. Patch tests were positive with bamboo shavings but no control results were recorded. Bamboo shoots are harvested in early spring and are used for food, particularly in Japan. Kitajima (1986) records erythematous plaques on the backs of the hands in a housewife who had handled the shoots 2 days previously. Further exposure led to a more extensive flare of the eruption. Patch tests were strongly positive to the 'head of leaves' (Kitajima 1986).

Kitajima T. (1986) Contact allergy caused by bamboo shoots. *Contact Dermatitis* **15**: 100–2.
Mitchell J. & Rook A. (1979) *Botanical Dermatology*. Greengrass, Vancouver.
Schiff B.L. (1951) Contact dermatitis caused by bamboo. *Archives of Dermatology and Syphilology* **64**: 66–7.

CYMBOPOGON

Common names: *C. citratus* : lemon grass.
C. martini : palmarosa. *C. nardus* : citronella

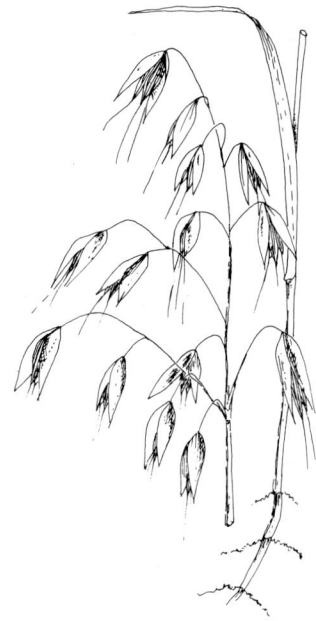

Fig. 7.5.136 *Avena fatua* (oat).

Patch test: Oils 1%, 10% in MEK or olive oil. Citral 1% pet. if available. Citronellal 1% pet. if available

Cymbopogon citratus is sometimes grown as a hot-house plant for its aromatic leaves. All three species are important sources of essential oils, derived by steam distillation. Oil of lemon grass and citronella are used in perfumery and as insect repellents. Palmarosa oil, with a rose-like perfume, is used in homoeopathic remedies. The oils may cause an irritant, even vesicular dermatitis (e.g. Mendelsohn 1946). Allergic contact dermatitis has been reported due to oil of citronella (Mendelsohn 1946, Keil 1947) and cross-reaction has been observed with palmarosa oil (Paschoud 1963). Allergic reactions may also occur to lemongrass oil (Mendelsohn 1946), which contains citral, a known sensitizer, although its effect may be 'quenched' by D-limonene, also found in lemongrass (Opdyke 1976). Oil of citronella contains geraniol and the aldehyde citronellal (Guenther 1950) (**7.L**).

Citronellal

7.L

Guenther E. (1950) *The Essential Oils*, Vol IV. Van Nostrand, New Jersey.
Keil H. (1947) Contact dermatitis due to oil of citronella. *Journal of Investigative Dermatology* **8**: 327–44.
Mendelsohn H.V. (1946) Lemongrass oil. A primary irritant and sensitizing agent. *Archives of Dermatology and Syphilology* **53**: 94–8.
Opdyke D.L.J. (1976) Inhibition of sensitization reactions induced by certain aldehydes. *Food and Cosmetic Toxicology* **14**: 197.
Paschoud J.M. (1963) Quelques cas d'eczema de contact avec sensibilisation de groupe. *Dermatologica* **127**: 349.

ORYZA sativa

Common name: Rice
Distribution: Tropics, widely cultivated

Irritant contact dermatitis is common among rice workers, due in part to the stagnant water in the paddy fields and mechanical irritation from the plants, as well as other hazards including schistosomiasis. Allergy to rice protein was recorded by Nasution *et al.* (1973) and Nakamura (1983) reported patch test positive dermatitis in a rice worker. Rice starch was removed from cosmetics because of its allergenicity (Schieffelin *et al.*, quoted in Mitchell & Rook 1979).

Mitchell J. & Rook A. (1979) *Botanical Dermatology*. Greengrass, Vancouver.
Nakamura T. (1983) Contact dermatitis to oryza. *Contact Dermatitis* **9**: 80.
Nasution D., Klokke A.H. & Nater J.P. (1973) A survey of occupational dermatoses in Indonesia. *Berufsdermatosen* **21**: 215–22.

PHLEUM pratense

Common name: Timothy grass
Distribution: Widespread, esp. Europe and Americas
Patch test: Pollen as is

This ubiquitous grass is an important cause of immediate hypersensitivity reactions (Brostoff & Roitt 1969). Positive patch test reactions have been reported using the pollen (Ramirez & Eller 1930) and an albumin fraction of the pollen (Mitchell & Mitchell 1945). Again, this may represent a 'hybrid' between atopic eczema and delayed hypersensitivity.

Brostoff J. & Roitt I.M. (1969) Cell-mediated (delayed) hypersensitivity in patients with summer hay fever. *Lancet* **ii**: 1269–72.
Mitchell J.H. & Mitchell W.F. (1945) Seasonal dermatitis due to the albumin fraction of Timothy pollen. *Journal of Allergy* **16**: 48–50.
Ramirez M.A. & Eller J.J. (1930) The 'patch test' in 'contact dermatitis' (dermatitis venenata). *Journal of Allergy* **1**: 489–95.

Ginkgoaceae

GINKGO biloba

Common names: Ginkgo, ginkyo. Maidenhair tree
Distribution: West China (probably extinct in wild). Cultivated in streets, parks, gardens, especially southern Britain and USA
Patch test material: 1 : 10 fruit pulp in acetone

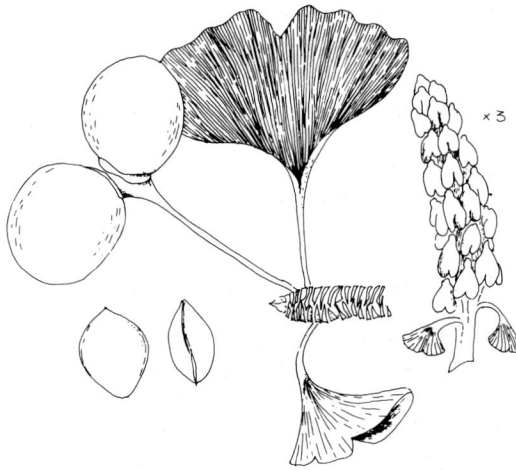

Fig. 7.5.137 *Ginkgo* in fruit.

Ginkgo is a 'living fossil', the sole remnant of its family. It was introduced to Europe in 1730 from specimens growing around Buddhist monasteries. It is deciduous, forming a roughly pyramidal branching tree between 10 and 30 m. The fan-shaped leaves (Fig. 7.5.137) individually resemble the pinnules of the maidenhair fern (*Adiantum capillus-veneris*) and are clustered on spurs. Male and female flowers are borne on different plants. Male plants bear cylindrical short-stalked catkins with green stamens. Female plants bear eventually a yellowish green plum-like fruit (drupe); the outer fleshy layer is malodorous and inedible. However, it surrounds an ovoid nut which has a sweet taste when roasted.

Allergic contact dermatitis occurs chiefly in eastern Asians who are aware of the culinary qualities of the nuts (Nakamura 1985, Tomb *et al.* 1988). A small epidemic occurred in 35 American schoolgirls who trampled the fallen fruit. Erythematous papules or a streaky papulovesicular erythema developed on the legs, resembling poison ivy dermatitis (Sowers *et al.* 1965). Children play marbles with the unripe fruit (Tomb *et al.* 1988). Ingestion of the fruit causes stomatitis and proctitis (Becker & Skipworth 1975) and preputial oedema has been recorded (Tomb *et al.* 1988).

The fruit pulp is irritant; thus Becker and Skipworth recommend a 10% dilution in acetone. The allergens appear to be ginkgolic acids I which are structurally similar to urushiol (**7.LI**) (Lepoittevin *et al.* 1989). Cross-sensitization to poison ivy is reported in humans (Sowers *et al.* 1965).

Ginkgolic acid

7.LI

An extract of *Ginkgo biloba* has numerous pharmacological actions, acting as a free-radical scavenger and reducing neutrophil chemotaxis. It may be useful for skin changes secondary to venous stasis (Cheatle *et al.* 1991).

Becker L.E. & Skipworth G.B. (1975) Ginkgo-tree dermatitis, stomatitis and proctitis. *JAMA* **231**: 1162–3.
Cheatle T.R., Scurr J.H. & Coleridge Smith P.D. (1991) Drug treatment of chronic venous insufficiency and venous ulceration: a review. *Journal of the Royal Society of Medicine* **84**: 354–8.
Lepoittevin J.P., Benezra L. & Asakawa Y. (1989) Allergic contact dermatitis to *Ginkgo biloba* L.: relationship with urushiol. *Archives of Dermatological Research* **281**: 227–30.
Nakamura T. (1985) Ginkgo tree dermatitis. *Contact Dermatitis* **12**: 281–2.
Sowers W.F., Weary P.E., Collins O.D. & Crawley E.P. (1965) Gingko tree dermatitis. *Archives of Dermatology* **91**: 452–6.
Tomb R.R., Foussereau J. & Sell Y. (1988) Mini-epidemic of contact dermatitis from ginkgo tree fruit (*Ginkgo biloba* L). *Contact Dermatitis* **19**: 281–3.

Ferns — Dryopteridaceae (Aspidiaceae)

ARACHNIODES adiantiformis (RUHMORA *adiantiformis*)

Common name: Leather leaf fern
Distribution: Australasia, South Africa, South America. Increasingly cultivated and used in floristry
Patch test: Fern frond as is

The fronds of this fern (Fig. 7.5.138) are sometimes imported from Central America,

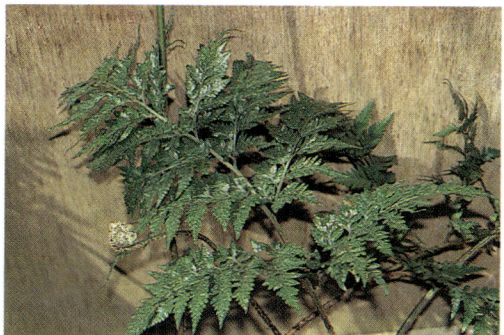

Fig. 7.5.138 *Arachniodes adiantiformis*.

mostly to continental Europe, as a substitute for *Asparagus plumosus* in florist's bouquets. Hausen and Schultz (1978) report two cases of allergic contact dermatitis affecting the fingers and palms after handling the fern. The allergen appears to be in the spores and is not yet determined, although 9(11)-fernen is suggested by Schmalle *et al.* (1980 in Hausen 1988) (**7.LII**).

9-(11)-fernen

7.LII

Hausen B.M. (1988) *Allergiepflanzen-Pflanzenallergene*. Ecomed, Landsberg/Munchen.

Hausen B.M. & Schultz K.D. (1978) Occupational allergic contact dermatitis due to leatherleaf fern *Arachniodes adiantiformis* (Forst.) Tindal. *British Journal of Dermatology* **98**: 325–9.

Ferns — Oleandraceae

NEPHROLEPIS exaltata

Common names: Sword fern. Ladder fern. Boston fern
Distribution: Tropics — widespread. A common house plant
Patch test: Crushed young frond as is

This popular fern (Fig. 7.5.139) is freely available in garden centres and is used as a pot plant or for hanging baskets. The wiry rhizomes produce numerous dark green fronds split into numerous narrow, linear segments arranged in parallel. Several cultivars are propagated intensively by meristem culture.

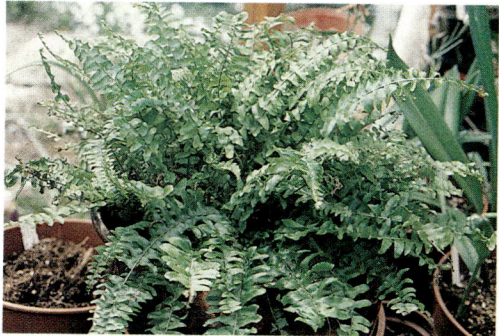

Fig. 7.5.139 *Nephrolepis exaltata*.

Two nursery employees developed erythema, vesicles and fissures, associated with micropropagation of several cultivars. Patch tests were positive with 'crushed young leaves' of 'Boston Orange Bell', 'Boston Blue Bell' and 'Teddy Junior'. Ethanol extracts of leaves and spores were negative (Stoof & Bruynzeel 1989). The allergen is unknown.

Stoof T.J. & Bruynzeel D. (1989) Contact allergy to *Nephrolepsis* ferns. *Contact Dermatitis* **20**: 234–5.

7.6 Allergenic conifers

Conifers are primitive trees which bear ovules naked on a scale (hence 'gymnosperm'), and not enclosed in an ovary. Several orders are of dermatological importance. *Pinus* species (Pinaceae) are the major source of colophony and X *Cupressocyparis leylandii*, the Leyland cypress, is a major source of elicitation of allergic contact dermatitis.

7.6.1 Pinaceae

Pinus species

Pinus species (pines) are evergreen conifers found across the northern hemisphere, crossing the equator to Java. The needles (leaves) are borne in bundles of two, three or five. The characteristic cones (Fig. 7.6.1) may take 2–3 years to develop. The Mediterranean, or cluster, pine (*P. haleppensis*) (Fig. 7.6.2) is of economic importance as the source of colophony, and turpentine is derived from several species. Although pine forestry is a major industry in temperate countries, dermatitis is rare in cutters and woodworkers (Mitchell 1970). Red deal is derived from the Scots pine (*P. sylvestris*) and has caused allergic contact dermatitis in wood workers (Woods & Calnan 1976). Burry (1969) has reported contact dermatitis to the Monterey pine (*P. radiata*) (Fig. 7.6.3), originating in California, but widely grown for timber in Australia and New Zealand. Japanese black pine (*P. thunbergii*) is rarely grown in larger gardens and arboreta; it is also allergenic (Nakamura 1986). Colophony 20% is a useful screening test. A 'pseudo-phytodermatitis' may be caused in pine foresters due to irritant hairs on the caterpillars of the pine processionary moth (*Thaumetopoea pityocampa*) (Katzenellenbogen 1955).

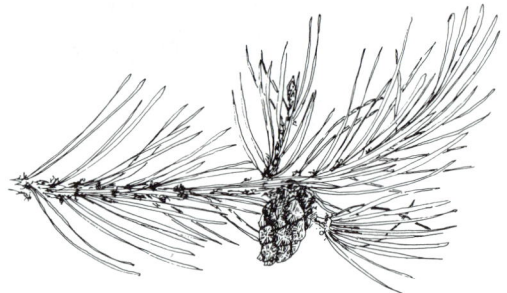
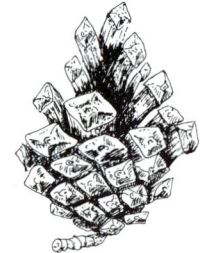

Fig. 7.6.1 Scots pine.

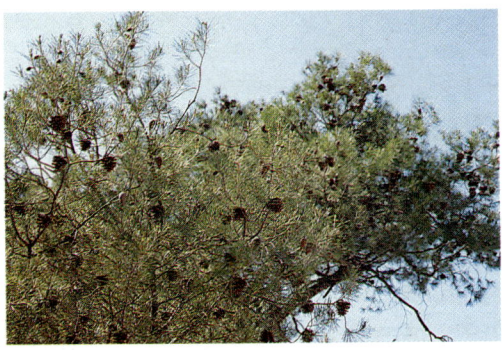

Fig. 7.6.2 *Pinus haleppensis* (Maritime pine).

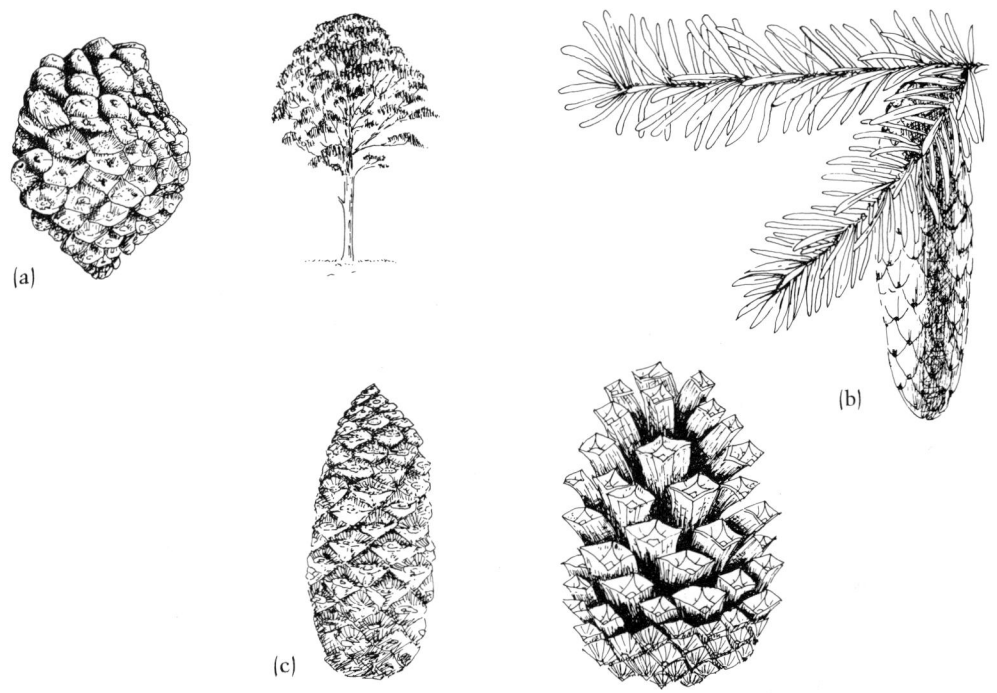

Fig. 7.6.3 Cones of (a) Monterey pine, also showing habit of tree, (b) Norway spruce and (c) Maritime pine (open and closed).

References

Burry J.N. (1969) Contact dermatitis from radiata pine. *Contact Dermatitis* **2**: 262–3.
Katzenellenbogen I. (1955) Caterpillar dermatitis as an occupational disease. *Dermatologica* **111**: 99.
Mitchell J.C. (1970) Patch testing results – screening set and plants. *Contact Dermatitis Newsletter* **8**: 177.
Nakamura T. (1986) Contact dermatitis to Japanese black pine. *Contact Dermatitis* **14**: 317.
Woods B. & Calnan C.D. (1976) Toxic woods. *British Journal of Dermatology* **95** (Suppl. 13): 1–97.

Picea species

Picea species (spruce) include the Christmas tree or Norway spruce, *Picea abies* (syn. *P. excelsa*) (Fig. 7.6.3), a native of northern Europe, although stunted forms are not uncommon in suburban gardens! Allergic contact dermatitis has been reported after decorating Christmas trees (Agrup 1969). The eruption affects the face, neck, forearms and hands, and patch tests are positive to 20% balsam of spruce in petrolatum (Fregert & Rorsman 1963), as well as to colophony. Diethylstilboestrol may be an allergen (Fregert & Rorsman 1963).

References

Agrup G. (1969) Hand eczema and other hand dermatoses in south Sweden. *Acta Dermato-Venereologica* **49** (Suppl. 61): 1–91.

Fregert S. & Rorsman H. (1963) Hypersensitivity to balsams of pine and spruce. *Archives of Dermatology* **87**: 693–5.

Colophony/turpentine

Colophony and turpentine are both derived from conifers. Colophony is a sticky, amber-coloured material of variable composition. It is named after Colophon, an ancient town on the west coast of Turkey. Synonyms are kolophonium (Germany), colophane (France), colofonia (Spain), kolofonium (Sweden) and gum rosin or wood rosin (USA). Gum rosin is derived from the oleoresin of living trees (notably *Pinus palustris* and *P. caribaea*). Wood rosin is obtained from distillates of pine stumps. Tall oil rosin ('tall' is Swedish for pine) is derived by fractional distillation of crude tall oil, a by-product of wood pulping in paper manufacture. Rosins contain roughly 90% resin acids, notably abietic acid and its isomers (pimaric acids).

In ancient civilizations of the eastern Mediterranean, exudates from conifers were cooked in open pots. A sheepskin was stretched across the pot to catch the vapour. Turpentine was obtained by wringing out the sheepskin manually. The residue in the pot, pitch, had many uses, particularly in the ship industry. It was valued greatly in medicine; Dioscorides recommended it to 'circumscarificate carbuncles and rotten ulcers' (quoted in Huxley & Taylor 1977). Now a million tons of colophony are produced every year (Karlberg 1988) and its major use is in sizing of paper and paper board. Some of its other uses are shown in Table 7.6.1.

Contact dermatitis has been reported from rosin in a soldering flux (Rivers & Rycroft 1987). Dermatitis due to colophony most commonly follows exposure to sticking plaster (Fig. 7.6.4), although there are

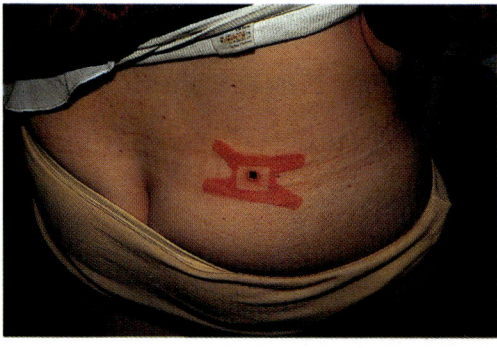

Fig. 7.6.4 Allergic dermatitis from sticking plaster.

Table 7.6.1 Sources of colophony contact allergy (based on Karlberg 1988).

Sawdust from pine trees: tapping and collecting exudate
Paper size (a finish to prevent ink spreading or 'feathering')
Soldering fluxes: e.g. Multicore®
Some printing inks and finishers
Varnishes
Cutting oils and anti-rust oils (tall oil fatty acids added to some soluble oils) (Fregert 1979, Matos et al. 1988)
Tranparent soaps
Glues, sealants and mastics
Adhesive plasters, stickers, price labels, black insulating tape, fly papers
Grip enhancer/anti-slip agent: e.g. fan and machine belts; bow rosin for stringed instruments; 'tackifier' for racquet handles, golf clubs, bowls; applied to dancers' shoes and dance floors
Shoe and floor polishes (rarely)
Eyeshadows, rouge and mascara (rarely)
Medicaments: e.g. herbal preparations (Lee & Lam 1990); wart paints — Cuplex® (Monk 1987), Verucid® (Veraldi & Schianchi-Veraldi 1990)
Dentistry: e.g. cements, cavity varnisher
Ostomy appliances
Chewing gum: e.g. Sportlife®, Mister Bubble® (Satyawan et al. 1990)
Depilatory powder
Shirt dirt and grease remover
Linoleum

many other sources of exposure, either following the use of cosmetics or medicaments or through the patient's occupation or leisure activities (Table 7.6.1). The history of exposure may be bizarre, as in a masseur to a ballet company who was sensitized by the anti-slip agent added to the dance floor and transferred to the dancers' shoes (Aberer 1987) or in a pastry cook who dipped pastries (used for exhibition) in hot rosin to provide a good finish (Hausen 1984).

Although abietic acid was traditionally held to be allergenic, detailed studies by Karlberg et al. (1985) indicate that the allergens include oxidation products of abietic acid, including 5-hydroperoxyabietic acid, and of dehydroabietic acid (**7.LIII**). Hydrogenation

Abietic acid

15-hydroperoxyabietic acid

Pimaric acid

7.LIII Allergens in colophony.

reduces the allergenicity of colophony (Karlberg 1988). Other reported allergens include hydroabietyl alcohol (abitol) in patch test tape (Cronin & Calnan 1978) and mascara (Dooms-Goossens *et al.* 1979).

Because of the multiplicity of sources, and biological variation, the sole use of a standard allergen (e.g. ICDRG colophony 10/20%) may not detect all cases. Where possible, it is important to test with the material handled by the patient. If available, it is useful to include 10/20% hydroabietyl alcohol, 20% hydroabietic acid and 10/20% pimaric acid as well as other types of colophony (e.g. Spanish colophony). Patients sensitized to colophony may develop allergic contact dermatitis after exposure to conifers, e.g. juniper (Dooms-Goossens *et al.* 1984) and X *Cupressocyparis leylandii* (Lovell *et al.* 1985). Cross-sensitivity occurs with balsams of benzoin, styrax and tolu (Fregert & Rorsman 1963).

Turpentine is an oleoresin derived from several conifer species, including *Pinus pinaster* and *P. palustris*, as well as silver firs (*Abies* spp.). The gum tapped from the trunk (Fig. 7.6.5) is separated by vacuum or steam distillation. Alternatively, turpentine is obtained via the sulphate extraction process, making paper pulp from pine wood. In ancient Greece, a good quality turpentine was extracted also from

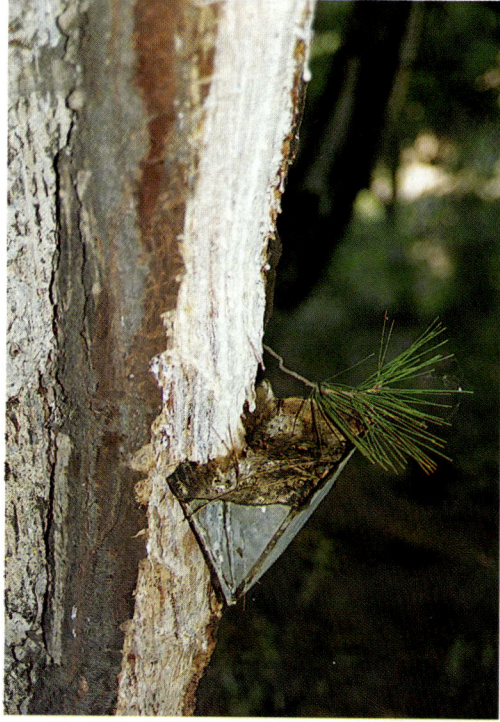

Fig. 7.6.5 Tapping *Pinus haleppensis* for turpentine (Greece).

Pistachia terebinthus, a member of the Anacardiaceae (Huxley & Taylor 1977).

Oil of turpentine was in the past used commonly as a paint thinner and brush cleaner, as well as in waxes, polishes and industrial soaps. Turpentine oil is irritant and also a potent sensitizer, typically causing facial dermatitis because of its volatility. It has also caused periungual dermatitis. It has mostly been supplanted by white spirit and the decline in its use is mirrored by decreased prevalence of allergic contact dermatitis. Like colophony, the composition of turpentine varies considerably. Swedish or Finnish turpentine, which contains a hydroperoxide of Δ3-carene, is more allergenic than French turpentine, which lacks it (Pirila *et al.* 1969). Other constituents, including α-pinene, are irritant. When necessary, patch testing with 0.3% turpentine peroxides in olive oil is recommended (Cronin 1980).

References

Aberer W. (1987) Allergy to colophony acquired backstage. *Contact Dermatitis* **16**: 34–6.
Cronin E. (1980) *Contact Dermatitis*. Churchill Livingstone, London.
Cronin E. & Calnan C.D. (1978) Allergy to hydroabietic alcohol in adhesive tape. *Contact Dermatitis* **4**: 57.
Dooms-Goossens A., Degreef H. & Luytens E. (1979) Dihydroabietyl alcohol (Abitol®). A sensitiser in mascara. *Contact Dermatitis* **5**: 350–3.
Dooms-Goossens A., Marstens M., van Lintd Ruys-Latlender C.M. & Scheffer J.J.C. (1984) Colophony-induced sensitivity in *Juniperus chinensis* L. 'Hetzii'? *Contact Dermatitis* **10**: 185–7.
Fregert S. (1979) Colophony in cutting oil and in soap water used as cutting fluid. *Contact Dermatitis* **5**: 52.
Fregert J. & Rorsman H. (1963) Hypersensitivity to balsams of pine and spruce. *Archives of Dermatology* **87**: 693–5.
Hausen B.M. (1984) Ungewohnliche Kontaktsensibilisierung im Konditorgewerbe. *Aktuelle Dermatologie* **10**: 13–16.
Huxley A. & Taylor W. (1977) *Flowers of Greece and the Aegean*. Chatto & Windus, London.
Karlberg A.T. (1988) Contact allergy to colophony. *Acta Dermato-Venerologica* (Suppl. 139).
Karlberg A.T., Bergstedt E., Boman A., Bohlinder K., Liden C., Nilsson J.L.G. & Wahlberg J.E. (1985) Is abietic acid the allergenic component of colophony? *Contact Dermatitis* **13**: 209–15.
Karlberg A.T., Boman A., Hacksell V., Jacobsson S. & Nilsson J.L. (1988) Contact allergy to dehydroabietic acid derivatives isolated from Portuguese colophony. *Contact Dermatitis* **19**: 166–74.
Lee T.Y. & Lam T.H. (1990) Patch testing of 11 common herbal topical medicaments in Hong Kong. *Contact Dermatitis* **22**: 137–40.
Lovell C.R., Dannaker C.J. & White I.R. (1985) Allergic contact dermatitis from X *Cupressocyparis leylandii* and shared allergenicity with colophony. *Contact Dermatitis* **13**: 344–5.
Matos J., Mariano A., Gonçalo S., Freitas J.D. & Oliveira J. (1988) Occupational dermatitis from colophony. *Contact Dermatitis* **18**: 53–4.
Monk B. (1987) Allergic contact dermatitis to colophony in a wart remover. *Contact Dermatitis* **17**: 242.

Pirilä V., Kilpio O., Olkonnen A., Pirilä L. & Siltanen E. (1969) On the chemical nature of the eczematogens in oil of turpentine V. Pattern of sensitivity to different terpenes. *Dermatologica* **139**: 183–94.

Rivers J.K. & Rycroft R.J.G. (1987) Occupational allergic contact urticaria from colophony. *Contact Dermatitis* **17**: 181–8.

Satyawan I., Oranje A.P. & van Joost T.H. (1990) Perioral dermatitis in a child due to rosin in a chewing gum. *Contact Dermatitis* **72**: 182–3.

Veraldi S. & Schianchi-Veraldi R. (1990) Allergic contact dermatitis from colophony in a wart gel. *Contact Dermatitis* **22**: 184–5.

7.6.2 Cupressaceae

Juniperus spp. (junipers) occur throughout most of the northern hemisphere. The leaves are generally sharp and awl-shaped (Fig. 7.6.6), particularly in immature plants. *Juniperus virginiana* wood is used to make 'red cedar' pencils. Many slow-growing spp., including forms of *J. communis*, the 'Noah's Ark' juniper, are grown in rock gardens. The berries of this species provide the distinct aromatic taste of gin. Contact sensitivity to *Juniperus* spp. occurs in gardeners who are previously sensitized to colophony (Dooms-Goossens *et al.* 1984). Oil of Cade is derived by destructive distillation of the wood of *J. oxycedrus*; it causes irritant and allergic contact dermatitis (Rothe *et al.* 1973).

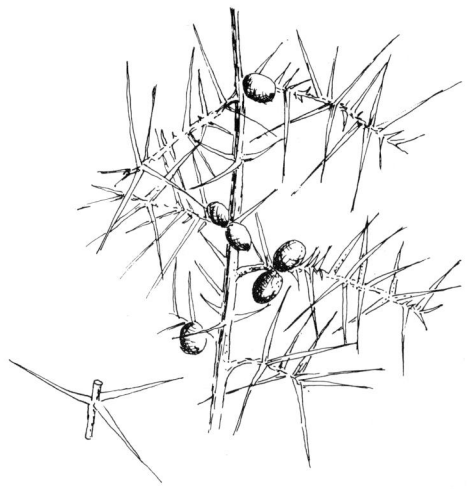

Fig. 7.6.6 Juniper.

References

Dooms-Goossens A., Marstens M., van Lintd Ruys-Latlender C.M. & Scheffer J.J.C. (1984) Colophony-induced sensitivity to *Juniperus chinensis* L. 'Hetzii'? *Contact Dermatitis* **10**: 185–7.

Rothe A., Heine A. & Rebohle E. (1973) Oil from juniper berries as an occupational allergen for the skin and respiratory tract. *Berufsdermatosen* **21**: 11–16.

X CUPRESSOCYPARIS leylandii

Common name: Leyland cypress.
Distribution: Man-made hybrid genus. Very common in gardens in temperate regions
Patch test: Ether extract of leaf (5–10%); colophony 20% screens most individuals

This hybrid genus is derived from *Cupressus macrocarpa* and *Chamaecyparis nootkatensis*. There are several cultivars, including 'Castlewellan', 'Haggerston Grey', 'Leighton Green' and 'Robinson's Gold'.

X *Cupressocyparis leylandii* (Fig. 7.6.7) is a columnar evergreen conifer. In the UK (and also in New Zealand and South Africa) it is used popularly for hedging and screening. Its ease of propagation makes it an ideal nursery gardener's plant. However, because it grows rapidly it requires frequent pruning in small gardens, leading to greater exposure than other garden conifers. Contact dermatitis may follow pruning or burning (Fig. 7.6.8). Sprigs are used for bouquets or wreaths in floristry.

Hindson *et al.* (1982) reported a 40-year-old man, known to react to

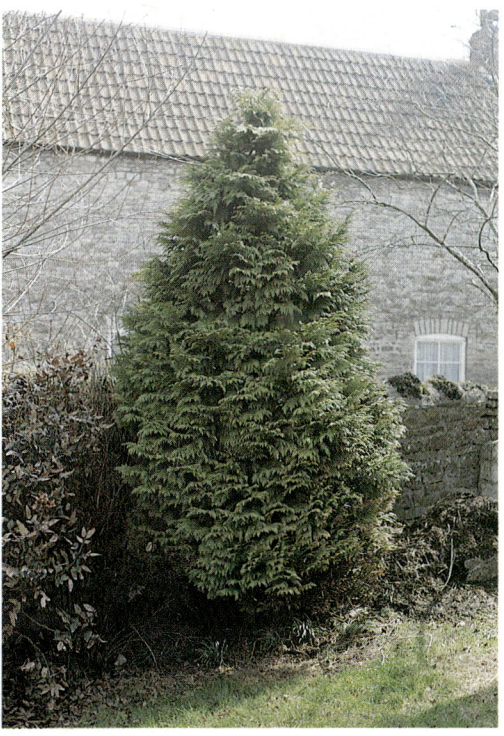

Fig. 7.6.7 X *Cupressocyparis leylandii.*

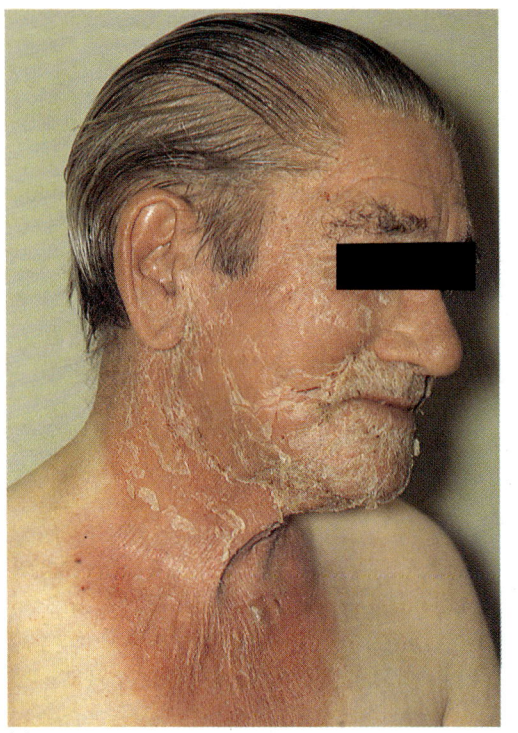 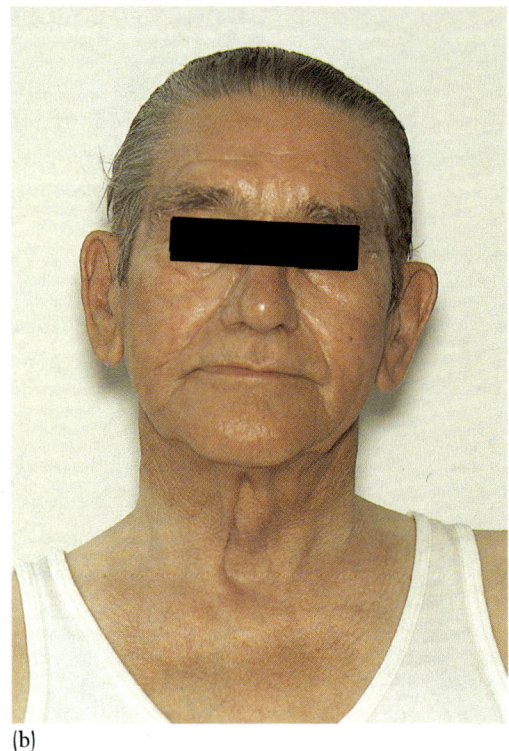

Fig. 7.6.8 Airborne allergic contact dermatitis after cutting down and burning X *C. leylandii*. (a) at presentation, (b) within 5 days after topical steroid therapy and avoidance of allergen.

zinc oxide plaster, who presented with acute eczema of the face, arms and hands after planting 100 X *C. leylandii*. Patch tests were positive to an ether extract of the leaf and to 20% Spanish colophony but negative using ICDRG colophony. In a later study (Lovell *et al.* 1985) of 17 patients with positive patch test reactions to a 10% 24-h ether extract of X *C. leylandii*, 15 also reacted to 20% ICDRG colophony. This 10% extract proved irritant in two other patients, and a 5% dilution may be preferable.

The constituents of X *C. leylandii* have not been identified although Watt and Bryer-Brandwijk (1982) describe the presence of carvacrol (methylisopropyl phenol), sesquiterpenes and terpenes in extracts from its parents. Most of the allergens are shared, or cross-react, with those of colophony.

It is possible that dermatitis is commonly elicited by this ubiquitous plant in individuals previously sensitized by sticking plaster. As yet, it is not clear whether the plant may itself sensitize.

References

Hindson C., Lawlor F. & Downey A. (1982) Cross-sensitivity between zinc oxide plaster and *Cupressus leylandii* shrubs. *Contact Dermatitis* **8**: 335.

Lovell C.R., Dannaker C.J. & White I.R. (1985) Allergic contact dermatitis from X *Cupressocyparis leylandii* and shared allergenicity with colophony. *Contact Dermatitis* **13**: 344–5.

Watt J.M. & Breyer-Brandwijk M. (1982) *Medicinal and Poisonous Plants of Southern Africa*. E. & S. Livingstone, Edinburgh.

Thuya

Thuya is a small genus of six species originally from North America and the Far East. The cones are urn-shaped with thin scales. *Thuya orientalis*, the Chinese thuya, has been reported to cause allergic contact dermatitis (Zubiri & Obras-Loscertales 1970). The western red cedar, *T. plicata* (Fig. 7.6.9), is a west American species, the leaves of which have a characteristic pineapple scent. It is commonly grown in parks and gardens. There are several reports of allergic dermatitis to the wood (Calnan 1972, Ishizaki *et al.* 1973). The allergens are thought to be tropolones (Bleumink *et al.* 1973).

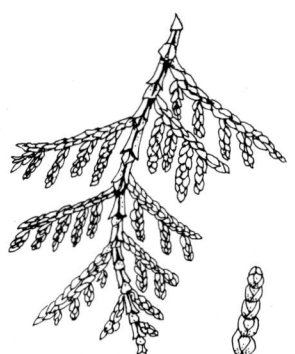

Fig. 7.6.9 Western red cedar.

References

Bleumink E., Mitchell J.C. & Nater J.P. (1973) Allergic contact dermatitis from cedar wood (*Thuya plicata*). *British Journal of Dermatology* **88**: 499.

Calnan C.D. (1972) Dermatitis from cedar wood pencils. *Transactions of the St John's Hospital Dermatological Society* **58**: 43.

Ishizaki T., Shida T., Miyamoto T., Matsumara Y., Mizuno K. & Tomaru M. (1973) Occupational asthma from western red cedar dust (*Thuya plicata*) in furniture factory workers. *Journal of Occupational Medicine* **15**: 580.

Zubiri A. & Obras-Loscertales J.M. de las (1970) Caso curioso de dermatitis por contacto. *Actas Dermosifilografias* **61**: 277.

7.7 Allergenic hardwoods

Many tropical hardwoods are highly allergenic and have caused dermatitis in tree fellers, loggers, sawyers, carpenters and joiners. Softwoods, such as pine and spruce, are considerably safer although allergic reactions can occur. Most temperate hardwoods appear to be blameless. The current, if perhaps belated, enthusiasm for conservation of rain forests and the prohibitive expense of tropical timbers has resulted in a reduced number of cases seen in Europe and USA. However, antique restorers, musical instrument makers and other specialists are still exposed to exotic woods. The major allergenic species are listed in Table 7.7.1. For a more detailed account, the reader is strongly urged to refer to the reviews by Woods and Calnan (1976) and more recently by Hausen (1986) as well as a textbook by Hausen (1981). Anatomical details of several tropical woods, including microphotographs, can be found in Benezra *et al.* (1985).

The terminology of woods is confusing: the name 'mahogany' or 'rosewood' is applied to several botanically totally unrelated species. Some of the commoner names are listed in Table 7.7.2. Beware 'rogue' logs of allergenic species as contaminants in a consignment of timber.

Several timbers have irritant properties; many have a crystalline bark. Others, notably members of the Euphorbiaceae (spurge family) and Moraceae (fig family), possess an irritant sap (latex) (see Chapter 5). A few species, including larch (*Larix decidua*), obeche (*Triplochiton decidua*) and Limba (*Terminalia superba*), rarely cause contact urticaria; other urticant species are noted in Table 4.3.1. Trees belonging to phototoxic families (Rutaceae and Flindersiaceae) are rarely used commercially. Inhalation of sawdust may cause severe respiratory problems (including rhinitis, asthma and even extrinsic allergic alveolitis) and wood dust may be carcinogenic (Wills 1982).

Allergic contact dermatitis typically begins in an airborne pattern, affecting the backs of hands, face and 'V' of neck, in those who are exposed to fine sawdust (Fig. 7.7.1). Later, the eruption spreads to the

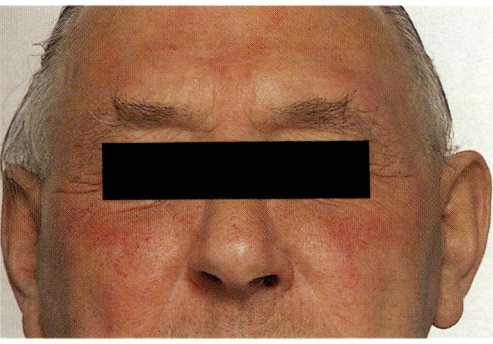

Fig. 7.7.1 Airborne allergic contact dermatitis from iroko wood dust.

areas where dust is trapped, i.e. groins, dorsa of feet, waist and axillae. More rarely, sensitization follows exposure to the finished product (e.g. musical instruments such as recorders, trinkets, knife handles, etc.). If the skin is previously damaged by irritants, e.g. water, detergents or perspiration, sensitization is more likely to occur since the toxin can more readily penetrate the epidermis. Initially symptoms are often mild and episodic; later a widespread persistent eczema may develop.

It is often necessary to patch test with the patient's own wood shavings or dust (including dust from other work areas and the dust that collects in undisturbed parts of the factory). Unfortunately, this carries the significant risk of active sensitization; in addition, many timbers cause highly irritant patch test reactions. Patch testing using a battery of purified allergens, although ideal, is for most dermatology departments a counsel of perfection. Hausen (1986) recommends the following technique to extract the allergens. Stir 1–10 g of wood dust overnight at room temperature in 50 ml ethanol. Filter. Evaporate the filtrate using a rotary evaporator or leaving on a windowsill; weigh residue and dissolve to 10% in ethanol. Further dilutions may be necessary if irritant reactions are obtained. Most of the allergens are quinones (e.g. dalbergiones); others include phenols related to poison ivy urushiols, stilbenes and terpenes. Some of the important allergens are illustrated below (**7.LIV**).

R-3,4-dimethoxydalbergione
(Rosewoods, p.a.o. Ferro)

Chlorophorin
(Iroko)

Grevillol
(Silk Oak)

7.LIV

Where possible, management should include primary prevention. The workforce should ideally be informed of the potentially dangerous woods and adequate exhaust ventilation, using extractor fans, should be provided. 'Damping down' the dust reduces allergenicity and the fire hazard. Barrier creams and protective clothing may only serve to increase contact with the dust. It may be possible to move an individual to another work area after patch testing has confirmed a specific sensitivity. Remember that allergic dermatitis may be due to liverworts or lichens rather than to the timber itself. Other potential allergens

Table 7.7.1 Allergenic timbers. See also *Eucalyptus*, pp. 139–40, *Olea*, p. 187 and *Juglans* & *Quercus*, p. 208.

Family	Genus	Species	Common name(s)	Distribution	Uses	Allergens	Comments/references
1 Dipterocarpaceae	*Shorea*	spp.	Meranti, lauan Philippine mahogany	Sri Lanka	Joinery, boat building. Lamella doors	?	Very rare sensitizer. Reported in foresters (Siregar 1975)
2 Sterculiaceae (Triplochitonaceae)	*Mansonia*	*altissima*	Mansonia, African black walnut, Bete	West Africa	As substitute for walnut	Mansonone A (a quinonoid)	Irritant and allergenic. Also systemic effects, including cardiotoxicity
3 Burseraceae	*Aucoumea*	*klaineana*	Gaboon mahogany, Okume	West Africa	As substitute for mahogany	?	Irritant and allergenic
4 Meliaceae	*Guarea*	*thompsonii*	Guarea, Bosse, Nigerian pear wood	West Africa (other spp. in tropical America)	As substitute for mahogany	?	? Entirely irritant
	4a *Khaya*	*anthoteca* (and other spp.)	African mahogany	Africa	The major source of mahogany. *Swietenia*, the American mahogany, is nearly extinct	Anthothecol ? + other allergens	Several reports of allergic contact dermatitis. Causes orange-brown discoloration of nails (Harris & Rosen 1989)
	4b *Turreanthus*	*africanus*	Avodire	Africa	Used in veneers	?	(Calnan 1970)
5 Anacardiaceae (see Chapter 7.4)	*Gluta* or *Melanorrhoea*	spp.	Rengas wood Singapore mahogany	Malaysia	Furniture. A durable wood but irritancy limits use	Thitsiol (an urushiol)	Irritant and allergenic. Other genera of Anacardiaceae also termed Rengas (Goh 1988)
6 Leguminosae (including Caesalpinioideae, Papilionideae and Mimosoideae)	6a *Acacia*	*melanoxylon*	Australian blackwood	Australia	A useful timber for furniture, boat building, handles, etc. Chiefly used in Australia	Acamelin 2,6-dimethoxybenzoquinone ? + non-quinoid allergens	Important sensitizer. Also causes respiratory symptoms (Clarke 1989)
	6b *Afzelia*	*africana*	Afzelia	West/central Africa	A durable timber, used for load-bearing floors, etc.	?	Several reports of allergic contact dermatitis

6c	*Andira*	*inermis*	Partridge wood	South America	Handles, turnery		
6d	*Bowdichia*	*nitida*	Sucupira	North Brazil	Frames, poles, stakes, etc.	2,6-dimethoxybenzoquinone Bowdichione	[Heyl 1966]. Cross-reaction with *Dalbergia*. Also causes rhinitis (Gonçalo 1992)
6e	*Brya*	*ebenus*	Cocus wood	South America West Indies	Musical instruments especially flutes in 19th century	?	A rare timber
6f	*Cassia*	*siamea*	Tagayasan	Japan	Various. Senna is derived from *Cassia* spp. including *acutifolia*	?	? Entirely irritant
6g	*Dalbergia*	*cearensis*	Kings wood, violet wood	South America	Marquetry	?	? Entirely irritant
		latifolia	East Indian rosewood Sissoo	Asia, India	Dark veneer for dining room and bedroom furniture. Mathematical instruments, etc.	(R)-4-methoxydalbergione + other quinones	A potent sensitizer. May cause systemic reactions. Dermatitis from chin rest (Haustein 1982)
		melanoxylon	African blackwood Grenadille African ebony (in part)	West Africa, esp. Senegal & Sudan	Musical instruments, inc. clarinets, recorders, bagpipes, knife handles, etc.	(R)- and (S)-4-methoxydalbergione (S)-4-hydroxy-4-methoxydalbergione	Chiefly affects instrument makers and musicians
		nigra	Brazilian rosewood 'Jacaranda' Rio-palisander	Brazil	Veneers for cabinet-making. Ornaments (e.g. wooden cross, Fisher & Bikowski 1981)	(R)-4-methoxydalbergione	A moderate sensitizer. The genus *Jacaranda* is an unrelated ornamental tree
		retusa	Cocobolo	Panama/Central America	In the past, musical instruments especially recorders. Cutlery, revolver stocks. A strong wood, uninfluenced by moisture	(R)-4-methoxydalbergione (S)-4-hydroxy-4-methoxydalbergione	Perioral dermatitis in recorder players
		stevensonii	Honduras rosewood	South America	Xylophones; handles	Dalbergiones	

Continued on p. 250

Table 7.7.1 Continued

Family	Genus	Species	Common name(s)	Distribution	Uses	Allergens	Comments/references
	6h Disteomonanthus	benthamianus	Ayan, Movingui Nigerian satinwood	West Africa	Cab bodies, coffins, handles, kitchen equipment. Flooring	Flavonoids ? Oxyayanins	Irritant bark. Allergic dermatitis reported (Gamboa et al. 1991)
	6i Erythrophleum	guineense	Tali, Missanda Doom bark, Ordeal Tree	West Africa	General		Cross-reaction with Disteomonanthus
	6j Gossweilerodendron	balsamiferum	Agba, Tola branca, Pink mahogany	Tropical west Africa	Construction, joinery		
	6k Machaerium	scleroxylon	Pao ferro Caviuna vermelha 'Santos rosewood'	Brazil	Hard, heavy timber Used as substitute for Brazilian rosewood. Instruments, including recorders. Kitchen utensils	(R) 3,4-dimethoxydalbergione (v. irritant on patch testing)	Strong sensitizer. Do not patch test with wood dusts or shavings — may actively sensitize. Logs may 'contaminate' shipments of Brazilian rosewood (Dalbergia) (Woods 1982). May induce erythema multiforme-like eruption (Irvine et al. 1988)
	6m Pericopsis	elata	Afrormosia	West Africa	Strong timber, joinery, boat-building. Furniture	Flavonoids ? 2,6-dimethoxyquinone	
	6n Prosopis	juliflora var. glandulosa	Mesquite	Southern USA	Furniture, construction		Rarely allergenic. Irritant gum (Sonova gum)
7 Sapotaceae	Tieghemella (Dumoria) (Mimusops)	heckelii	Makore Baku	West Africa	Veneers, furniture	? Not a saponin	? Entirely irritant

#	Family	Genus	species	Common names	Origin	Uses	Active compounds	Notes
8	Ebenaceae	*Diospyros*	*crassiflora* *ebenum*	African ebony East Indian ebony	Africa Far East	Hard black metal-like woods. Piano keys, tool handles, ornaments	Naphthoquinones	*D. methanoxylon* (coromandel) ? also allergenic
			celebica	Macassar	Celebes	Black wood with grey streaks, used in ornaments, knife handles, brushes, etc.	Naphthoquinones	
9	Apoyanaceae	*Aspidosperma*	spp.	Brazilian box tree Peroba rosa	Brazil Argentine	Construction, keyboard instruments	?	Irritant. Reported to cause allergic dermatitis in an organist and in a beautician who used 'orange sticks' made of the wood (Jemec & Hausen 1991)
10	Bignoniaceae	*Paratecoma*	*peroba*	Peroba do Campos Peroba amarella	East Brazil	Rot-resistant. Furniture, doors and window frames. Substitute for teak	Lapachonone and other quinones	
	10a	*Tabebuia*	*avellanedae* (and other spp.)	Lapacho Ipe amarello Mayflower	Brazil	Framework, joinery, ship building	Deoxylapachol (+ lapachenole)	
11	Verbenaceae	*Tectonia*	*grandis*	Teak	India Malaysia	Boat building, flooring, furniture. A highly valued wood	Deoxylapachol – variable concentration. Some cultivated stands contain reduced concentration of allergen	One of the oldest trade timbers: used in ancient Egyptian & Indian temples. An important sensitizer. Also causes contact urticaria. *Do not patch test with dust or shavings*
12	Lauraceae	*Nectandra*	*rodiae*	Greenheart Paracoto Brazilian walnut	West Indies	Light construction	? Berberine	Crystalline material in bark. ? Irritant
		Phoebe (Octoea)	*porosa*	Imbuia Brazilian walnut	South America	Light construction	"	Causes mucocutaneous effects

Continued on p. 252

Table 7.7.1 Continued

Family	Genus	Species	Common name(s)	Distribution	Uses	Allergens	Comments/references
13 Hernandiaceae	*Hernandia*	*sonora*	Topolite Jack-in-the-box	Trinidad and other neo-tropical regions	Joinery	? Podophyllotoxin	
14 Proteaceae	*Grevillea*	*robusta*	Silk oak	Australia; cultivated in Africa, Sri Lanka, India and southern USA	Flooring, plywood, furniture	Grevillol (5-n-tridecylresorcinol)	See also pp. 203–4
15 Thymelaeaceae	*Gonystylus*	*bancanus* (and other spp.)	Ramin Melawis	Malaysia	Furniture, joinery	?	Bark highly irritant. Also causes urticaria [Beck 1982]
16 Moraceae	*Chlorophora*	*excelsa*	Iroko, Kambala, African teak	West Africa	Joinery, esp. window frames; lab benches	Chlorophorine (a stilbene)	Used as a teak substitute and now often itself replaced by mahoganies. A moderate sensitizer
17 Pinaceae	*Pinus*	spp.	Pine	Temperate zones	Widely used in construction, furniture, etc.	Terpenes	Rare allergens in woodwork. See pp. 235–41
17a	*Picea*	spp.	Spruce	"	"	Tropolones	
18 Cupressaceae	*Thuya*	*plicata*	Western red cedar			Thuyaplicins Thymoquinone, etc.	Also causes allergic rhinitis, allergic asthma and extrinsic allergic alveolitis. See p. 245

Table 7.7.2 Some common names used for hardwoods. (Number denotes position in Table 7.7.1.)

Afrormosia	*Pericopsis elata* (6m)
Blackwood	
Australian	*Acacia melanoxylon* (6a)
African	*Dalbergia melanoxylon* (6g)
Ebony	*Diospyros* spp. (8)
Iroko	*Chlorophora excelsa* (16)
Jacaranda	*Dalbergia nigra* (6g) (not the genus *Jacaranda*)
Mahogany	
African	*Khaya* spp. (4a)
Gaboon	*Aucoumea klaineana* (3)
Philippine	*Shorea* spp. (1)
Pink	*Gossweilerodendron balsamiferum* (6j)
Singapore	*Gluta/Melanorrhoea* spp. (5)
Oak, silk	*Grevillea robusta* (14)
Palisander	*Dalbergia* spp. (6g)
Pao ferro	*Machaerium scleroxylon* (6k)
Peroba	*Aspidosperma* spp. (9) or *Paratecoma* spp. (10)
Ramin	*Gonystylus* spp. (15)
Rengas	*Gluta/Melanorrhoea* spp. (5)
Rosewood	
East Indian	*Dalbergia latifolia* (6g)
Brazilian	*Dalbergia nigra* (6g)
Honduras	*Dalbergia stevensonii* (6g)
'Santos'	*Machaerium scleroxylon* (6k)
Teak	*Tectonia grandis* (11)
Walnut	
African black	*Mansonia altissima* (2)
Brazilian	*Nectandra/Phoebe/Octoea* spp. (12)

include chemical preservatives and binders (Gan *et al.* 1987) encountered by wood handlers.

References

Beck M.H. (1982) A case of ramin wood sensitivity. *Contact Dermatitis* **8**: 74–5.
Benezra C., Ducombs J., Sell Y. & Foussereau J. (1985) *Plant Contact Dermatitis.* B.C. Decker, Toronto.
Calnan C.D. (1970) Avodire wood sensitivity. *Contact Dermatitis Newsletter* **8**: 190.
Clarke P.S. (1989) Allergic reactions to blackwood (*Acacia melanoxylon*). *Medical Journal of Australia* **150**: 222–3.
Fisher A.A. & Bikowski J., Jr. (1981) Allergic contact dermatitis due to a wooden cross made of *Dalbergia nigra*. *Contact Dermatitis* **7**: 45–6.
Gamboa P.M., Jauregui I., Gonzalez G., Fernandez J.C. & Antépara I. (1991) Allergic contact dermatitis from tali (missanda) wood (*Erythrophleum guianense*). *Contact Dermatitis* **24**: 309.
Gan S.L., Goh C.L., Lee C.S. & Hui K.H. (1987) Occupational dermatoses among sanders in the furniture industry. *Contact Dermatitis* **17**: 237–40.
Goh C.L. (1988) Occupational allergic contact dermatitis from Rengas wood. *Contact Dermatitis* **18**: 300.

Gonçalo S. (1992) Allergic contact dermatitis from *Bowdichia nitida* (sucupira) wood. *Contact Dermatitis* **26**: 205.

Harris A.O. & Rosen T. (1989) Nail discoloration due to mahogany. *Cutis* **43**: 55–6.

Hausen B.M. (1981) *Woods Injurious to Human Health*. De Gruyter, New York.

Hausen B.M. (1986) Contact allergy to woods. *Clinics in Dermatology* **4**(2): 65–76.

Haustein U.F. (1982) Violin chin rest eczema due to E. Indian rosewood (*Dalbergia latifolia* Roxbg.). *Contact Dermatitis* **8**: 77–8.

Heyl U. (1966) Kontakt ekzem bei Überempfindlichkeit gegen Sucupira und Palisanderholz. *Berufsdermatosen* **14**: 239–44.

Irvine C., Reynolds A. & Finlay A.Y. (1988) Erythema multiforme-like reaction to 'rosewood'. *Contact Dermatitis* **19**: 224–5.

Jemec G.B.E. & Hausen B.M. (1991) Contact dermatitis from Brazilian box tree wood (*Aspidosperma* sp.). *Contact Dermatitis* **25**: 58–60.

Siregar R.S. (1975) Occupational dermatoses among foresters. *Contact Dermatitis* **1**: 33.

Wills J.H. (1982) Nasal cancer in woodworkers: a review. *Journal of Occupational Medicine* **24**: 526–30.

Woods B. (1982) Contact dermatitis from Santos rosewood. *Contact Dermatitis* **17**: 249–50.

Woods B. & Calnan C.D. (1976) Toxic woods. *British Journal of Dermatology* **95** (Suppl. 13): 1–97.

8 Epilogue

8.1 Therapeutic uses of some plant products in dermatology

Inevitably, the previous chapters convey a negative impression of the effects of plants on the skin. It should be noted that relatively few plants are frequent causes of allergic contact dermatitis. Irritant reactions, although commoner, are often trivial. With sensible precautions, phototoxic reactions can be avoided or exploited therapeutically, as in PUVA (see p. 64). Humans, like other mammals, depend on the plant kingdom directly or indirectly as a source of food. In addition, even apparently primitive societies have developed sophisticated knowledge of the pharmacological properties of the plants which surround them. The current popularity of 'natural' medicines has tended to overshadow the fact that many conventional medicines are derived from plants. The cardiac glycoside digoxin is a classical example; although derived from foxglove (*Digitalis* spp.) the dosage of the purified drug is easier to control than crushed leaves of the plant.

Relatively few plant products are used in orthodox dermatological practice although 'alternative' practitioners, including homoeopaths and naturopaths, employ a much wider range. Several naturally derived fragrant and emollient oils are used by aromatherapists. Coconut oil forms the basis of many pomades used on scalp psoriasis and seborrhoeic dermatitis. It liquefies at body temperature, enhancing the penetration of keratolytics and other substances. Arachis oil and olive oil are used by nurses to reduce 'dry skin' particularly in the elderly.

Evening primrose oil is particularly rich in unsaturated fatty acids, notably gamma-linolenic acid. When taken orally it has been shown to reduce pruritus and other features of atopic eczema. It appears to be effective in only a proportion of individuals and may perhaps select for those with an inherent abnormality of fatty acid metabolism; it is derived from the seed oil of varieties of *Oenothera biennis* (Fig. 8.1.1). Although popularly termed 'evening primrose', the plant is botanically unrelated to *Primula*, being a member of the fuchsia family (Onagraeeae). It does *not* contain quinones such as primin.

Synthetic pyrethroids, related to the natural insecticide Pyrethrum (see p. 177) are valuable in the eradication of scabies and lice. Tea tree oil, derived from *Melaleuca alternifolia*, has antimicrobial effects and has been used successfully in the treatment of acne (see p. 139).

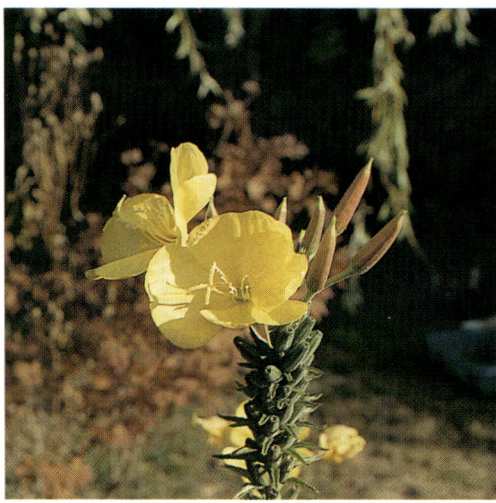

Fig. 8.1.1 *Oenothera biennis* (evening primrose).

The allergenic properties of plants can occasionally be put to good use. Induction of allergic contact dermatitis may stimulate regrowth of hair in patients with alopecia areata. The leaf of *Primula obconica* has been used with success, although a more rarely encountered allergen is generally favoured.

The irritant chemical constituents of several plants are used therapeutically. Thus the rhizomes of the American May apple (*Podophyllum peltatum*) (Fig. 8.1.2) and the allied Indian species, *P. emodi*, contain an irritant resin which includes C18 lignans such as podophyllotoxin and B-peltatin. Podophyllotoxin inhibits cell division in metaphase and induces epidermal necrosis. It has proved invaluable in the treatment of genital warts. Etoposide, a semi-synthetic derivative, arrests the cell cycle in carcinomata; it shows promise in the treatment of some leukaemias with cutaneous involvement and in histiocytosis X.

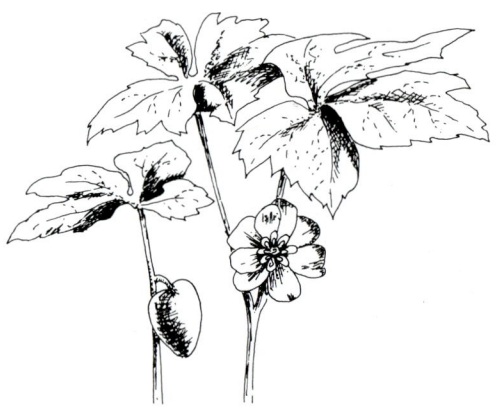

Fig. 8.1.2 *Podophyllum peltatum* (May apple).

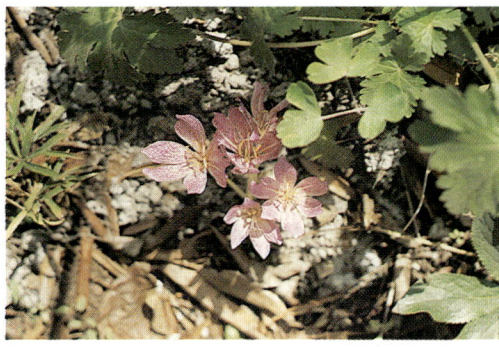

Fig. 8.1.3 *Colchicum bivonae*, an attractive species from Greece.

Colchicine is an alkaloid derived from *Colchicum* species (Fig. 8.1.3) (so called 'autumn crocus'). Although it has an antimitotic action when applied topically it is chiefly administered systemically. It has been used in the treatment of gout since ancient times, although highly toxic in overdose (Dioscorides states that 'it killeth by choking like to ye mushrumps') it has stood the test of time as a relatively safe drug in therapeutic doses. Colchicine suppresses polymorph chemotaxis, hence its use in gout. In dermatological practice it is used chiefly in Behçet's syndrome although it may also be of value in pustular psoriasis, Sweet's syndrome and leucocytoclastic vasculitis. Colchicine may also inhibit excess collagen deposition in systemic sclerosis and related syndromes.

A basic tenet of herbal medicine is that the selection of herbs should be flexible, blended for an individual patient and varied at different stages of the disease. A combination of herbs may have a synergistic effect greater than its constituents. Scientific assessment of

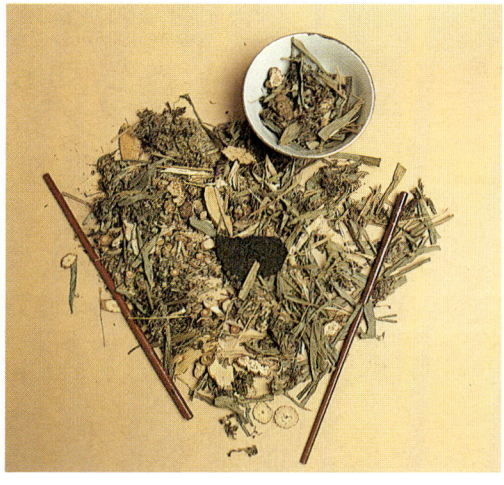

Fig. 8.1.4 Chinese herbs.

this type of therapy is therefore fraught with difficulties! In spite of this, a recent study of a specific mixture of traditional Chinese plants (Fig. 8.1.4) indicates a beneficial role in a sub-group of children with atopic eczema. Further studies are needed to exclude toxicity and to confirm these encouraging results.

Even today, new plant species await discovery, not only in tropical rainforests but also in relatively accessible regions such as Europe. Sadly several species are already extinct through human intervention. The therapeutic potential of the plant kingdom is great, and has only been realized in part. For this reason, if for no other, it is essential that we respect and preserve the habitats of the wealth of plants remaining on this planet.

Index

Page numbers in bold type indicate the principal reference

abietic acid, 239
Acacia species, 136
Aceraceae, 135
acetylcholine, 30
10-acetoxy-8, 9-epoxy-thymolisobutyrate, 155
Achillea millefolium, 84, **151–2**
acne, cosmetic-induced, 22
Acokanthera species, 188
actinomycosis, 49
Aeschynanthus pulcher, 195
Aesculus hippocastanum, 18, **135**
aftershaves, 16
Agave species, 216
  A. americana, 36, 216
  irritant chemicals in, 53
agricultural workers, 6–15
agrimony (*Agrimonia eupatoria*), 52, 86
airborne dermatitis
  to chrysanthemum, 162
  to dahlia, 161
  to feverfew, 178
  to marigold, 176
  to ragweed, 152–3
  to stinkwort, 164
  to sunflower, 166
  to wormwood, 156
alantolactone, 96, 159, **168**, 173, 199
alfalfa, 36
algae
  delayed hypersensitivity, 121–2
  lichens and, 122
  type I hypersensitivity, 36
Allamanda species, 188
allergic contact dermatitis, 96–254
  mechanisms, 96–7
  occupational, 6–13
  patch testing, 97–101
  photoallergies, 64, **75**
  plant extract preparation, 101–5
  to Aceraceae, 135
  to Agavaceae, 216
  to algae, 121–2
  to Alliaceae, 217–19
  to Aloeaceae, 215–16
  to Alstroemeriaceae, 222–4
  to Amaryllidaceae, 220–2
  to Anacardiaceae, 106–21
  to Annonaceae, 127
  to Apocyanaceae, 188
  to Araceae, 228–31
  to Araliaceae, 143–6
  to Arecaceae *see* allergic contact dermatitis to Palmae
  to Asclepiadaceae, 188–9
  to Asparagaceae, 216
  to Asteraceae *see* contact dermatitis to Compositae
  to Begoniaceae, 141
  to Brassicaceae (Cruciferae), 9, **128–9**
  to Burseraceae, 134
  to Buxaceae, 207
  to Cannabaceae, 207
  to Capparidaceae, 129–30
  to Caryophyllaceae, 130–1
  to Cistaceae, 130
  to citrus fruits, 11, **133–4**
  to Commelinaceae, 227
  to Compositae (Asteraceae), 7, **147–81**
  to conifers, 8–9, **235–46**
  to Cruciferae *see* allergic contact dermatitis to Brassicaceae
  to Cupuliferae *see* allergic contact dermatitis to Fagaceae
  to Dioscoraceae, 214–15
  to Ericaceae, 181–2
  to Euphorbiaceae, 205–7
  to Fagaceae (Cupuliferae), 208
  to ferns, 234–5
  to fragrance materials, 20
  to Geraniaceae, 132
  to Gesneriaceae, 195–6
  to Ginkgoaceae, 233–4
  to Gramineae (Poaceae), 229, **232–3**
  to Hamamelidaceae, 138
  to hardwoods, 246–54
  to Hippocastanaceae, 135
  to Hyacinthaceae, 217
  to Hydrangeaceae, 137–8
  to Hydrophyllaceae, 189–91
  to Illiciaceae, 127
  to Jubulaceae (liverworts), 7, **125–6**
  to Juglandaceae, 208
  to Labiatae (Lamiaceae), 196–200
  to Lauraceae, 201–3
  to Lecythidaceae, 141
  to Leguminosae, 136–7
  to lichens, 7, **122–5**
  to Liliaceae, 224–5
  to Linaceae, 131
  to Liverworts *see* allergic contact dermatitis to Jubulaceae
  to Lythraceae, 141
  to Magnoliaceae, **126–7**, 149
  to Malvaceae, 131
  to Myristicaceae, 200–1
  to Myrtaceae, 139–41
  to Oleaceae, 186–8
  to Orchidaceae, 210–13
  to Palmae (Arecaceae), 227
  to Papaveraceae, 127–8
  to Pedaliaceae, 196
  to Poaceae *see* allergic contact dermatitis to Gramineae

259

to Polygonaceae, 200
to Primulaceae, 182–5
to Proteaceae, 11, **203–4**
to Rubiaceae, 146–7
to Rutaceae, 11, **133–4**
to Salicaceae, 208–9
to Santalaceae, 204–5
to Saxifragaceae, 137
to Scrophulariaceae, 194–5
to Solanaceae, 191–4
to Styraceae, 185–6
to Umbellifereae, 142–3
to Vitaceae, 134
to Zingiberaceae, 213–14
to Zygophyllaceae, 132
allicin, 219
Allium species, 9, **217–19**
allylisothiocyanate, 128
almond nut, 36
Aloe species, 215–16
alpha-terthienyl, 65, 73
Alpinia species, 213
Alstroemeria sensitivity, 222–4
  occupational exposure, 7–8, 222
  protective gloves and, 13
Althea species, 131
amaranth feathers (*Humea elegans*), 167
Amaryllidaceae, 219–21
ambary plant (*Hibiscus cannabinus*), 131
Ambrosia species, 152–3
  A. acanthicarpa, 165
Ammi majus, 64, 69, 70, **89**
amylcinnamaldehyde, 20, 98, 186
Anacardiaceae sensitization, 8, **106–21**
  see also poison ivy/poison oak dermatitis
Ananas comosus see pineapple
anaphylactoid reactions, **38–9**
Anemone species, 58
anethole, 127
Anethum graveolens, 89
Angelica species, 64, 67
  delayed hypersensitivity, 142
  phototoxic reactions, 64, 67, 89
angelicins, 69, 93
angel's tears (*Narcissus triandus*), 221
animals, phototoxic reactions in, 65, 83–4
aniseed, 127, 142
Annonaceae, 127
anthecotulide, 153
Anthemis species, 171
  A. arvensis, **153**, 171
  A. cotula, 52, 86, **153–4**, 171
  A. nobilis, 157–8
anthraquinones in *Aloe*, 216
Anthriscus sylvestris, 83, 86–7
Apium graveolens see celery
Apocyanaceae, 188
apple mint (*Mentha rotundifolia*), 198
apples, 36, 39
apricots, 22, 36
Aracae
  delayed hypersensitivity, 228–31
  irritant properties, 53, 54, 56
arachis oil, 255
Arachniodes adiantiformis, 234–5
Araliacae, 143–6
arbusculin-A, 179

Arctotheca calendula, 154
Arctium lappa, 52
Arecaceae, 227
Arnica species, 154–5
Aroids
  delayed hypersensitivity, 228–31
  irritant properties, 53, 54, 56
aromatherapy, 19, 255
arteglasin A, 162
Artemisia species, 156
artichoke (globe), 160–1
arum lily (*Zantedeschia aethiopica*), 228, 231
Asclepiadaceae, 188–9
asiatic acid, 143
asiaticoside, 143
asparagus, 216
Aspidiaceae, 234–5
Asteraceae *see* Compositae
atranorin, 98, **122–3**
Atropa belladona, 191–2
atropine, 191–2
autumn crocus, 59, 99, **256–8**
azathioprine, use in Compositae dermatitis, 149, 173

bachelor's buttons (*Tanacetum parthenium*), 148, **172–3**
ball everlasting (*Helichrysum diosmifolium*), 167
balsam of Peru, 20, 36, **136–7**
  contact urticaria, 137
balsam of Tolu, 136–7
bamboo, 232
banana, 36
barberry (*Berberis* species), 49
barley
  actinomycosis lesions, 49
  mechanical irritation, 46
  sensitization to, 10, 36
barrier creams
  in dermatitis prevention, 13
  in poison ivy/oak prevention, 118
  sensitivity to, 16
bathurst burr (*Xanthium spinosum*), 181
bavachee (*Psoralea corylifolia*), 67, 91, 136
bay leaves (*Laurus nobilis*), 149, **202–3**
beach apple (*Hippomane mancinella*), 60–1
beans, 36
bee glue (propolis), 208–9
beggars' ticks, 52, 86
Begonia species, 141
benzylisothiocyanate, 129
Berberis species, 49
bergamot oil, 69, 83, 133
bergapten, 72, 75, 93
berlock (breloque) dermatitis, 22, 65, **83–4**
Bertholletia excelsa (brazil nut), 36, 141
Betula verrucosa, 36
Bhilawa (marking nut tree), 113
bindii (*Soliva pterosperma*), 46, 175
bindweed (*Convolvulus arvensis*), 86
birch (*Betula verrucosa*), 36
  pollen cross-reactivity, 39
bishop's weed (*Ammi majus*), 64, 69, 70, **89**
bithienyl, 176
bitterweed, 165–6
black bryony (*Tamus communis*), 215
black mustard (*Brassica nigra*), 52, 86, **128–9**
black nightshade, 191

black-eyed Susan (*Rudbeckia hirta*), 174
blackberries, 49
blackthorn (*Prunus spinosus*), 48
blackwood, 136, 253
blanket flower (*Gaillardia*), 165
blazing star (*Liatris spicata*), 170
bleeding heart (*Dicentra spectabilis*), 127
blessed thistle (*Cnicus benedictus*), 160
blister bush (*Peucedanum galbanum*), 90
blister plant (*Phlebalium argentuem*), 91
bloodtwig dogwood (*Cornus sanguineus*), 36
Blumea gariepina, 36
Blumenbachia species, 32
Boraginaceae, 43
borneol, 213, 214
Boswellia species, 134
Bougainvillaea species, 36
box elder (*Acer negundo*), 135
boxtree (*Buxus sempervirens*), 53
Brassicaceae (Cruciferae)
   B. nigra (black mustard), 52, 86, **128–9**
   B. oleracea (cauliflower), 9, 36, **129**
   chemical irritants, 52, 59
   delayed hypersensitivity, 9, **128–9**
   Raphanus sativus (radish), 52, 129
brazil nut
   contact urticaria, 36
   delayed sensitivity, 141
Brazilian pepper tree, 114
breloque dermatitis, 22, 65, 83–4
bromelin, 53, 56
bryony, 215
buckwheat, 65, 200
buffalo bean, 52
bulbs, irritant dermatitis, 55–6
   Narcissus species, 220–1
   Tulipa species, 224–5
burdock (*Arctium lappa*), 52
burnet saxifrage, 91
burning bush (*Dictamnus albus*), 70, 81, 91, **93**
Burseraceae, 134
buttercup family *see* Ranunculaceae
Buxaceae, 207
Buxus sempervirens, 53

cabbage, 36
cacti
   irritant crystals, 54
   spines and hooks, 46–8
cajuput oil, 139
caladium, 230
calcium oxalate crystals, 42–3, 53, **54–6**
Calendula species, 156
   in cosmetics, 18
   in herbal ointments, 147
Californian bluebell (*Phacelia*), 189
Calomeria amaranthoides, 167
Calotropis species, 52, 188
Cananga odorata, 127
Canary date palm, 48
cane pepper, 192
Cannabaceae, 207
   C. indica, 36, **207**
cape primrose (*Streptocarpus* species), 195–6
caper bush (*Capparis spinosa*), 129–30
capeweed (*Arctotheca calendula*), 154
Capparidaceae, 129–30

capsaicin, 52, **59**, 192
Capsicum species, 36, 52, **192**
caraway (*Carum carvi*), 36, 142
cardamom (*Elletaria cardoma*), 213–14
△-3-carene, 153
carnations, 130–1
carnauba wax, 133
carotene, 133
carrot weed (*Parthenium hysterophorus*), 148, **172–3**
carrots, 87
   delayed hypersensitivity, 143
   phototoxic reactions, 86, 89
   type I hypersensitivity, 36
carthamin, 157
Carthamnus tinctorius, 157
Carum carvi, 142
carvacrol, 200
D-carvone, 40
L-carvone, 199
Caryophyllaceae, 130–1
Caryota mitis, 55
cashew nut tree, 112
   cashew nut shell oil, 8
   cashew nut workers, 8, 112
   poison ivy dermatitis and, 110–11
cassia (*Cinnamomum cassia*), 201–2
castor oil plant (*Ricinus communis*), 36, 39, 206–7
caterpillars (irritant), 2
cauliflower
   dermatitis, 9, 129
   type I hypersensitivity, 36
cayenne, 192
cedar poisoning, 123
celandine (*Ranunculus ficaria*), 59
celery (*Apium graveolens*)
   celery harvesters, 10, 87
   delayed hypersensitivity, 142
   distribution, 89
   phototoxic reactions, 69, 70, 80–1, 84, 87
   type I hypersensitivity, 36
cement sensitivity, 2
Centella asiatica, 143
century plant (*Agave americana*), 53, **216**
Cephaelis ipecacuanha, 146
Cephalocereus senilis, 54
cereals, 10
   mechanical irritation, 46
   type I hypersensitivity, 36
Cetraria species, 124
Chamaemelum nobile, 157–8
chamomiles, 171
   chamomile lawns, 157
   corn chamomile, **153**, 171
   field chamomile, **153**
   German chamomile, **170–1**
   stinking chamomile, **153**
   sweet chamomile, **157–8**, 171
   wild chamomile, **170–1**
chefs *see* food handlers
chemical plant irritants, 50–63
   see also contact urticaria
cherry pepper, 192
chervil (*Anthriscus* species), 89
chick peas, 36
chicory (*Cichorium intybus*), 9, 52, **158–9**
child abuse, phototoxicity misdiagnosed as, 81
chili peppers, 59, **192**

Chimaphila species, 181
chimaphilin, 181
chives
    delayed hypersensitivity, 9, 218, 219
    type I hypersensitivity, 36
Chlorella (algae), 122
chlorochrymorin, 163
chlorophorin, 247
Christmas trees, 9, 237
chrysanthemum (*X. Dendranthema*), 147, 158, **161–4**, 169
    C. cinerariifolium, 177
    C. coronarium, 158
    C. leucanthemum, 158, **169**
    C. parthenium, 178
    C. segetum, 158
    contact urticaria, 162
    delayed hypersensitivity, 158, **161–4**
    occupational exposure, 7, 147, 162
    sensitivity screening, 99
Cichorium species, 158–60
    C. endivia (endive), 159–60
    C. intybus (chicory), 9; 52, **158–9**
    C. intybus var. *foliosum*, 9
cigar/cigarette workers, 10, **193–4**, 199
Cinchona species, 146
cinnamic acid, 136
cinnamic alcohol, 20, 98
cinnamic aldehyde, 20, 98, **201**
Cinnamomum species, 201–2
cinnamon (*Cinnamomum zeylanicum*), 36, **201–2**
Cistaceae, 130
citral, 213
citronellal, 213, **233**
Citrus species
    C. aurantifolia, 92
    C. aurantium, 133
    C. bergamia, 69, 70, 83
    C. deliciosa, 133
    C. limon, 36, 91, 133
    C. paradisi, 133
    C. sinensis, 133
    citrus oil extraction, 19
    delayed hypersensitivity, 11, 133–4
    phototoxic reactions, 69, 70, 91–2
    type I hypersensitivity, 36
Cladonia species
    C. alpestris, 7
    delayed sensitivity, 123, 124
    occupational dermatitis, 7, 123
classification of plants, **23–8**, 121
    poison ivy/oak confusion, 106–7
Clematis species, 52, 58
Clostridium tetani infection, 48
clotbur, 181
cnicin, 160
Cnicus benedictus, 160
CNSO (cashew nut shell oil), 8
coast daisy bush (*Olearia axillaris*), 171
cocklebur (*Xanthium strumarium*), 181
cocobolo, 136
coconut, 227–8
coconut oils
    in cosmetics, 17
    therapeutic uses, 227, 255
Codiaeum variegatum, 8
Coffea species, 146

coffee
    delayed hypersensitivity, 146
    type I hypersensitivity, 36
colchicine, 59, 99, **256–8**
Coleon O, 197
Coleus species, 197
collection of plant material, 25–6
Collins Pocket Guide to Wild Flowers, The (McClintock & Fitter 1965), 27
cologne water, 19, 65, 83
colophony, 8, 236, **238–42**
comfrey (*Symphytum officinale*), 43
Commelinacaeae, 227
Compositae (Asteraceae)
    allergen extraction, 102
    chemical irritants, 52, 86, **147–8**
    contact urticaria, 148
    delayed hypersensitivity, 7, **147–81**
    dermatitis screening test, 98–9
    dermatitis treatment, 149–50
    patch testing, 149
    photosensitization, 74–5, 148
    taxonomy, 121
    see also under individual plant
Concise British Flora in Colour, The (Keble Martin 1965), 27
coneflower (*Rudbeckia hirta*), 174
congress grass (*Parthenium hysterophorus*), 148, 172–3
conifer allergy, 8–9, 235–46
Conservation of Wild Creatures and Wild Plants Act (1975), 25
contact dermatitis *see* allergic contact dermatitis; irritant contact dermatitis
contact urticaria, 29–35
    immunological, 29, **35–41**
    occupational exposure, 11
    to chrysanthemum, 162
    to Compositae, 148
    to fragrance materials, 20, 137
Convolvulus arvensis, 86
Conyza bonariensis, 160
Copernicia cerifera, 18
copperweed (*Oxytaenia acerosa*), 171
coriander
    delayed hypersensitivity, 142
    type I hypersensitivity, 36
corn chamomile (*Anthemis arvensis*), 153
Cornus species
    C. sanguineus, 36
    mechanical irritants, 46
corticosteroid therapy, 117, 149, 173
cosmetics, 15–22, 206
    checklist, 4
    type I hypersensitivity, 36
costunolide, 174, **203**
costus root, 174–5
Cotoneaster species, 36
cotton (*Gossypium* species), 36, 131
cow parsley (*Anthriscus sylvestris*), 83, 86–7, 90
cow parsnip (*Heracleum sphondylium*), 11, 70, 83, 87, 90
cowhage (*Mucuna pruriens*), 52, 136
Crataegus monogyna, 36
creosote bush (*Larrea tridentata*), 132
creosote plant (*Dictamnus albus*), 70, 81, 91
crimson shower (*Humea elegans*), 167

crocuses
    autumn crocus (*Colchicum*), 59, 99, 256–8
    Prairie (*Pulsatilla patens*), 52, 58
cross-sensitivity, 100
    testing for, 38
Croton, 8
croton (*Codiaeum variegatum*), 8, 205
crown flower (*Calotropis gigantea*), 52, 188
Cruciferae *see* Brassicaceae
Cryptocarya pleurosperma, 53
cryptopleurine, 53
Cryptostegia species, 188
Cryptostemma, 154
crystals (irritant), 54–6
cucumber, 36
cumin, 89
Cupressaceae, 242–5
    C. leylandii, 9, **243–5**
Cupuliferae, 208
Curcuma longa, 213
curcumin, 213
Cyclamen persicum, 185
Cymbidium species, 211
Cymbopogon species, 232–3
Cymopterus watsonii, 70
Cynara scolymus, 160–1
cynaropicrin, 161
cypress, 243–5
cypripedin, 211
Cypripedium species, 210–11

daffodils
    daffodil itch, 7, **220**
    delayed sensitivity, 55, **220–2**
    irritant crystals, 53, 55, 56
    occupational exposure, 7, 8
Dahlia species, 161
daisy family *see* Compositae
Dalbergia latifolia, 36
dalbergiones, 184, 247–9
dandelion (*Taraxacum officinale*), 179–81
daphnane orthoesters, 62
date palms, 48
Daucus carota see carrots
De materia medica libri quinque (Dioscorides), 5
2-deacetoxyxanthinin, 164
deadly nightshade (*Atropa belladona*), 191–2
death
    due to anaphylaxis, 38
    from *Dendrocnide cordata*, 34
    from dumb cane (*Dieffenbachia*), 54
    from *Nerium oleander*, 188
    from *Parthenium hysterophorus*, 172
    from *Urtica ferox*, 32
debbeltje, 65
debromoaplysiatoxin, 121
dehydroabietic acid, 239
dehydrocostus lactone, 174
Dendrocnide species, 32–4
deodorants, 16
desacetyl laurenobiolide, 203
desacetyl matricarin, 171
desensitization
    to poison ivy/oak, 118–19
    see also hyposensitization
desert heliotrope, 189
devil's ivy, **228–9**, 231

dhobie mark dermatitis, 113
diallydisulphide, 219
Dianthus caryophyllus, 130–1
Dicentra spectabilis, 127
Dictamnus albus, 70, 81, 91, 93
didehydrofalcarinol, 145
Dieffenbachia, 9, 228, 230
    irritant crystals, 53, 54, 56
diethylstilboestrol, 237
Digitalis purpurea, 195
digoxin, 195
dill (*Anethum graveolens*)
    delayed sensitivity, 142
    phototoxic reactions, 89
    type I hypersensitivity, 36
2,6-dimethoxy-1,4-benzoquinone, 196, **211**
dimethoxygeranyl benzoquinone, 191
1,1-dimethylallyl-caffeic acid ester, 209
Dioscoraceae, 214–15
    D. batatas, 214
Dioscorides (Greek physician), 5
    on Euphorbiaceae, 59
    on fig tree, 94
    on garden rue, 92
    on gum storax, 185
    on *Nerium oleander*, 188
    on pitch, 238
diterpene (diphorbol) esters, 205
Dittrichia viscosa, 164–5
dock leaves, 32
dog fennel (*Anthemis cotula*), 52, 86, **153–4**, 171
Dogger bank itch, 121
dogwoods (*Cornus* species), 46
drying of plants, 26
Dryopteridaceae, 234–5
dumb cane (*Dieffenbachia*), 9, 53, **54**, 230

eau de cologne, 19, 65, 83
Echium species, 43
eczema (childhood), 12
elecampane, 167
elephant's ears, 230
Elletaria cardoma, 213–14
emollient creams, 13
endive (*Cichorium endivia*), 9, 36, 159–60
English ivy, 143–5
English marigold (*Calendula officinalis*), 18, 147, 156
English Names of Wild Flowers (Dony, Perring & Rob 1980), 24
Englishman's Flora, The (Grigson 1975), 24
Epipremnum pinnatum, **228–9**, 231
Equisetum arvense, 36
Ericaceae, 181–2
Erigeron bonariensis, 160
Erwinia carotovora (bacterium), 10
escarole (*Cichorium intybus*), 9, 52, **158–9**
esculin, 135
essential oils *see* oils
etoposide, 256
Eucalyptus species, 36, 139–40
eugenol, 20, 98, 131, **140**, 201
Euphorbiaceae
    chemical irritants, 59–62
    Codiaeum, 205
    delayed sensitivity, 205–7
    E. marginata, 9
    E. pulcherrima, 205–6

stinging (urticating) hairs, 31
evening primrose oil, 255
'everlasting' flowers
    Helichrysum species, 166–7
    Ixodia species, 168
Evernia prunastri (lichen), 123, 124
evernic acid, 122–3
'Expert' series (Hessayon), 27
extract (plant) preparation, 101–5
eye problems
    due to crown flower, 188
    due to dumb cane (*Dieffenbachia*), 54
    due to *Euphorbia tirucalli*, 60
    due to *Grevillea robusta*, 203
eye-shadows, 16

Fagaceae, 208
Fagara xanthoxyloides, 69, 70
Fagopyron species, 65, 200
falcarinol, 102, 143–5
falcarinone, 145
false ragweed, 165
farnesylhyroquinone, 190
fatal reactions *see* death
fennel, 89, 142
9-(11)-fernen, 235
ferns, 234–5
feverfew (*Parthenium hysterophorus*), 148, **172–3**
feverfew (*Tanacetum parthenium*), 147, 178
field mayweed/chamomile (*Anthemis arvensis*),
    153, 171
fig plant (*Ficus carica*), 64, 70–1, 91, **94**
fishtail palm (*Caryota mitis*), 55
flamingo plant, 230
flax (*Linum usitatissimum*), 36, **131**
fleabane (*Conyza bonariensis*), 160
Flora of the British Isles (Clapham, Tutin & Moore
    1987), 27
Florida holly, 114
florists/floristry, 1, 4, **6–15**
    Alstroemeria dermatitis, 222–3
    daffodil dermatitis, 55
Flower Expert, The (Hessayon), 27
flower petals, oil extraction from, 19
Foeniculum vulgare, 89, 142
folliculitis, cosmetic-induced, 22
food handlers, 1, 4, 9
    atopic history, 39
    protein contact dermatitis, 11, 29, 35, 36, **38**
forestry workers *see* woodworkers/forestry workers
forget-me-not (*Myosotis* species), 43
foxglove (*Digitalis purpurea*), 195
fragrance materials, 19–22
    see also perfumes
fragrance mix, 19–20, 98
Franseria acanthicarpa, 165
friars balsam, 185
fruit handlers, 11, 36
fruit salad plant, 231
Frullania species, 7, **125–6**, 149
    lichen allergy and, 123
frullanolide 125–6
fumarprotecetraric acid, 123
fungal sensitivity, 2
    phototoxicity and, 69
    Sclerotinia sclerotiorum, 10, 69, 86
    Septoria apii, 10

see also lichens
furocoumarins (psoralens), 10, 21–2, 65, **66–78**

Gaillardia species, 165
galangal, 213
Galium aparine, 44
garden rue *see* rue
Gardeners Encyclopedia of Plants and Flowers, 27
Gardenia jasminoides, 146
gardening, 1
    professional gardeners, 1, **6–15**
    see also weeds/weeding
garlands
    of *Cananga odorata*, 127
    of crown flower, 188
    of *Grevillea*, 203
    of jasmine, 186
    of *Pelea anisata*, 80, 82
garlic
    delayed sensitivity, 9, **217–19**
    type I hypersensitivity, 36
gas plant (*Dictamnus albus*), 70, 81, 91, **93**
geeldikkop, 65
Geraea viscida, 165
Geraniaceae, 132–3
geraniol, 20, 98, 127, **132–3**, 198
geranium, 132–3
geranyl geranylhydroquinone, 190
geranyl hydroquinone 189–90
Gerard's herbal, 2, 5, 178
Gesneriaceae, 195–6
giant hogweed (*Heracleum mantegazzianum*)
    distribution, 90
    furocoumarins in, 69
    phototoxicity, 10, 70, 80–1, 87
    strimmer dermatitis, 83
ginger (*Zingiber officinale*), 214
gingerol, 214
gingkolic acid *see* ginkgolic acid
Ginkgoaceae
    delayed hypersensitivity, 233–4
    Ginkgo tree, 114
    poison ivy cross-reactivity, 114
ginkgolic acid, 100, **234**
Girardinia species, 30
globe artichoke (*Cynara scolymus*), 160–1
glochids as mechanical irritants, 46–9
gloves
    protective, 12–13
    sensitivity to, 1–2, 13, 39
glucocapparin, 129
golden rod (*Solidago* species), 175
Goodyer, John, 5
goosegrass (*Galium aparine*), 44
gordolobo, 194
Gossypium species, 36, 131
Gramineae *see* grasses
grape vine (*Vitis vinifera*), 134
grapefruit
    delayed hypersensitivity, 133
    phototoxic reactions, 91
    type I hypersensitivity, 36
grasses
    animal disorders due to, 65
    delayed hypersensitivity, 229, **232–3**
    type I hypersensitivity, 36
green pepper, 36

Grevillea species, 203–4
  G. juniperifolia, 36
  Robyn Gordon cultivar, 114, **204**
grevillol, 247
guayulins A and B, 171
gum arabic, 136
gum rosin (colophony), 238–42
gum trees (*Eucalyptus* species), 36

hair colourants/styling agents, 16, 22, 38, 141
hairs as mechanical irritants, 43–6
Hakea suaveolens, 36
halva (ground sesame), 196
Hamamelidaceae, 138
hardwoods (allergenic), 246–54
hawthorn (*Crataegus monogyna*), 36
hazelnuts, 36
heather (*Erica* species), 181
Hedera species
  allergen extraction, 102, 145
  delayed sensitivity, 143–5
helenalin, 155
Helenium species, 165–6
Helianthus species
  H. annuus, 166
  H. tuberosus, 160
Helichrysum diosmifolium, 166–7
Helleborus species, 52
hemp (*Cannabis indica*), 36
henna (*Lawsonia inermis*)
  delayed hypersensitivity, 141
  type I hypersensitivity, 22, 36, 38
5-heptadecatri-8(Z), 11(Z), 14(Z)-enylresorcinol, 229
Heracleum species, 90
  H. laciniatum, 70, 75, 82, 90
  H. mantegazzianum see giant hogweed
  H. sphondylium, 11, 83, 87, 90
herbalism/herbal medicine, 17, 67, 239, 255, 257
  Angelica leaves, 64
  feverfew, 178
  mullein, 194
  pot marigold, 156
  tansy, 179
herbals, 2, 5
  see also Dioscorides; Gerard
herbs
  checklist, 3
  type I hypersensitivity, 36
  see also specific type
Hevea brasiliensis, 36
Hibiscus species, 131
hightaper, 194
Hippocastanaceae, 135
Hippomane species, 60–2
histamine 30–31, 35
hives see urticaria
hogweed see giant hogweed; *Heracleum* species
hollyhock (*Althea* species), 131
homolycorin, 221
Hooker's gaertneria, 165
hooks as mechanical irritants, 43–6
hoop-petticoat, 220, 221
hop (*Humulus lupulus*), 36, 207
hop tree (*Ptelea* species), 91
horse chestnut (*Aesculus hippocastanum*), 18, 135
horseradish, 59
horsetails, 36

horseweed (*Conyza bonariensis*), 160
hortensia (*Hydrangea macrophylla*), 137–8
horticultural workers, 6–15
hound's tongue (*Cynoglossum* species), 43
House Plant Expert, The (Hessayon), 27
Hoya carnosa, 188–9
Humea elegans, 167
humulone, 207
Humulus lupulus, 36, **207**
hyacinths, 217
  irritant crystals, 53, 55
hydrangea, 137–8
hydrangenol, 138
hydroabietyl alcohol, 240
Hydrocotyle asiatica, 143
15-hydroperoxyabietic acid, 239
Hydrophyllaceae, 189–91
  stinging (urticating) hairs, **31–2**, 189
hydroxycitronellal, 20, 98
5-hydroxytryptamine, 30
hymenin, 173
hyoscine, 191–2
hypericin, 65
Hypericum species, 65, 84
hypersensitivity reactions
  delayed see allergic contact dermatitis *and* specific allergens
  immunological contact urticaria, 29, 35–41
Hypogymnia physodes, 124
hyposensitization
  dangers of, 13
  oral, 97, 149–50, 173
  to *Frullania*, 126
  to *Parthenium hysterophorus*, 173
  to urushiol, 118–19
  in weed dermatitis, **149–50**, 173

icterogenic acid, 65
identification of plants, 23–8
Illiciaceae, 127
immunological contact urticaria, 29, 35–41
imperatorin, 70
incense, 134
incense bush (*Humea elegans*), 167
Indian hemp (*Cannabis*), 36, 207
Indian rosewood (*Dalbergia latifolia*), 36
insects
  CNSO sensitivity and insecticides, 8
  insect repellants, 81, 93
  irritant insects, 2
Inula species, 164–5, 167–8
inuviscolide, 164
ipecacuanha powder, 146
Iris species, 36, 226–7
irritant contact dermatitis, 42–63
  chemical irritants, 50–63
  mechanical irritants, 43–50
  occupational, 6–13
  see also contact urticaria
isobergapten, 71, 75
isoeugenol, 20, **141**
isopimpinellin, 71
isopsoralen, 71
isothiocyanates, 128–9
IVA xanthifolia, 168
ivy (*Hedera* species)
  allergen extraction, 102, 145

delayed sensitivity, 143–5
ivy (*Toxicodendron radicans*) *see* poison ivy dermatitis
Ixodia achillaeoides, 168

Jackman's blue, 92
Japanese lacquer tree (*Rhus/Toxicodendron verniciflua*), 8, 112
jasmine (*Jasminum officinale*), 186–7
jasmine tea, 146
Jerusalem artichoke, 160
jo-jo (*Soliva pterosperma*), 46, **175**
jojoba oil, 207
jonquils, 220–1
   irritant crystals, 53
   jonquil handlers, 7
Jubulaceae (liverworts), 7, 123, **125–6**, 149
Juglans species, 208
junipers, 242

kahili flower, 203
Kamillosan, 158
khaki weed (*Tagetes minuta*), 176
khellin, 74
kiwi fruit, 35, 36
Klaber, Robert, 64
knotweeds (*Polygonum* species), 52, **200**
Kokardenblume, 165

Labiatae, 196–200
lactopicrin, 159, **169**
Lactuca sativa see lettuce
lactucin, 159, **169**
ladanum (aromatic gum), 130
lady's slipper, 210–11
Lamiaceae, 196–200
Laportea species, 32
larch (*Larix decidua*), 36
Larrea tridentata, 132
latex (irritant), 57–62
Lauraceae, 201–3
Laurus nobilis, 149, 202–3
laurenobiolide, 203
Lavatera species, 130
lavender (*Lavendula* species), 197–8
lawsone, 149
Lawsonia inermis (henna), 22, 36, 38, **141**
Lecanora species (lichens), 123, 124
Lecythidaceae, 141
leeks
   delayed hypersensitivity, 9, 218, 219
   type I hypersensitivity, 36
Leguminosae, 136–7
   see also under specific plant
leis *see* garlands
lemon-grass, 232–3
   geraniol cross-reactivity, 133
lemons
   delayed sensitivity, 133
   phototoxic reactions, 91
   type I hypersensitivity, 36
lent lily, 221
lettuce
   contact urticaria, 9, 11, **169**
   delayed hypersensitivity, 168–9
   type I hypersensitivity, 36, 169
Leucanthemum vulgare, 158, 169

Levisticum officinalis, 142
leyland cypress, 243–5
Liatris spicata, 170
lichens
   delayed hypersensitivity, 122–5
   occupational dermatitis, 7
   type I hypersensitivity, 36
Liliaceae
   delayed hypersensitivity, 224–5
   occupational dermatitis, 7
   type I hypersensitivity, 26
   see also tulips
lilies, arum, 228, 231
lily rash, 7
limba tree (*Terminalia superba*), 36
limes
   Citrus aurantifolia, 92
   Citrus bergamia, 69
   phototoxic reactions, 69, 91–2
   in shampoos, 36
   type I hypersensitivity, 36
D-limonene, 20, 127, **133**
Linaceae, 36, 131
linalool, 127, **198**
linalylacetate, 198
Linnaeus, Carl, 23–4
linseed oil plant (flax), 36, **131**
Linum usitatissimum, 36, **131**
Lippia species, 65
lipsticks, 16, 206
Liquidambar orientalis, 138
liverworts, 7, **125–6**, 149
   lichen allergy and, 123
Loasaceae
   Loasa species, 31, 32
   stinging (urticating) hairs, 31, 32
lovage, 142
ludovicins, 156
lumber *see* wood(s)
lungwort (*Pulmonaria officinalis*), 43
lupulone, 207
Lycopersicon lycopersicum see tomato plant
Lyngbya majuscula (algae), 36, **121–2**
lyngbyatoxin A, 121
Lythraceae, 141

mace (*Myristica fragrans*), 200–1
madder (*Rubia tinctoria*), 146
madecassic acid, 143
Madecassol ointment, 143
Magnoliaceae, **126–7**, 149
mahogany, 248, 253
maize, 36
Malphigia urens, 43–4
malt flour, 10
Malvaceae, 131
manchineel tree (*Hippomane mancinella*), 60–1
mandarin (*Citrus deliciosa*), 133
mangos
   delayed sensitivity, 111
   occupational exposure, 8
   type I hypersensitivity, 36, 111
maple tree (*Acer negundo*), 135
marguerite (*Leucanthemum vulgare*), 158, 169
marigolds
   pot marigold (*Calendula* species), 18, 147, 156
   Tagetes species, 176–7

marking nut tree, 113
marshelder (*Iva xanthifolia*), 168
masonin, 221
masterwort (*Peucedanum ostruthium*), 86, 90
Matricaria species, 170–1
meadow elecampane, 167
mechanical plant irritants, 43–50
medicinal uses of plants, 255–8
    Aloe species, 215–16
    Arnica species, 154–5
    autumn crocus (*Colchicum*), 59, 99, **256–8**
    chamomile, 158
    Compositae, 147
    garden rue, 92–3
    Madagascar periwinkle, 188
    Ranunculaceae, 58–9
    Rubiaceae, 146
Melaleuca species, 139
melons, 36
Mentha species, 198–9
menthol, 199
Mesonia chinensis, 199
5-methoxypsoralen, 70, 93
8-methoxypsoralen (8-MOP), 70, 73, 83, 93
1-0-methyl 1-4,5-dihydroniveusin A, 166
Mexican rubber plant, 171
milfoil (*Achillea millefolium*), 86, **151–2**
mimosa of florist (*Acacia*), 136
mint (*Mentha* species), 198–9
mite sensitivity, 2
mokihana, 82, 91
monarch of the east, 231
Monstera deliciosa, 36
mother-in-law's tongue, 53
motherwort, 156
mountain tobacco, 154
Mousse de Chene, 124
moyu (*Amorphophallus*), 230
Mucuna pruriens, 52, 136
mucunain, 52
mudarin, 52
mugwort (*Artemisia vulgaris*), 156
mullein, 194
musk ambrette, 134
mustard, 59, 86
    Brassica nigra, 52, 86
    mustard oil sensitivity, 9
    type I hypersensitivity, 36, 39
mutterkraut (*Tanacetum parthenium*), 148, **172–3**
Mycobacterium infections, 49
Myosotis species, 43
myristates, 201
Myristica fragrans, 200–1
Myroxolon species
    M. pereirae, 20, 136–7
    M. toluiferum, 136–7
Myrtaceae
    clove tree, 140–1
    delayed sensitivity, 139–40
    Eucalyptus species, 36, **139–40**
    Melaleuca species, 139

nail varnishes, 16
Narcissus species
    chemical irritants, 53
    delayed sensitivity, 220–2
    occupational exposure, 7, 8

Nephrolepis exaltata, 235
Nerium oleander, 188
nettle rash, 29, 32
niaouli oil, 139
nickel sensitivity, 2
Nicotiana tabacum, 10, 52, **193–4**
nicotine, 52, 193
nobilin, 158
nomenclature of plants, 23–8
Norway spruce, 237
nurserymen
    daffodil dermatitis, 55
    see also florists/floristry
nutmeg (*Myristica fragrans*), 200–1
nuts, type I hypersensitivity, 36

oak moss, 20, 98, 123, 124
oak (poison) *see* poison ivy/poison oak dermatitis
oak tree (*Quercus* species), 208
oat bran, 232
occupational contact dermatitis, 1–2, 6–15
    dhobie mark dermatitis, 113
    to carrots, 143
    to chicory, 158–60
    to coffee beans, 146
    to flax, 131
    to gum arabic, 136
    to lettuce, 169
    to poison ivy/poison oak, 106, 119
Oenothera biennis (evening primrose), **255–6**
oils
    arachis oil, 255
    cashew nut shell oil, 8
    castor oil, 206
    clary oil, 199
    coconut oil, 17, 227, 255
    in cosmetics, 17–22
    costus root oil, 174
    eucalyptus oil, 140
    evening primrose oil, 255
    hyacinth oil, 217
    jojoba oil, 207
    lavender oil, 198
    marigold oil, 176
    oil of anise, 142
    oil of bay, 203
    oil of Cade, 242
    oil of cardamom, 213
    oil of cassia, 201
    oil of citronella, 233
    oil of cloves, 140
    oil of lemon-grass, 233
    oil of niaouli, 139
    olive oil, 187, 255
    palm nut oil, 17
    Palmarosa oil, 233
    peppermint oil, 198
    sandalwood oil, 204–5
    sesame seed oil, 36, 196
    sunflower seed oil, 166
    Tagetes patula oil, 176
    thyme oil, 200
    turpentine oil, 241
okra, 131
ol (*Amorphophallus*), 230
old man's beard, 124
Oleaceae, 186–8

oleander (*Nerium oleander*), 188
Oleandraceae (ferns), 235
Olearia axillaris, 171
olive (*Olea europaea*), 187
onions
    delayed sensitivity, 9, **217–19**
    lachrymatory properties, 59
    type I hypersensitivity, 36
Opopanax species, 142
Opuntia species
    glochids of, 9, 46–7
    O. ficus-indica, 46–7
    O. lingularis, 48
oranges
    delayed sensitivity, 133
    type I hypersensitivity, 36
Orchidaceae, 210–13
orris root, 226
Oryza sativa, 233
osier (*Salix vimminalis*), 53
Oviedo (Spanish explorer), 61
ox-eye daisy (*Leucanthemum vulgare*), 158, 169
oxypseudanin, 73
oxytaenia acerosa, 171

palm nut oil, 17
Palmae, 227
Panicum species, 65
pao ferro, 136
Papaveraceae, 127–8
paper-bark tree, 139
paperwhite (*Narcissus papyraceus*), 221
Paphiopedilum species, 211
paprika, 192
Parmelia species (lichen), 123, 124
parsley
    delayed sensitivity, 142
    phototoxic reactions, 80–1, 87, 89
    type I hypersensitivity, 36
parsnips
    delayed sensitivity, 142
    phototoxic reactions, 70, 72, 87, 90
    type I hypersensitivity, 36
    wild parsnip phototoxicity, 81, 90
parthenin, 172–3
Parthenium species
    P. argentatum, 171
    P. hysterophorus, 148, **172–3**
    photoallergy to, 64, 173
parthenolide, 102, **178**, 179
pasque flower (*Pulsatilla vulgaris*), 52, 58
Pastinaca species *see* parsnips
patch testing, 43, 97–101
    for chrysanthemum sensitivity, 162–3
    for citrus peel sensitivity, 133
    for Compositae dermatitis, 149
    in hardwood allergy, 247
    for lichen sensitivity, 123
    in occupational cases, 11
    plant extract preparation, 101–5
    for *Primula* sensitivity, 183–4
pea family (Leguminosae), 136–7
Pedaliaceae, 196
Pelargonium species, 132–3
Pelea anisata, 82, 91
pennyroyal (*Mentha pulegium*), 198
pentadecylcatechol, 204
    see also urushiol
pentadecylresorcinol, 204
pepper (*Capsicum* species), 36, 52, 192
peppermint (*Mentha x piperita*), 198
perfumes, **15–22**, 65, 83
    balsam of Peru, 20, 136–7
    clary oil, 199
    compositae extracts and, 174
    costus root oil, 174
    geranium oil, 132–3
    jasmine, 186
    lichens and, 123, 124
    marigolds and, 176
    oak moss sensitivity, 123, 124
    oil of cardamom, 213
    oil of sandalwood, 204
    ylang ylang, 127
periwinkle (*Vinca*), 188
permethrin, 177
α-peroxyachifolide, 151
Persian lime (*Citrus aurantifolia*), 92
peruvian lily *see* Alstroemeria
pesticide sensitivity, 1
petals, oil extraction from, 19
Petroselinum crispum see parsley
Peucedanum species, 86, 90
Phacelia species, 189–91
pheasant's eye (*Narcissus poeticus*), 53, 221
phellopterin, 70
Phellopteris littoralis, 90
phenolic resins, 8
pheophorbide A, 84
Philippine red mahogany (*Shorea*), 36
Philodendron scandens, 189, **229**, 231
Phlebalium argenteum, 91
Phleum pratense, 233
photopatch testing, 100–1
phototoxicity *see* phytophototoxic reactions
phycocyanin, 121
phylloerytherin, 65
Physcia species, 124
phytoalexins, 87, 92
phytophototoxic reactions, 64–95
    in animals, 65
    clinical features, 78–85
    mechanisms of, 72–5
    occupational phytophotodermatitis, 10–11
    photopatch testing, 100–1
    plants causing, **86–95**, 148, 173
    to Compositae, 148
    to cosmetics/perfumes, 21–2
    to lichens, 123
    treatment of, 84–5
Picea species, 237–8
pick-a-back plant (*Tolmiea menziesii*), 137
pigmentation of skin
    from cosmetics/perfumes, 21
    from phototoxicity *see* phytophototoxic reactions
pimaric acid, 239–40
Pimpinella species
    P. anisum, 127, 140
    phototoxic reactions, 91
pimpinellin, 70, 72, 74
Pinaceae allergy, 8–9, **236–42**
    to pine trees, 236–7
    to spruce trees, 237–8
Pine Processionary moth, 2, 236

pineapples
    irritant crystals, 53, 56
    type I hypersensitivity, 36
pinene, 127
pipsissewa, 181
piss-a-bed (*Taraxacum officinale*), 179–81
pissenlit (*Taraxacum officinale*), 179–81
plant press, 26
Platismatia glauca, 124
Plectranthus barbatus, 197
plume bush (*Humea elegans*), 167
Plumeria species, 188
Poaceae *see* grasses
podophyllotoxin, 256
poinsettia (*Euphorbia pulcherrima*), 205–6
poison ivy/poison oak dermatitis, 1, 7, **105–21**
    clinical features, 114–16
    cross-reacting plants, 111–14
    treatment and prevention, 13, **116–19**
    versus phototoxicity, 80, 93
poison sumac, 109–10
poison walnut (*Cryptocarya pleurosperma*), 53
pollen
    of ragweed, 152–3
    of timothy grass, 233
    of wormwood, 156
polyanthus, 184
Polygonaceae, 52, 200
poplar (*Polulus* species), 208–9
pot marigold (*Calendula officinalis*), 18, 147, 156
potassium dichromate sensitivity, 1–2
potatoes, 11, 36
Pothos, 228–9, 231
pottery workers, 136
prairie crocus (*Pulsatilla patens*), 52, 58
prairie sage (*Artemisia ludoviciana*), 156
Prangos species, 91
pressing of plants, 26
prick tests, 37, 38
    to cactus glochids, 48
prickly pear (*Opuntia ficus-indica*), 46–7
primetin, 184
primin, 96, **183–4**
primrose, *see Primula*; evening primrose, *see Oenothera biennis*
Primula species, 7, 8, **182–5**, 211, 255
propenylsulphenic acid, 59
propolis (bee glue), 208–9
Proteaceae, 203–4
    Grevillea species, 36, 114, 203–4
protein contact dermatitis, 11, 29, 35–6, **38**, 39
protoanemonin, 52, **57–58**
Prototheca (algae), 121
Prunus spinosus, 48
Pseudevernia furfuracea, 123, 124
pseudo-phytodermatitis, 2, 135
Psoralea corylifolia, 67, 91, 136
psoralen 67, 70
psoralens (furocoumarins), 10, 21–2, 65, **66–78**, 133
psoriasis, 64
Pulmonaria officinalis, 43
Pulsatilla, 52, 58
puncture vine, 65
PUVA therapy, 64, 83–4
    use in Compositae dermatitis, 149
Pyemotes (mite) sensitivity, 2
pyrethrosin, 177

pyrethrum (*Tanacetum cinerariifolium*), 147
Pyrolaceae, 181–2

Queen Anne's lace (*Ammi majus*), 64, 69, 70, **89**
'quenching', 20
Quercus species, 208
quinine sensitivity, 146

radioallergosorbent (RAST) test, 38
radish (*Raphanus sativus*), 52, 129
ragweeds, 152–3
    false ragweed, 165
Ranunculaceae
    chemical irritants, 52, **57–9**, 86
    medicinal uses, 58–9
    not phototoxic, 86
ranunculin, 57
rapeseed, 36
Raphanus sativus, 52, 129
RAST test, 38
red clover (*Trifolium pratensis*), 36
rehmannic acid, 65
reindeer moss, 124
Rengas tree, 8, 113
resins, CNSO sensitivity, 8
rheumatism weed, 181
Rhododendron, 181
rhubarb (*Rheum rhaponticum*), 200
Rhus species
    classification problems, 106–8
    R. typhina, 110
    R. verniciflua, 8, 112
    see also poison ivy/poison oak dermatitis
rice, 233
ricinoleic acid, 206
Ricinus communis, 36, 39, **206**
rock rose (*Cistus creticus*), 130
rolled oats, 10
Rosaceae
    chemical irritants, 52
    rose thorns, 48
rose geranium (*Pelargonium graveolens*), 132
rosehips, 46
rosewoods, 136, 249
rubber latex
    fatal anaphylaxis, 38
    glove sensitivity, 1, 13, 39
rubber plant (Mexican), 171
rubber tree (*Hevea brasiliensis*), 36
Rubiaceae
    delayed sensitivity, 146–7
    mechanical irritant plants, 44
Rudbeckia hirta, 174
rue (*Ruta graveolens*), 91
    Culpeper on, 92–3
    delayed sensitivity, 134
    medicinal use, 92–3
    phototoxic reactions, 78, 81, 85, 93
Ruhmora adiantiformis, 234–5
runner beans, 36
Rutaceae
    delayed sensitivity, 133–4
    occupational exposure, 10
    phototoxic reactions, 91–3
    R. chalepensis, 91, 134
    R. corsica, 10, 93
    R. graveolens see rue

type I hypersensitivity, 133
see also Citrus species
rye, 36

sabra dermatitis, 9, 46
safflower (*Carthamnus tinctorius*), 157
safrole, 127
sage (*Salvia officinalis*), 199
St John's Wort (*Hypericum* species), 65, 84
Salicaceae, 208–10
Salicylic acid, 53
Salix vimminalis, 53
Salsola kali, 35, 36, 46
Salvia officinalis, 199
sandalwood (*Santalum album*), 204–5
sandwich makers see food handlers
Santalaceae, 204–5
Santalol, 205
sap (irritant), 57–62
Saussurea species, 174–5
sawdust inhalation, 246
Saxifragaceae, 137
Schefflera actinophylla, 145–6
Schinus terebinthifolius, 114
Scindapsus aureus, 228–9, 231
Sclerotinia sclerotiorum (fungus), 10, 87
scorpion weed, 189
Scots pine, 236
scratch test, 37, 38
Scrophulariaceae, 194–5
seabather's itch, 121
seaweeds (algae), 121–2
Semecarpus species, 8, 36, 113
Septoria apii (fungus), 10
sesame (*Sesamum indicum*), 196
  sesame seed oil, 36, 196
sesamin, 196
sesamolin, 196
sesquiterpene lactone mix, 98, **149**
sesquiterpene lactones, 102, 125–6, **148–9**
shallots, 36
shampoos, 16, 36
Shorea, 36
Siam benzoin, 185–6
silk oak, 203
Simmondsia species, 207
sinigrins, 52, 128
sisal (*Agave sisalana*), 216
skimmia, 91
skin care preparations
  in dermatitis prevention, 13
  sensitivity to cosmetics/perfumes, 15–22
skin pigmentation
  from cosmetics/perfumes, 21
  see also phytophototoxic reactions
slimes (algae), 121–2
sneezeweed (*Helenium*), 165–6
snow-on-the-mountain (*Euphorbia marginata*), 9
snowbell, 185
soaps, 16
sodom apple (*Calotropis procera*), 188
Solanaceae
  chemical irritants in, 52, 59
  delayed sensitivity to, 191–4
  see also under specific plant
soleil d'Or (*Narcissus bertolonii*), 221
Solidago species, 175

Soliva pterosperma, 46, 175
spathulin, 165
spearmint (*Mentha spicata*), 198
sphondin, 70, 74
spices
  caraway, 36, 142
  cinnamon, 36, 201–2
  galangal, 213
  ginger, 214
  green cardamom, 213–14
  star anise, 127
  turmeric, 213
spider flower, 203
spinach, 36
spines as mechanical irritants, 43–9
sporotrichosis, 49
spring onions, 218
spring parsley (*Cymopterus watsonii*), 70
spurge family see Euphorbiaceae
stalkless soliva (*Soliva pterosperma*), 46, 175
Staphylococcus aureus infections, 48
star anise (*Illicium verum*), 127
sticky elecampane (*Dittrichia viscosa*), 164–5
stinging nettle (*Urtica dioica*), **29–31**, 32
stinging tree (*Dendrocnide excelsa*), 32
stinking mayweed/chamomile (*Anthemis cotula*), 52, 86, **154–5**, 171
stinking Roger (*Tagetes minuta*), 176
stinkwort (*Dittrichia viscosa*), 164–5
storax
  from *Liquidambar orientalis*, 138
  from *Styrax officinalis*, 185
straw flower (*Helichrysum diosmifolium*), 166–7
strawberries, 11, 36
Streptocarpus species, 195–6
strimmer rash, 65, 83, 87
string-trimmer's dermatitis, 65, 83
Styrax species, 36, **185–6**
suncreams
  bergapten concentrations, 22
  ultraviolet barrier creams, 16, 85
sunflower (*Helianthus annus*), 166
sweet bay (*Laurus nobilis*), 149, **202–3**
sweet flag (*Acorus gramineus*), 230
sweet myrrh, 142
sweet pepper, 192
sweetheart vine (*Philodendron scandens*), **229**, 231
Swiss cheese plant, 231
Symphytum officinale, 43
Synadenium grantii, 60

Tagetes species, 176–7
Tamus communis 215
tanacetin, 179
Tanacetum species, 147
  T. cinerariifolium, 36, 177
  T. parthenium, 178–9
tanning promoters, 85
tannins, 208
tansy (*Tanacetum vulgare*), 179
Taraxacum officinale, 179–81
taraxinic acid β-glucopyranoside, 102, **180–1**
taxonomy of plants, 23–8, 121
tea-tree, 139
teak (*Tectona grandis*), 36, 251, 253
Terminalia superba, 36
α-terthienyl, 65, 73, 86

testing
  in occupational dermatitis, 11–12
  for type I hypersensitivity, 37–8
  see also patch testing
Thamnosa montana, 91
thatchers (occupational hazards), 48
Thevetia species, 188
thiocyanates, 52, 59
thioglucosides, 128
thistles, Salsola kali, 35, 36, 46
thiuram sensitivity, 1, 39
thorns, 43, **46–9**
Thuja plicata, 36
Thuya, 245
thyme (Thymus vulgaris), 199–200
Thymelaceae, 62
thymol, 200
tigliane polyol esters, 61
timothy grass, 233
tincture of Arnica, 154
tincture of benzoin, 185–6
tobacco (Nicotiana tabacum), 10, 52, **193–4**
toiletries, 15–22
  checklist, 4
Tolmiea menziesii, 137
Toluifera pereirae see balsam of Peru
tomato plant
  allergic dermatitis, 192
  irritant contact dermatitis, 42, 192
  type I hypersensitivity, 36, 193
toothpastes, 16, 20, 21, 142
Toxicodendron species, 106–21
  T. verniciflua, 8, 112
  see also poison ivy/poison oak dermatitis
tradescantia (Zebrina pendula), 227
trans-jasmone, 186
Tree and Shrub Expert, The (Hessayon), 27
trees
  conifer allergy, 8–9, **235–46**
  hardwood allergy, 246–54
  type I hypersensitivity, 36
  see also wood(s)
Tribulus terrestris, 65
tridecylresorcinol, 204
Trifolium pratensis, 36
Triplochiton scleroxylon, 36
Tromsø palm (Heracleum laciniatum), 70, 75, 81–2, 90
tropolones, 245
tulip tree, 149
tulipalin A, 13, 219, **222–3**, 225
tulipinolide, 203
tuliposide A, 13, 100, **222–3**, 225
tulips
  delayed sensitivity, 224–5
  protective gloves and, 13
  tulip finger, 7, 46, 224–5
  type I hypersensitivity, 36
tumbleweed (Salsola kali), 35, 36
turmeric (Curcuma longa), 213
turpentine, 238–42
turpentine broom, 91
Turricula parryi, 190
Tyroglyphus farinae (mite), 212

ultraviolet screening creams, 16, 85
Umbelliferae
  basic plant structure, 86–7

delayed hypersensitivity, 142–3
phototoxic reactions, 10, 69, 70, 86–90
plant identification, 26
  see also under specific plant
Umbilicaria species (lichens), 124
umbrella tree (Schefflera actinophylla), 145–6
unsaturated fatty acids, 225
Urtica species, 29–31, 32
urticaria, 29–41
  due to toxin injection, 29–35
  immunological contact, 29, **35–41**
  types of, 29
  see also contact urticaria
urushiol, 100, **110–11**
  see also poison ivy/oak dermatitis
Usnea species (lichen), 123, 124
usnic acid, 98, **122–3**, 126, 208

vanilla (Vanilla planifolia), 210–13
vanillaism/vanillism, 212
vanillin, 136, 212
varnishes, CNSO sensitivity, 8
vegetables
  sensitivity to, 9, 11, 36, 87, 128–9
  see also under specific type
Verbascum species, 194–5
vinca alkaloids, 188
Vinca species, 188
viper's bugloss (Echium species), 43
vision see eye problems
Vitaceae, 134
vitiligo, 64, 67, 69, 82–3

walnut trees, 251, 253
  Juglans species, 208
  poison walnut tree, 53
water mint (Mentha aquatica), 198
wax flower (Hoya carnosa), 188–9
Wedelia trilobata, 181
weeds/weeding
  Compositae dermatitis, 147–81
  occupational risks, 10–11
  string trimming, 10–11
  weeds checklist, 3
  see also under specific plant
western red cedar (Thuja plicata), 36, **245**
wheat, 36, 232
white bryony (Bryonia), 215
Wigandia species, 31, 190–1
wigandol, 191
wild carrot (Daucus carota), 87
Wild Flowers of Britain and Northern Europe (1974), 27
Wild Fower Key, The (Rose 1981), 27
wild parsnip (Pastinaca sativa), 81
wintergreen (Pyrola), 181
witloof (Cichorium intybus), 9, 52, **158–9**
wolf's bane, 154
wood rosin (colophony), 238–42
wood(s)
  of Hippomane mancinella, 61
  identification problems, 99
  mahogany, 248, 253
  oak wood, 208
  olive wood, 187
  patch testing of, 100
  teak, 36, 251–3

terminology confusion, 246
type I hypersensitivity to, 36
walnut, 208
woodworkers/forestry workers, 4, **6–15**
   conifer allergy, 8–9, **235–46**
   Frullania sensitivity, 125
   hardwood allergy, 246–54
   lichen allergy, 123
   tulip tree allergy, 126
woody nightshade, 191
wormwood (*Artemisia absinthum*), 156
wurmkraut (*Tanacetum vulgare*), 179

X. Cupressocyparis Leylandii, 243–5

X. Dendranthema, 147, 158, **161–4**
Xanthium species, 181
xanthotoxins, 93

yams (*Dioscorea* species), 214
yarrow (*Achillea millefolium*), 86, 151–2
ylang ylang perfume, 127
Yucca species, 48–9

Zebrina pendula, 227
Zingerone, 213, **214**
Zingiberaceae, 213–14
   Z. officinale, 214
Zygophyllaceae, 132